DOCTORS AND ETHICS: THE EARLIER HISTORICAL SETTING OF PROFESSIONAL ETHICS

THE WELLCOME SERIES IN THE HISTORY OF MEDICINE

The *Clio Medica* series editors are
V. Nutton, C. J. Lawrence and M. Neve.
Please send all queries regarding the series to Michael Laycock,
The Wellcome Trust Centre for the History of Medicine at UCL,
24 Eversholt Street, London NW1 1AD, UK.

DOCTORS AND ETHICS: THE EARLIER HISTORICAL SETTING OF PROFESSIONAL ETHICS

Edited by
Andrew Wear, Johanna Geyer-Kordesch
and Roger French

Rodopi

Amsterdam – Atlanta, GA 1993

First published in 1993
by Editions Rodopi B. V., Amsterdam – New York, NY 1993.

2nd edition, 2003

Design and Typesetting by Christine Lavery,
The Wellcome Trust.
Printed and bound in The Netherlands by Editions Rodopi B. V.,
Amsterdam – New York, NY 1993.

The series editors for this volume are W.F. Bynum and Roy Porter

British Library Cataloguing in Publication Data
A catalogue record for this book is available from the British
Library
ISBN 90-5183-553-1 (Bound)

'Doctors and Ethics:
The Earlier Historical Setting of Professional Ethics –
Amsterdam – New York, NY:
Rodopi. – ill.
(Clio Medica 24 / ISSN 0045-7183;
The Wellcome Series in the History of Medicine)

Front cover:
Physicians attending a patient.
Woodcut from Pliny, *Aureum opus et sublime*, Pavia 1516.
Courtesy: *Wellcome Library*, London.

Transferred to digital printing 2003
Printed in The Netherlands

All titles in the Clio Medica series (from 1999 onwards) are available to
download from the CatchWord website: http://www.ingenta.com

Contents

Acknowledgements

We would like to thank the Wellcome Trust for generously funding the conference at Corpus Christi College, Cambridge that gave rise to this book. The Wellcome Unit for the History of Medicine at Cambridge provided invaluable administrative help in organising the conference.

We would also like to thank Jenni Crisp of the Wellcome Institute for helping to prepare the text and Dr Kim Cross and her colleague Christine Lavery at The Wellcome Trust for their technical skill and expertise in getting this work to the press.

Notes on Contributors

Michael J. Clark is a former Research Fellow of the Department of History, University of Lancaster and the Centre de Recherche en Histoire des Sciences et des Techniques, La Villette, Paris. He has published a number of articles on aspects of the history of psychiatry in the nineteenth and twentieth centuries, and is currently working on an outline history of English forensic medicine during the past 150 years. Since 1990 he has managed the Wellcome Trust's collections of medical and medical-historical films and videos.

Roger French taught History and Philosophy of Science in the universities of Leicester and Aberdeen, after a D.Phil in Oxford, and since 1975 has been Director of the Wellcome Unit for the History of Medicine in Cambridge, where he is the University Lecturer in the History of Medicine. He has published on a range of topics from Greek texts to nineteenth century reform in medicine. He is General Editor of a series of books on science in antiquity with Routledge and part editor of a series on history of medicine with Cambridge University Press. Current research interests include William Harvey and medieval natural philosophy.

Luis Garcia-Ballester, MD, Ph.D., is a member of the CSIC (Unit of the History of Science), Barcelona, and professor of the History of Medicine. He is now working on the social and intellectual history of medicine in medieval and renaissance medicine. He is co-editor (with J.A. Paniagua and M.R. McVaugh) of the critical edition of the medical corpus of Arnau de Vilanova.

Johanna Geyer-Kordesch is Director of the Wellcome Unit for the History of Medicine, University of Glasgow, Scotland. Her area of expertise is eighteenth-century European Medicine. She was general secretary to the Cambridge Medical Ethics Forum 1989-92. She is continuing work on forensic and medical case histories both in regard to witchcraft and infanticide. Currently she is also interested in case histories as life narratives and their relation to periodical writings and literary forms in the Enlightenment.

Ole Peter Grell is a Carlsberg Fellow at the Wellcome Unit for the History of Medicine at the University of Cambridge. He has published several articles on religion and medicine and has recently co-edited the volume, *Medicine and the Reformation* (Routledge, 1993). He is at present completing a study of the Bartholin circle and the Danish Medical Renaissance.

Andreas-Holger Maehle, born 1957 in Siegen, Germany, studied medicine at the University of Bonn (Dr. med. 1983) and worked then as a Research Fellow at the Institute for the History of Medicine of the University of Göttingen (Dr. med. habil. 1990). He is now a Lecturer in the History of Medicine at this Institute. Since 1991 he has been working as a Wellcome Research Fellow at the Wellcome Institute for the History of Medicine in London. His publications include *Johann Jakob Wepfer (1620-1695) als Toxikologe* (Aarau: Sauerländer, 1987) and *Kritik und Verteidigung des Tierversuchs: Die Anfänge der Diskussion in 17. und 18. Jahrhundert* (Stuttgart: F. Steiner, 1992).

Vivian Nutton is a professor in the Academic Unit at the Wellcome Institute for the History of Medicine, London. His interests cover the classical tradition of medicine from the Greeks to the seventeenth century. Among his books are: *Galen: On Prognosis* (1979); *From Democedes to Harvey: Studies in the History of Medicine* (1988); and *Essays on the History of Therapeutics* (1991).

Roy Porter is professor of the Social History of Medicine at the Wellcome Institute for the History of Medicine. He is currently working on the history of hysteria. Recent books include *Mind Forg'd Manacles. Madness in England from the Restoration to the Regency* (Athlone, 1987); *A Social History of Madness* (Weidenfeld and Nicolson, 1987); *In Sickness and in Health. The British Experience,* 1650-1850 (Fourth Estate, 1988); *Patient's Progress* (Polity, 1989) – these last two co-authored with Dorothy Porter; and *Health for Sale. Quackery in England 1660-1850* (Manchester University Press).

Andrew Wear is a lecturer in the History of Medicine at the Wellcome Institute. He has research interests in early modern medicine and in colonial and empire medicine.

Introduction

This book is not so much a search for definitive answers to the question of how history can inform present-day medical ethics but is more an attempt to begin such a history. It shows that a history of medical ethics does in fact exist and that medical ethics were a constant part of the history of medicine in the period between those often-cited 'origins' of medical ethics, the Hippocratic Oath and Thomas Percival's *Medical Ethics* of 1803. This book tackles the gap on the subject that exists between these two works.

A number of themes emerge from these studies. The first shows that the perception of what was 'ethical' changed greatly in the past. At different periods and in different groups, practices like infanticide and abortion and the doctor's refusal to take hopeless cases were ethically unproblematic. At other times they met with the severest of censure.

Also of significance is the great complexity of interpretation. Hippocratic ethics have been seen as an expression of the loftiest moral philosophy, but it is also possible to view them as professional rules of thumb designed to protect one group of physicians against competition from another. Moreover, in the medical market-place one group might usefully evolve a system of ethics that appeared to benefit the patient at the expense of the doctor thus giving a competitive edge to that group of practitioners. Apart from the influences of market forces, it is clear that the practising physician derived his ethics from his religion and also from his education (for moral philosophy was a central part of the course in arts of the medieval and Renaissance university). In other cases an ethic was imposed on him by the state or his professional body: it is not always easy to separate these sources.

In this way we can recognise, although not always isolate, some of the sources of medical ethics. These chapters reveal these sources. Within medicine, in one example, it was claimed that the most ethical form of practice was that derived from the most learned and hence most advanced medicine. Sources outside medicine offered, in other examples, the framework for the ethical treatment of the insane and for the medical use of animals. Other chapters discuss cases where different ethical systems met and clashed. Taken together the chapters show that in contrast to present codified guidelines more weight rested on the doctor as an individual in deciding ethical issues. He was faced with less regulation than the modern doctor, less technology, fewer administrators and no ethical committees. What was central to medical ethics in the period before the present century was the personal conduct, behaviour, manners and knowledge of the practitioner.

Our book begins with Greek medical ethics. As with much else, one must look to the ancients in order to trace the beginnings of Western medical ethics or medical deontology. The text that connects present-day medical ethics to the classical period is the Hippocratic Oath. However, as Vivian Nutton notes in his chapter, 'Beyond the Hippocratic Oath', it was only in the Renaissance that the Oath achieved the authoritative and normative status which today it is assumed it had from the beginning. There were many classical texts other than the Oath which dealt with medical ethics. It is thus possible to envisage a code of medical ethics being drawn up before the Renaissance without having recourse to the Oath.

In his discussion of these texts Nutton emphasizes that it was the medical practitioners themselves who laid down ethical norms. Not only was the medical market-place a competitive one, but the State was absent from it. Greek medical ethics did not come from State regulation of medicine, nor, as was the case in some later instances in our volume, did they reflect the needs of the State or of civil society. In the situation of an open unregulated medical market place with competing groups of practitioners who produced ethical rules for themselves, uniformity in these rules could not be expected. Moreover, between the fifth century BC when the first Hippocratic treatises were produced and the death of Galen around AD 200 there were changes in the religious and philosophical influences that helped to shape medical ethics and, of course, the social worlds of the practitioners. Nutton discusses these changes and a significant point that emerges is how morality and technical competence came to be closely associated. It was felt that the morally good doctor must practise to the best of his ability. In the absence of licensing or of diplomas morality was, in a sense, a sign to the patient of medical competence. Galen, who after Hippocrates came to be the authority in medicine for the Middle Ages and the Renaissance, integrated Hippocratic rules of bedside conduct into medical practice by pointing out that they made the practitioner a more effective healer – they helped the patient to believe in him. As Nutton indicates, Galen was less interested in discussing morality *per se* and was more concerned with the practitioner's competence. This was achieved by experience and by learning from previous writers. For Galen the moral goodness of his ideal doctor was guaranteed by competence in the art.

Much of the ethical content of the learned medicine of the Middle Ages and Renaissance was supplied by the Hippocratic and Galenic texts. There was a continued emphasis on a good moral character, on confidence-boosting behaviour at the bedside, and on the prohibition of harming the patients. Luis García-Ballester discusses the medical ethics of Latin medicine in the thirteenth and fourteenth centuries. The texts of Galen were incorporated in a more sophisticated and detailed manner in the teaching of the newly created universities, and they were joined to Aristotelian natural philosophy. The substantial reform in medical knowledge tied to 'humanist medicine' gave university trained physicians and surgeons a claim for being the best type of medicine. It was through a new and high level of technical competence that the learned practitioners believed their medicine to be safer than that of the empirics. García-Ballester points out that the doctor-patient relationship was affected by the increased complexity of the doctor's technical competence (derived from books as well as from experience). Moreover, discussion of how to charge fees and of medical etiquette was integrated into the new synthesis of Galenic practical medicine undertaken by Arnau de Vilanova and others, and this again emphasizes the close connection between ethics and technical competence.

The new Galenic medicine spread to the Courts and to the newly emerging cities. Urban growth and commercial trade affected the ethical and social basis of medicine. Medicine could now be defined as a pecuniary occupation with its practitioners allowed to charge extra for their scholarly knowledge. Towns and cities saw it as their civic duty to contract learned physicians to treat their inhabitants. Medical practices began to be integrated with civic issues and made to take on the burden of civic responsibilities.

García-Ballester explores how the duties of town physicians were defined, for instance, in cases of plague. He also indicates how Christianity mitigated some of the commercial instincts of the physicians with those of charity and philanthropy. Nevertheless, for many, the mark of a learned physician and of his professional success was the ability to make money. García-Ballester's chapter shows how in the new society that was being forged in Europe a new medicine was also coming into existence, and 'how medical, intellectual, social and ethical matters overlapped'.

The Renaissance saw the first lengthy texts that dealt solely with medical ethics. The Oath was very brief and other classical passages on medical ethics were scattered in the writings of Hippocrates and Galen. Gabriele de Zerbi's *De Cautelis Medicorum (Concerning the Precautions of Medical Men)* published in 1495 explored in detail how the physician should behave at the bedside and with colleagues. In his study of Zerbi's medical ethics Roger French argues that they were designed (like other medical ethics) to help the group of practitioners to which Zerbi belonged to survive in its competitive struggle with other groups in the medical market-place. A sign of this is the stress laid by Zerbi on the reputation of the doctor. The physician is advised on the need for a solemn demeanour, warned not to mix with the lower classes and shown how to get on with his social superiors. Group solidarity was emphasized in Zerbi's advice that physicians should not criticize their colleagues in public when brought in to give a second opinion (a point that keeps recurring and can be found in Percival's advice on medical etiquette in his *Medical Ethics*).

Zerbi, as with most other writers who produced medical ethics for their type of practitioner, felt that his kind of medicine – rationalist, based on Galen and on Aristotelian natural philosophy, taught in the universities – was the best and therefore safest kind of medicine. However, Zerbi also included Christian ethics as a guideline for the medical practitioner. Zerbi saw no distinction between learned medicine and the moral claims of religion. He instructed the physicians to pray to God, reminding all that it is in essence God who cures and not the physician. French thus describes how Zerbi constructs a picture of the faithful, righteous physician who followed the canons of both medicine and religion.

The learned physicians were not the only group to incorporate Christian values into their ethics. In his chapter on 'Medical Ethics in Early Modern England' Andrew Wear discusses how the learned physicians and those hostile to establishment medicine brought into play two opposing sets of values. The former argued like Zerbi from the rightness, efficacy and safety of their learning. The latter, as well as advocating alternative medical systems, stressed the Christian values of charity and of neighbourly help which they felt were lacking in their opponents. Christ was the model for the proper physician, because he was the Divine example for healing the sick, the lame and the blind.

A specific issue which involved religion, medicine and also governments was the question of whether to flee or stay during plague. Ole Grell in his chapter 'Conflicting Duties: Plague and the Obligations of Early Modern Physicians Towards Patients and Commonwealth' shows how Lutheran and Calvinist teaching in England and The Netherlands shaped two contrasting views of the duties of physicians and of magistrates during a plague visitation. The earlier, Lutheran, opinion held that physicians and ministers should stay with the afflicted, whilst the later, Calvinist, view was that they and other godly worthies were too valuable for the commonwealth to lose – they should flee from the danger of contagion. Two different concepts of community are here at stake, one relating to the obligation of the ministry to an afflicted community, whilst the second seeks to preserve the community through preserving the continuity of its leadership. Grell's chapter focuses on the interplay between community and government policy and shows how these affect specific ethical behaviour in the medical sphere, whose normal obligation is to minister to the sick in times of plague.

The change from the seventeenth century to the Age of Reason, or Enlightenment, naturally conditioned changes in the approach to ethics from the end of the seventeenth century to the mid-eighteenth century. The Aristotelian and Galenic hold on natural philosophy and medicine was broken and the rivalry of different approaches to medical knowledge became evident. Two contributors to the volume attempt to look at the realignment of religious and legal perspectives under the pressure of these changes, on the one hand a new push towards secularisation, and on the other the attempt to separate natural law theory from the pervading moral concepts of a biblically orientated Protestant Christianity. Geyer-Kordesch and French both look at one of the centres of radical change, namely the University of Halle, where both Pietist Christian activism and medico-legal secularisation determined the agenda.

Roger French's chapter 'Ethics in the Eighteenth Century: Hoffmann in Halle' allows us to trace the changes and the continuities from the past. Friedrich Hoffmann's *Medicus Politicus* echoed some of Zerbi's advice to the aspiring physician: do not put any diagnosis or prognosis down on paper (it could later be used against the physician), do not appear hard-hearted in asking for fees. Hoffmann saw fees as honoraria which could not be insisted upon, but could be received. A particularly propitious time for a generous honorarium was when the patient was in pain. French shows how the new Enlightenment views of the prudent, urbane physician, cynical and skilful in the art of dissimulation, were influential in Hoffmann's treatise. In both Zerbi and Hoffmann ideas of honour and propriety were present, but in Hoffmann they were related more to the needs of civil society. Moreover, in Zerbi's Italy the difference between physicians and surgeons was not great, if the surgeon, as he could, had also been educated at a university. However, in Hoffmann's Halle the physicians deemed themselves superior to the surgeons and apothecaries who had been trained through apprenticeship. Hoffman, with the authority of State decrees behind his words, insisted on the separation of physicians, surgeons and apothecaries, and on an overall supervisory role for the physicians over the other two groups. In a sense, the physicians validated their practice. The greatest difference between Zerbi and Hoffmann, however, lay in Hoffmann's new learning. Like other contemporaries he rejected traditional authority and insisted that medicine should be based on experiment and reason, the new Authority. The old scholarly learned physician was slowly changed into the medical scientist, and as medical knowledge changed, so a new set of ethical imperatives would be formed.

Halle is also the focus for Johanna Geyer-Kordesch and her chapter on 'Infanticide and Medico-legal Ethics in Eighteenth Century Prussia'. She shows how the medical profession was influenced by the secular moral virtues of civic duty with the ideals of *honestum, justum et decorum.* Civic duty was one of the central reference points for a vision of man as an independent and rational human being, who was able to decide how to act properly for the best of society. In the medical legal cases that Geyer-Kordesch discusses it is possible to see, on the one hand, how the experts of these newly emerging professions of the Enlightenment saw expert opinion become the arbitrator for judging human conduct. Observation and experiment now invested with competence the secular professions of law and medicine. They could rightly claim to detach themselves from traditional authority. In other words, the major change introduced by the leading professions of the Enlightenment pertained to their rejection of traditional authority, including Galenic and scholastic medicine, as well as the legal influence of codified law. The change in approach to ethical issues in medicine centred on their use of cases rather than the authority prescribed in the literature of law and medicine.

Geyer-Kordesch then focuses on infanticide cases, because this particular issue indicates extremely well how an overall pattern of ethical assessment can change within the narrow scope of the medico-legal prosecution. The self-legitimising knowledge of the professional can define the crime. He judges according to obligations and duties legitimised by empirical experts. However, the establishment of a new authority through the professions in the case of infanticide clashed with an overall social reassessment of the plight of women. Therefore, Geyer-Kordesch focuses on how the duties and obligations of the doctor and the lawyer can find a substantial opposition in the public discussion of social values. It is through the arts that women came to be seen as the victims of social discriminations.

As with the essentially powerless group of women known as infanticides so too the issue of animal rights presents a matter of continuous debate. From classical times the law and medicine had agreed that the patient should not be harmed. This was not the case with animals. On this basic issue the major intellectual, philosophical, religious and legal traditions of western Europe were brought into play on one or the other side. Andreas-Holger Maehle's chapter on 'The Ethical Discourse on Animal Experimentation, 1650–1900' represents a major study of this debate. From early in the history of western medicine (the Alexandrians, Galen) animal experimentation formed part of medical research. In the seventeenth century when anatomy was seen as the foundation of medicine, the anatomists frequently employed vivisectional techniques. From the seventeenth century onwards there was debate on vivisection. Arguments used to justify the practice included those from natural theology (the intricate bodily structure of animals gave evidence of God's workmanship and indeed supported physico-theological arguments) and from utility (the greater good of mankind outweighing the pain caused to the animals). Those against ranged from the danger of the animal experimenters becoming brutalised and then practising cruelly on their human patients to the view that animals had souls, could feel pain and had rights. In a sense the arguments were about power and rights, and it is not until the medical profession begins to have *de facto* monopoly powers over their human patients that there is anything approaching the ethical debates over animal rights.

In England such a point did not come until at least the mid-nineteenth century, even though, as with the medical men of Halle, medicine was being integrated into a new civic order and given a sense of civic duty. On the whole, in England 'regular' medical men lacked confidence. Their social status was often low and they faced competition from various groups on the medical market-place. Thomas Percival's *Medical Ethics* reflects this lack of confidence. The treatise was designed to clear up problems of precedence amongst the different medical practitioners who worked in that new medical institution, the infirmary. As Roy Porter notes in his chapter, historians have taken *Medical Ethics* to be about medical etiquette. Therefore, Percival should be seen as writing at the end of a long tradition and should not be taken as a new start in medical ethics. It was only when a near monopoly was achieved by the university-educated practitioners with the Medical Act of 1858 and the Medical Register that medical etiquette and the personal behaviour and character of the practitioner were given less emphasis. At the end of the eighteenth century the character of the physician was still important. Thomas Gisborne, a noted Church of England clergyman, and friend of Percival gave an outsider's view of the ideal physician. In his *An Enquiry into the Duties of Men in the Higher and Middle Classes of Society in Great Britain* (1794) he noted down the character of the good physician. As Porter points out in his essay on Gisborne, the Christian gentleman was the example of the good physician. He should treat all classes with compassion, he should not stoop to the tricks of his competitors to get trade, he should not be avaricious and he should have the interest of his patients rather than of his career uppermost in his mind. Unlike Percival, Gisborne was more critical of the medical profession. He warned against experimenting on poor hospital patients and he pointed out how in the minds of the poor experimentation and hospital doctors had become linked. In this Gisborne is pointing to the future. As medicine became more powerful, not only in its hold over the poor, but also over the articulate middle classes, through its new institutions, through professionalization and finally through its association with science and technology, so ethical problems such as experimentation on patients came to the fore.

Gisborne's work probably had little influence on the future development of medical ethics, but it shows that the Christian gentlemanly ideals still had some meaning at the same time as Percival's rules of interprofessional behaviour were being publicised.

An area where medicine was given increasing power by the State in the nineteenth century was in the certification, control and treatment of the insane. Michael Clark's chapter 'Does a Certificate of Lunacy Affect a Patient's Ethical Status?' analyses psychiatric paternalism and its critics in Victorian England, and explores a theme which would appear to be ripe for a lengthy discussion of ethical implications. Certification meant a huge loss of rights and the reduction of an adult to the legal status of a minor, as well as loss of liberty and the possibility of forcible treatment. However, Clark shows it was not psychiatrists but lay organizations founded by former patients which pointed to ethical pitfalls and pressed for safeguards of those about to be certified or already in asylums. The medical profession did not doubt the medical rightness of involuntary confinement; instead psychiatrists were more concerned with justifying their new authority to other groups, such as the law profession, and to each other. But Clark goes on to show that ultimately the failure to develop patients' rights for the insane was due to a combination of factors: the power of social conformity which exacted retribution in the form of certification, the failure of the Lunacy Commissioners to press for patients' rights (because they feared alienating the medical profession) and the increasing authority of the 'science' of psychiatry which drowned the voices of the insane. Clark takes us closer to the present-day world of medical ethics. In his chapter the interplay between the government, the public and the medical profession shapes the problems and answers of medical ethical issues. We are far from the classical emphasis on the individual doctor and his character.

1

Beyond the Hippocratic Oath

Vivian Nutton

The Hippocratic *Oath* is arguably the most mysterious as well as the most influential of all the treatises that are associated with the name of Hippocrates of Cos, fl. 450–370 BC. No other document from the ancient world, save for the Bible, has undergone so many transformations and yet still retains authority today. Its provisions, at least in part, are still appealed to as normative, especially in the debate on abortion, and it is still viewed by the public at large as setting the proper standards for medical behaviour. Yet there is much that remains obscure about the *Oath,* not least the process whereby it came to achieve this status. The meaning of several of its clauses remains open to dispute, and the whole context in which it was produced has provoked considerable controversy. Above all, the later normative status of the *Oath* has given it a preeminence in discussions of ancient medical ethics that it did not have until centuries after it was composed, and which has tended to distort, at least in the public mind, perceptions of the medical ethics, or deontology, of Antiquity. This chapter attempts to restore the balance by drawing attention also to other ethical texts from Antiquity, and by outlining the transformations of this material from Antiquity to the Renaissance.

Hippocratic Ethics

The collection of medical writings that is commonly called the Hippocratic Corpus is linked together only by a reputed origin in the teaching of Hippocrates. Yet, as even the most cursory glance reveals, they differ considerably in doctrine, language, style, audience and intention. Some are written for public consumption, others for a private group; some are mere notes, others highly finished prose; some attack philosophy, others accept it wholeheartedly. To determine which, if any, is a genuine work of the great Hippocrates has been a topic of academic and medical debate for centuries, and agreement is still far from being reached on even the most basic of facts. There are few external criteria for judgement. Few traces remain of what Hippocrates' contemporaries thought of him and his beliefs, and although certain treatises obviously fit very closely together and may even be by the same author, this cannot of itself prove that their author was Hippocrates. The texts themselves can rarely be dated, or even put into a relative chronological order, and the researcher must frequently rely on linguistic and stylistic criteria or on impressions of doctrinal development that rarely permit a dating within half a century. The temptation (and the opportunity) is there to select a group of treatises as genuinely Hippocratic, and to reduce the extent of the problem by discarding the rest as unworthy of scholarly attention. Certain texts, for instance *Prognostic* and *Epidemics I* and *III*, are thus viewed as exemplary, while others on related themes, *Diseases* or *Epidemics II* and *IV*, are neglected and not even given the honour of a translation. On the other hand, for those who express a certain scepticism about the historical Hippocrates, there is the prospect of being able to consider all the texts in the Corpus as equally valid in the information they give about medicine and its practice in Ancient Greece.

It is thus no coincidence that the first major study to give the same weight to the Hippocratic *Oath* as to the other ethical statements and treatises in the Corpus was by Ludwig Edelstein, whose robust refusal to ascribe for certain any surviving text to the historical Hippocrates had earlier provoked a bitter controversy.[1] He distinguished the *Oath* and such contemporary treatises as the *Law*, the *Art*, and *Aphorisms* from the considerably later *Precepts* and *Decorum*, and these in turn from the ethical comments by authors of the Roman period.[2] He suggested that there was a change over this time away from the self-interest of the doctor-craftsman towards a more humanitarian approach to ethics. Just as the medical art turned into medical science, so too the new physician adopted a more philosophical attitude towards his responsibilities. The restricted quasi-familial instruction in the *Oath* was replaced by public lectures in a town gymnasium and by multiple consultations.[3]

That there is an increasingly philosophical component in the pronouncements by Greek doctors on medical ethics can hardly be doubted. *Precepts*, for example, begins with several sentences on the nature of reasoning and sense perception before passing on to the duties of a doctor, and its language recalls that of Hellenistic philosophy. A similar discussion on wisdom *(sophia)* opens *Decorum*, and is followed in Chapter 4 by speculations on nature *(physis)*.[4] But whether the incentive to change came from within medicine or from within philosophy is a more difficult question to answer, and not everyone would now accept Edelstein's simplistic model of a switch from art to science as an explanation. Besides, as he himself showed, there is a substantial philosophical component even in the early texts, albeit expressed less overtly and in a less specialized philosophical vocabulary. The author of the *Law* compares the learning of medicine to the natural growth of plants, for 'nature herself points the way to what is best'.[5] Nor can the *Oath* be understood properly without a background knowledge of fifth-century philosophical developments.[6] The fact that later treatises reveal the influence of Stoicism or Epicureanism, both philosophies with a strongly ethical bias, parallels the influence of Democritus and Heraclitus on earlier texts in the Hippocratic Corpus, and may indicate nothing more than that Stoicism in general superseded Democriteanism over the centuries. Even on more pragmatic topics there are distinct overlaps. The long sections on dress and behaviour in *Precepts* and *Decorum* may well be seen as expansions of hints in *Epidemics VI*, now modified to fit new social circumstances. The smooth physician of *Decorum*, Chapter 3, and his gaudy opponents recall the polite world of Menander's plays or Theophrastus' *Characters* rather than Aristophanic comedy, and there is a danger of mistaking these general social changes for specific developments within the ethical tradition.

Edelstein himself was too good a scholar not to notice this trap and disregard these continuities. He was well aware that the authors of *Law*, *Oath*, and the *Physician*, each in their own way, asserted that the morality they were advocating was a useful weapon in the struggle for patients. They were better able to treat the sick because they possessed ethical standards as well as more effective therapies, and were hence on both counts superior to the diviner, the quack, or the travelling-salesman. The practical advantages of an openly moral stance were theirs, even if they did not express them as blatantly as the author of *Precepts*, whose discussion in Chapter 4, on when and how to charge fees, avowedly stresses the benefits to be gained by acting ethically. A reputation for good conduct, however much it might occasionally cost in financial terms, would assuredly in the end bring in substantial profits.

The pragmatic tone of *Precepts*, with its details of appropriate dress and bedside manner (no luxurious headgear and strange perfumes, flowery language or loud talking), and of *Decorum*, with its advice to avoid gossip and always to carry an emergency set of instruments, even on a journey, would appear to contrast with the religious injunctions of the *Oath* and the *Law*. The conclusion of *Decorum*, that the practitioner should follow its author's recommendations because he would thereby obtain glory and respect, is a far cry from that of the *Law*, which states that 'the things which are holy are revealed only to the holy' and which thus implicitly associates the study of medicine with initiation into a mystery cult. Similar religious language ends the *Oath*, which begins with an oath sworn to the healing deities.[7] But it would be wrong to conclude from this that a professional and philosophical ethic displaced entirely a religious sanction for medical practice. The situation at Elea/Velia in S. Italy in the first century AD, where doctors participated in a *pholeon*, a word that can characterize a religious as well as an intellectual association, resembles that envisaged in the *Oath* far more than it does the open market-place of *Precepts*.[8]

Recent studies have, if anything, only confirmed another of Edelstein's qualifications to his general schema of the development of medical ethics in Antiquity. There was no monolithic medical profession, but rather a competing variety of healers; there was no state or professional examination before practice, and the fact that, on occasion, a healer might be sued successfully for incompetence by an individual patient was small consolation if one had been left after treatment worse off than before. In the doctor/patient relationship the state scarcely intervened at all, and never to lay down precise ethical standards. In other words, there were few, if any, organized constraints on what a healer could or could not do. It is thus remarkable, as Edelstein himself said, that some healers should have themselves thought it in their own interests to lay down rules for practice. Not that these rules were always accepted in every detail. On abortion, euthanasia, and the duty to attend to those thought incurable, there could be a variety of views, and the *Oath* is not the only text in which one can find traces of a debate over the necessity for a doctor to practise surgery himself or leave this dangerous procedure to others more skilled than he. Just as there were many ways of becoming a healer, and many, at times conflicting, opinions on the first principles of medical science, so there were no fixed rules for ethical practice. The Hippocratic *Oath* was thus one of a series of writings that attempted to lay down the manner in which a doctor should behave towards his patient. It was neither unique in this nor universally acknowledged as the standard.[9] Although, as we shall see, it was adapted in various ways to fit a Christian, Muslim or Jewish environment, the very fact that it could be so adapted proves that its validity rested in its ideas rather than in its words, and, equally, that there was no universal authority that demanded strict adherence to it in every detail. It was at best a signpost to a variety of destinations.

The Patient's Expectations

The deontological texts in the Hippocratic Corpus at the very least imply that the healer who practises ethically will have a return on his moral investment. 'Where there is love of man [on the part of the doctor] there also is love of the art [on the part of the patient and doctor]'.[10] Adherence to a medical ethic differentiates the good healer from the less good; it is both a selling-point, and an insurance policy. How far, then, were its claims bought by the patient?

An answer to this question is far from easy. Attitudes towards a doctor might range the whole way from total dependence to total rejection.[11] Besides, there is very little evidence contemporary with Hippocrates to give us the patient's view. Nonetheless, the hints given by Plato and Aristophanes of the doctor's appropriate behaviour do suggest that there was a general belief in a link between morality and sound practice, even if there was disagreement over the precise nature of that link.[12] For better indications of the patient's attitude towards medical morality, however, one must wait until the Hellenistic period, and, for the most extended discussion, until the Roman Empire.

Then, in the course of a splendidly rhetorical attack on his competitors in Rome *c.* AD 177, Galen contrasted the criminal incompetence of the doctors of the metropolis with those of his home town.[13] In his view, the anonymity of the big city offered an incentive for the quack literally to commit murder, whereas the face-to-face society of an Asia Minor city acted as its own guarantee of sound practice. In a town where 'we all know one another, our families, our education, and our way of life', the incompetent is swiftly unmasked and driven out. One may well wonder at the truth of this characterization, especially as Pergamum, Galen's home, was no village, but had a population of tens of thousands, yet his point has a certain validity. A doctor resident in a small community did have his whole life, both private and professional, open to public scrutiny, and his abilities could be assessed well before his services were called on. By contrast, the population of the countryside had to rely on their own resources or on the chance arrival of a healer, whereas those who lived in a big city, such as Ephesus, Alexandria, or Rome, might be faced with a bewildering choice of healers, each promising success. Unless the patient could rely on the testimony of others, or, best of all, was as learned in medicine as his potential physician and had the time to examine him, he had to entrust himself blindly to the mercies of his chosen healer.[14] When assailed by such potentially fatal uncertainty, the patient needed to find in his healer not only competence as a therapist but also morality, in order to escape being cheated in some way. For Galen, the two are tightly linked. Not only is the good doctor in therapeutic terms also a morally good man, but his outward morality also offers a clear insight into his possible skill as a therapist. His lifestyle, his honesty and his application, are all sound indications of at least potentially good practice, and these public virtues can be recognised as such by the intending patient.

This interdependence can be seen also at work on the side of the patient, in the series of near-contemporary legal decisions conferring tax immunity and similar privileges on healers. The lawyer Ulpian, writing around AD 200, declared that the choice of civic physician was to be left to the local town council, who would then make it on the basis of moral probity and scientific skill (*'probitas morum et peritia artis'*)[15] A similar combination is hinted at by Ulpian's contemporary, Modestinus, who ruled that those healers who did their job 'neglectfully', a word with strong moral overtones, were not eligible for tax immunity. The wording of honorary decrees, which span the period from *c.* BC 300 to *c.* AD 150., tells a similar message. Moral virtue accompanies professional skill; 'a life of sobriety and responsibility was allied to a sound, effective and blameless practice drawing on consummate experience.'[16] The same combination was sought by the highest of patients: Tiberius Claudius Tyrannus was 'approved by the emperors for his skill in medicine and for the beauty of his manners'.[17] The abundance of commendatory moral adverbs and adjectives found in such testimonials, and on the tombstones of healers, is, of course, a feature of the epigraphic genre, and should not be pressed too far. Yet two points are significant here. The first is that the moral and the professional are linked; and, secondly, the epigraphic language fits very closely with that of texts such as *Decorum* (especially Chapter 5) and *Precepts* in a shared moral universe of doctor and patient.[18] This suggests that the claims of the ethical texts and of

Galen would be very likely to have met with acceptance on the part of the patient.

The emphasis on the need for morality as well as skill is not confined to healers. Rather, it is a commonplace in Antiquity, for the best orator, the best teacher, the best architect – and even, in Lucian's satire *On dancing*, the best dancer – are also declared to be virtuous as well as competent. Their moral virtue is seen as an essential element in their practice, for it not only controls the uses to which their arts are put, but, much more importantly, ensures that what is done is done to the best of their ability.[19] Indeed, in the somewhat artificial situation in which a choice has to be made between virtue and competence, the theorists whole-heartedly come down on the side of virtue. In a passage preserved only in a late Latin author, the Hellenistic Greek physician Erasistratus, fl. 280 BC, is reported as saying that it is better to choose a good man without learning (whatever '*doctrina*' means exactly in this context) than a consummate healer who is wicked and immoral.[20] Whether this dilemma, and indeed this choice, corresponds to the reality of medical life in Antiquity must, however, remain uncertain.

Medical Ethics in the Roman Empire, from Scribonius to Galen

Although, as has just been argued, there was a shared understanding and expectation of medical morality between doctor and patient, the development of medical ethics in Antiquity must also be set against a background of marked individualism. The doctor-patient relationship was essentially between individuals, untroubled by guild or state regulations. True, from time to time, groups of doctors might meet to agree on proper practice, including the level of fees, but there is no proof that their decision was binding even on the healers of their own community.[21] Save for the choice of civic doctor, the state's intervention was confined almost entirely to questions of finance, not of ethics or competence, and even in this apparent exception the interests of the state arguably did not always coincide with those of the population at large. In one notorious case, a healer was allowed by a provincial governor to keep his tax immunity and to call himself a doctor despite being accused by his patients of bad practice.[22] Besides, as everybody knew, the denomination 'healer' could cover a multitude of specialties, competences and statuses, legal and otherwise.[23] It is thus in no way surprising that there should be an equally varied collection of deontological prescriptions, dealing with surgeons and midwives as well as with doctors *(medici/iatroi)*, or that attempts to relate them to a single Hippocratic source have all foundered.[24]

This is not to say that, over time, certain texts, most notably the Hippocratic *Oath,* did not achieve canonical status, or that this process of canonization does not go back a long way. How far back is impossible to determine, for our fragmentary Hellenistic sources scarcely permit any reconstruction at all of the four hundred years of medicine that separate the Hippocratic Corpus from the age of Celsus, Scribonius Largus and the elder Pliny in the first century AD By this time, Hippocrates has become a familiar, if somewhat legendary, figure, but by no means the dominant father of medicine he was later to become. Hippocratism in medicine was an option, not a universal rule.

One healer who followed Hippocratic medical ethics was Scribonius Largus, a Sicilian-trained doctor, who came to Britain in AD 43 with the invading Roman forces, and who dedicated his book of *Drug recipes* perhaps four or five years later to a leading member of the emperor's household. In his *Preface,* and elsewhere in his book, Scribonius interprets the Hippocratic *Oath* in Roman military terms.[25] The 'profession' or the 'discipline' of medicine has its ethical foundations in the Hippocratic *Oath* and in some of the incidents believed to have happened to Hippocrates. Just as the soldier submits to military discipline and declares his loyalty to the Emperor by taking the *oath* of allegiance, so by following the Hippocratic Oath and openly making a *'professio',* a declaration, the healer is automatically accepting a series of ethical presuppositions and commitments, both positive and negative. Certain treatments and remedies fall 'outside the profession of medicine', although they are known to have been advocated and adopted by others, while, in turn, the healer, whatever his philosophical or doctrinal stance, must always display a charitable and compassionate attitude towards the sick, and towards his fellow healers. His commitment is to healing, and hence he will never give a noxious drug even to the enemy, although he is perfectly at liberty to kill the enemy in war by non-medical means as a soldier and good citizen.[26]

If Scribonius gives to the *Oath* a very military flavour, its reworking by an Athenian doctor-philosopher half a century later bears all the hallmarks of the contemporary Greek literary renaissance. The *Oath* is in part transmuted into a poem, complete with choice vocabulary and a tinge of philosophy. The doctor must provide his god-like ministrations for all alike, slave, rich, poor, and princes, 'in all (or "to all") a brother'. He is a participant in a sacred rite, and will cure with virtue and morality, in no way 'contrary to divine laws and the oath'.[27] The author of the poem, Sarapion, came from a wealthy and intellectual Athenian family, and the poem tells us perhaps more about his education and his interests than it does about his medicine. The Hippocratic basis for its moral injunctions is, however, clear – as is its status as a literary *tour de force*.

Neither Scribonius nor Sarapion can, however, compare in their Hippocratism with Galen (AD129-*c*.199/216), whose interpretation of the great doctor from Cos came to dominate much of medieval medicine. Galen was both philosopher and physician, and his whole massive oeuvre can be seen as an attempt to reconcile these two traditions as represented by Plato (and to a lesser extent Aristotle) and Hippocrates. His task was made easier by the well-known fact that Plato had mentioned Hippocrates in his *Dialogues*, on one occasion specifically commending him for his expertise in logical division. Equally, Plato in the *Timaeus* had described diseases and their causes in terms which had their equivalents in the Hippocratic Corpus. The philosopher's interweaving of anatomy and physiology in his discussion of the tri-partite soul as an explanation for morality also allowed Galen to take back to Hippocrates theories that ascribed moral as well as strictly physical failures of the mind to changes occurring in the body – and, vice versa, to consider some physical ailments as the direct result of mental or emotional changes.[28] But, as Wesley Smith argued, the resulting synthesis, Galen's reconstruction of Hippocrates as the model for medical practice, is far removed from the historical reality, and tells us far more about Galen than it does about the fifth century BC.

A good example of Galen's reworking of the Hippocratic physician in his own image comes in a little tract entitled *The best doctor is also a philosopher*.[29] In it Galen attacks his opponents for a multitude of sins, not least their avarice, contentiousness and failure to grasp the fundamentals of Hippocratic medicine, most notably prognosis. To them Galen opposes his model physician, who like Hippocrates will despise the blandishments of Artaxerxes and Perdiccas and instead go out of his way to treat the poor and those who need him. He will leave his family and pupils in Cos and travel around the small towns, thereby gaining first-hand experience of airs, waters and places. He will have a knowledge of the stars and the order of the seasons, and his therapies will be guided above all by a sound logical, scientific method. His behaviour, too, will be 'philanthropic', fairminded, and restrained, for he will reject and despise pleasure and money (beyond what suffices to avoid hunger and thirst). In short, by following this mode of practice he will become, whether or not he knows it, a true philosopher, an accolade that, in another treatise, *On prognosis,* Galen proudly records as bestowed on him by no less a philosopher than the Emperor Marcus Aurelius.[30]

Galen thus turns Hippocrates into a philosopher, whose modern adherent not only possesses the three parts of philosophical knowledge, logical, ethical, and natural, but also can put them into practice. This appeal to the authority of philosophy is only too typical of Galen's day, and was, indeed, parodied by the contemporary satirist Lucian, who claimed similar status and similar benefits for the art of dancing.[31] Equally characteristic of the priorities of the second century is Galen's complaint that his opponents clearly have no desire to emulate Hippocrates' 'ability of expression', for they otherwise would not have been seen so often to commit two errors in a single word.[32] His ideal physician is a scholar as well as a sage.

This exaltation of the Hippocratic physician is not entirely without foundation. Galen assembles a cento of Hippocratic statements to back up his case, and thereby accuses his antagonists of ignorance of past literature as well as of immorality. Yet his choice of texts to prove that the Hippocratic doctor was indeed a philosopher demands attention. It is no surprise to find quotations from *Airs, waters, and places, Prognostic, On the nature of man,* and *Epidemics I* and *III*, for these form the basis of Galen's whole view of the historical Hippocrates, and are frequently cited throughout his writings.[33] Nor should the presence of an allusion to *Epidemics II,* which Galen took as in some way Hippocratic, cause alarm. Similarly, the biographical details of Hippocrates' career given by Galen in Chapter 3 can be easily explained on the supposition that Galen is drawing on a familiar 'life of Hippocrates' like that attributed to Soranus.[34] In all this, Galen's reconstruction of the Hippocratic physician is little different from that of a modern scholar, with one significant omission. In his description of the proper behaviour of the physician Galen makes no allusion at all to any of the deontological tracts in the *Corpus.* His failure to quote either *Precepts* or *Decorum,* texts which had entered the Corpus by the first century AD but which are not cited elsewhere by Galen, is hardly surprising, for he may not have known them or recognised them as Hippocratic, but his silence on the earlier texts and, in particular, the *Oath* is worth pursuing.[35]

Throughout his writings, Galen sets himself up as the very model of a moral healer. In a naughty world, he stands almost alone in his righteousness. In Rome, above all, he, and others like him, are assailed by quacks, charlatans, crooks, thieves, and murderers. He looks on in pained anger as incompetents rise high and fast in society, while honest men who have simply had bad luck are forced out into the backwoods.[36] He is consoled only by philosophy and his own success. Every day, so he says, he reads twice over the *Golden verses* of Pythagoras (an appropriately ethical text), and his dreams occasionally bring him direct messages from his god-protector, Asclepius.[37] Against such a background, the rarity of his references to the Hippocratic *Oath* is somewhat surprising, not least because substantial fragments of a commentary on the *Oath* survive under his name in Arabic. The authenticity of this commentary, however, is open to question. As good an Arabist as Max Meyerhof thought that it might be a later forgery, and its first editor and translator, Franz Rosenthal, scrupulously refrained from identifying its author with Galen, although, equally, he allowed that there was nothing in the fragments that could not have been said by Galen.[38] Even if we had not the explicit statement of the author that he came from Pergamum, frag. 1c, the argument against authenticity would be weak, for, as Gotthard Strohmaier has shown, the description of Asclepius given by the *Oath* corresponds closely to that of the cult-statue at the Pergamene Asclepieion, and its sentiments and the range of learning displayed fit Galen exactly.[39]

To reconstruct the lost commentary from scattered quotations in a variety of authors is an almost impossible task, and any conclusion is likely to be based on extremely fragile and hazardous foundations.[40] Certainly, Galen lavishes on the *Oath* all his store of knowledge, historical as well as medical, and treats the opening invocation to the gods with as much care as he elsewhere deals with Hippocrates' medical aphorisms. Whether the resulting impression of an overall antiquarian rather than a moralising interpretation of the *Oath* is valid is more questionable, since the process of selection may well have focused on the rarer flowers of Galen's learning rather than on his more commonplace moral injunctions. Nonetheless, I regard it as significant that in none of the passages so far revealed is there any suggestion that the *Oath* was administered in Galen's day or that he regarded it as possessing overriding authority. If this supposition is correct, it offers an explanation for Galen's neglect of the *Oath* in his picture of the ideal doctor. The Oath gave at best historical sanction to what could be derived from other, more authoritative Hippocratic texts. In other words, Galen's Hippocratic morality was not dependent on the *Oath.*

In part, this is because of the very practical way in which Galen regards the duties of the doctor. What might be thought moral dilemmas in the *Oath,* suicide, abortion, euthanasia, the use of the knife, take very much second place in Galen to the doctor's behaviour when in the presence of the sick. So, for instance, when Galen discusses the injunction that the doctor should help, or at any rate not harm, the sick, he admits that to a beginner this might seem a trivial commonplace.[41] But his own observations of the reckless practice of others have shown him just how important and overwhelmingly sensible this advice was and is. Thus, by laying down practical guidelines, Hippocrates was showing the physician at the same time how to treat the patient and how to behave morally.[42] He was not acting as a moral casuist but providing the most effective way of restoring the patient to health.

Nowhere in the Galenic Corpus is this non-moralising approach to the doctor's duties more clearly expressed than in Galen's commentary on *Epidemics VI.*[43] The original author, at the end of a section that briefly mentions treatments and the like that will 'gratify the patient', added nine words: 'entrances, words, appearances, dress, to the patient, hair, nails, smell'. On this Galen built an impressive edifice of medical deontology, describing in considerable detail how the doctor should behave towards the patient. True, at times his advice seems banal: for instance, he explains at length that the doctor should adjust the time and frequency of his visits to cause least inconvenience to the patient. But even these 'commonsense' prescriptions are not always followed, and the horror stories that Galen tells, although in part amusing, are intended to show that mistakes can be made, and the patient put at risk. What motivates Galen throughout is his conviction, deriving from the Hippocratic *Epidemics* and *Prognostic,* that in the battle against illness the patient's cooperation is essential for success. What might, in other circumstances, be termed the doctor's moral standing is here used for a specifically practical purpose, to convince the patient that the Hippocratic healer who stands before him or her is the person who can cure. By acting in a proper manner, with appropriate speech, dress, and deportment, the doctor is being true to the Hippocratic ideal and, at the same time, being an effective healer. The sentiments in the Hippocratic oath add little or nothing to this, as well as importing a series of prohibitions which, as both Edelstein and Danielle Gourevitch have pointed out, were at variance with the medical and social practices of the ancient world.[44]

Galen being Galen, it is hardly surprising to find that his interpretation of his Hippocratic deontological heritage develops it in ways that would have been impossible in the time of Hippocrates. His image of the doctor as possessed of both reason and experience, 'the two legs of sound practice', is not far removed from that of the Corpus, even if his emphasis on logical analysis owes more to Plato and Aristotle than it does to Hippocrates. But his delineation and evaluation of 'experience' goes beyond even that of his predecessors in the Hellenistic world. Above all, as a recent discovery reveals, Galen's model physician is a man of learning, to be judged on what he knew as well as on what he could do.

Written *c.* AD 178, his tract *On examining the best physicians* is intended as a guide for the prospective patient.[45] Reliance on the word of friends or on a healer's social success is, for Galen, illusory. Quacks and charlatans are, if anything, more likely to succeed in Rome than elsewhere, and the reasons for their attendance on the rich and powerful reside as much in their social skills as in their medical. The patient in search of a doctor must, according to Galen, rely on his own resources, and on what he himself can discover about his prospective attendant. This falls into two parts, his way of life and his practical ability. On the first Galen says relatively little, except by way of contrast. The good physician is not going to spend his time in drinking, social climbing, salutations and similar frivolities, but in hard work and study.[46] Indeed, it is self-study that, in this tract, marks out the good doctor from the bad, for Galen nowhere in it mentions any teacher or place of study, or discourses on the ethical qualities expected of the doctor. Instead, he expects his doctor (and, indeed, his patient) to have read a whole series of books, and to be familiar with the opinions of a range of physicians, from Hippocrates onwards. Only if the doctor passes the tests of his theoretical knowledge should he be examined in his practical skills, and, even so, at one point, Galen may well be saying that sound book learning is a more than adequate substitute for experience.[47] How far any physician could come up to Galen's own expectations is an open question, and, even in this treatise, Galen realises that his definition of what a healer should be able to do is well beyond the capacities of the average competent practitioner. Besides, his ideal physician, the encyclopaedic autodidact, bears a suspicious likeness to Galen himself, both in his emphasis on the priority of Hippocratic ideas and in his stress on books. In this treatise the Hippocratic sage turns into the Hippocratic bookworm, and both can be identified with the historical Galen.

The Fate of Hippocratic Deontology

Galen's ideal of the learned doctor, well-versed in all the literature of the past, remained exactly that – an ideal. Although doctors might be occasionally portrayed among their books, what is known about their private libraries suggests that they remained small until the sixteenth century.[48] Yet Galen's prescriptions on the overriding need for book-learning continued to be repeated in the Arab world among writers on the duties of the doctor or of the *muhtasib,* the market inspector, who had the oversight of medical practitioners.[49] Even if not everyone went as far in their adherence to books as the autodidact (and ferocious Galenist) Ibn Ridwan (998–1068), or expressly acknowledged their inheritance of ancient learning, there can be little doubt that the physician in the Islamic world was expected to be familiar with at least some of the writings of Galen and Hippocrates.[50] The Hippocratic *Oath* in particular was seen as in some way normative, for, after its translation into Arabic in the ninth century, it was frequently discussed both in separate tracts and in introductions to medicine. In at least two of the tracts on the duties of the *muhtasib,* that official is advised to administer the *Oath* to any medical practitioner coming under his jurisdiction.[51] Whether this advice was actually carried out is less certain, and perhaps less significant, than the fact that the *Oath* was believed to have been applied in the past to all or to most doctors.[52]

Evidence for the truth of this belief, which, as we have seen, was shared by Scribonius Largus and by Plutarch, is notoriously hard to come by. Galen himself makes very little reference to the *Oath* outside his commentary, and, as I have argued, he regarded it even there as an antiquarian document or, at the very least, as an oath that was no longer to be sworn. Better, if still somewhat fragile, evidence for its use comes in the late fourth century. In one of his letters, St Jerome mentions in passing that Hippocrates 'made all his students swear an oath', illustrating his view of the ideal physician with an allusion to *Decorum.*[53] This comment is probably to be taken simply as a statement about the past, correctly derived from the words of the *Oath* itself, although Jerome clearly implies that such a procedure might well be followed in his own day. More controversial is an allusion to the *Oath* by Gregory of Nazianzus in an oration in praise of his brother Caesarius. This brilliant student had gone off to Alexandria to study medicine, to the consternation of his pious family. They need not have worried about a possible lapse into paganism, for, so his brother proudly declared, Caesarius 'did not swear the Hippocratic *Oath*'.[54] A variety of possible reasons for this omission may be suggested. The *Oath* may not have been compulsory; it may, indeed, never have been administered at all, and Gregory's reference would thus be a piece of antiquarian learning put to good rhetorical use; Christians may, by this date, *c.* 366, have been exempted from taking the *Oath;* or, finally, Caesarius may have taken the *Oath* but in a Christian form.

That the *Oath* was occasionally sworn – and late-Antique Alexandria would have been an appropriate medical centre for such a ceremony[55]– is evident from the various modifications to its wording found in the Greek manuscripts and translations, for a purely dead document would have been left in peace. The earliest text, preserved on a papyrus from Oxyrhynchus in Egypt, shows considerable differences from the norm of the Greek manuscripts; dialect and archaic forms of words are replaced by simpler ones.[56] But even in the later manuscripts there are also substantial divergencies, not least on religious grounds. In some manuscripts, the invocation to the pagan gods is replaced by a version acceptable to Christians; the first section on teaching is drastically cut; and, in one manuscript at least, the operation-clause is replaced by one that strengthens the prohibition of abortion a few lines earlier. In two manuscripts, Vatican, Urbinas gr. 64, and Milan, Ambrosianus B. 113 sup., the words are laid out in the shape of a cross, and in the latter to the confident 'I shall teach the art' is added the cautious 'as it is needful, right, and fitting for Christians to learn it'.[57] Such a tinkering with the text implies that some people at least thought that the *Oath* would be actually administered to a prospective doctor, and that its wording should be brought into line with the prevailing religious morality and linguistic practice.[58]

Of the Classical, ethical or deontological texts that have been mentioned so far in this survey, few, save for the *Oath,* exerted any influence on the Middle Ages. Although, as Professor Garcia Ballester shows, the Galenic image of the physician as a man of reason, experience and learning came to the fore with the rise of the Universities, the texts in which Galen set out his claims in the greatest of detail remained almost unknown. *On prognosis,* which was first translated into Latin around 1340 in S. Italy by Niccolò da Reggio, seems rarely to have been read,[59] while *The best doctor is also a philosopher* and the *Exhortation to medicine* never enjoyed a medieval translation at all. Only in 1525, with the printing of the Aldine Galen in Greek, and perhaps not until Latin translations were published on the basis of the newly discovered Greek, did these works become easily accessible. For the rest, Galen's *Commentary on the Hippocratic Oath* was lost until the nineteenth century, when the translation of large sections into French went almost unnoticed, while *On examining the best physicians* had to wait until 1988 for its *editio princeps.* The treatises in the Hippocratic Corpus were likewise largely forgotten. *Precepts, Decorum,* and the *Physician* were not translated into Latin until the sixteenth century, and although allusions to the *Law* have been detected as early as the ninth century, there is no evidence for a Latin translation until the fourteenth.[60]

What takes the place of these 'genuine' works from the Greek is a series of tracts composed perhaps in late Antiquity and basing themselves on themes, hints, and statements from Hippocrates, Galen and Cassiodorus, and ascribed in the manuscripts to a variety of classical authors or to none. Although the *Oath* is mentioned or implied in several of these treatises, some of which masquerade under the authorship of Hippocrates, the relationship with any Greek original in the Hippocratic Corpus is somewhat remote.[61] In one group of manuscripts a version of the Hippocratic *Oath* is supplemented by a quotation from *Precepts,* and preceded by rules for the need for preliminary instruction in grammar, rhetoric, geometry and astronomy.[62] In another text, which is ascribed to Hippocrates only in late copies, the intending medical student is given advice on how to visit the sick and the questions he should ask. In this document close parallels can be found with the *Medical questions* of Rufus of Ephesus (fl. AD 110) and with statements in Galen, but direct copying from either source is unlikely.[63] Behind some of these texts may lurk the practical advice of Galen. So, for example, in a letter ascribed to Hippocrates, Galen, or, more misleadingly, Isidore of Seville, the physician is warned always to read and to shun indolence; to avoid quarrels and instead to praise the cures of others, since thereby one will obtain a better reputation. It is less clear whether the original version of this little guide contained the injunctions to refrain from getting involved with incurable or certainly fatal cases and to claim half the agreed fee at the outset, for 'when the pain ceases, your services also cease'.[64]

Possibly the most influential of all these later 'Hippocratic' treatises goes under the name of the *Testament of Hippocrates.* It is found in Latin, in Arabic, and also in Greek, where it forms a little paragraph headed 'What the medical student ought to be like'. He is to be of free birth and noble character, young, of medium stature, sturdy, capable in everything, sound in body and mind, resourceful, modest, brave, slow to anger and full of energy. Besides these and many other personal qualities, he should not indulge in abuse, or have his hair close-cropped or too long. His nails, clothing, gait, should all be appropriate, and he should adjust the time and manner of his visit to the patient to suit each case.[65] In some versions, he must also have had a preliminary training in grammar, astronomy, music, and geometry, but not in rhetoric, for this only leads to vaniloquence. Philosophy he will learn alongside medicine.[66] As Deichgräber argued, although the sentiments and language in this *Testament* are Hippocratic, their ultimate source is the section in Galen's commentary on *Epidemics VI* that we have already singled out as his major reinterpretation of the practical duties of the doctor.[67] It is thus not surprising that the advice that is recounted here is independent of the *Oath*, despite, in some manuscripts and versions, its claims to the authorship and authority of Hippocrates.

Conclusion

The Hippocratic *Oath*, as this survey has shown, is not the only text on medical ethics or deontology surviving or purporting to survive from Antiquity, nor did it have the overriding authority sometimes imputed to it by modern medical ethicists. Both in Antiquity and in the Early Middle Ages it was perfectly possible to devise a code of medical practice that was ostensibly Hippocratic without involving the moral choices implied in the *Oath*. Whether the result is to be classified as medical ethics or medical deontology is a question of terminology rather than of substance, for the advice given to the doctor in these treatises is couched in moral language and, implicitly or explicitly, touches on moral actions. But these moral actions are subordinated to the needs of effective practice, since all parties were agreed on the need to gain the patient's confidence and co-operation in the battle against disease. Kindness, courage, a refusal to cheat the patient, a willingness to set a fair fee, a lifestyle that lacked ostentation and extravagance, all would suggest that here was a healer who would act to the best of his ability and whose treatment was likely to be successful (for both sides). From such a practical perspective, the Hippocratic *Oath* was less useful than *Precepts* or even than the rules for medical practice that could be derived from other therapeutic texts in the Corpus. Its injunctions to help the sick and respect the art of medicine, and, negatively, to refrain from poisoning, gossip, and sexual misdemeanours with patients, can all be seen as acting towards a practical end, the cure of the sick. Hence they fit easily into the more general picture of medical behaviour, whether in Antiquity or in the Middle Ages, for the therapeutic relationship between doctor and patient hardly changes, and there are few technological advances that open up radically new possibilities for medical intervention. The other recommendations of the *Oath*, on abortion, euthanasia, and surgery, as Edelstein and Gourevitch have both shown, presuppose a series of answers to moral dilemmas that were not accepted in society at large in Antiquity, and hence they figure rarely, if at all, in the medical writings of Antiquity. Indeed, it might be argued that it was precisely because these sections fitted more neatly a Christian, Muslim, and Jewish moral code, that the Hippocratic *Oath* gained in authority over the other texts in the Corpus, and came ultimately to be seen as possessing an overriding validity. Even then, as we have seen, texts that defined the duties of the healer narrowly in terms of what was most conducive to healing continued to figure largely in discussions of appropriate medical practice.

It should not be forgotten also that the function of a medical *oath* might vary from place to place, and that it served as much to bind the members of a medical group together as to compel them to follow specific therapies and practices. True, the Hippocratic *Oath* can be interpreted in both senses, but it is dangerous to assume that in Antiquity or in the Middle Ages the same priorities operated that today invite both layman and physician to invoke the authority of the *Oath*. The Early Middle Ages, as we have seen, possessed a whole series of deontological texts that were presumed to derive from the great doctor of Cos. Whether short or long, they helped to foster a model of medical behaviour that could co-exist alongside that of the *Oath*. Indeed, their existence both confirmed the validity of the Hippocratic model of medical practice and, at the same time, removed the *Oath* from any position as the unique purveyor of medical ethics. The Hippocratic tradition of proper medical behaviour did not flow in a single channel.

Against this background, it is not surprising to find that very few of the medical oaths that were sworn by medical students in the mediaeval universities (and beyond) incorporated sections from the Hippocratic *Oath*, although several are recognisably 'Hippocratic' in spirit.[68] Indeed, far from being universally sworn by all medical students, the *Oath* as such does not appear to have been used at all until the sixteenth century, first in a somewhat altered form at Wittenberg in 1508, and then in the revised humanist statutes of the University of Basle in 1570.[69] The concentration in medical literature on the *Oath* as the prime, not to say unique, ethical document from Antiquity is thus a relatively recent phenomenon, the product of a Renaissance which purified itself of its medieval accretions. The decline of Galenism from the mid-sixteenth century and the consequent exaltation of the 'historical' Hippocrates only confirmed the superiority of the *Oath*, and led to the neglect of other similar texts. But, as Edelstein argued, the medical ethics of Antiquity are far too complex – and far too interesting – to be confined to a single document. Indeed, the appeal to a text whose wording and interpretation are assumed to possess a universal and unchanging validity may reveal far more about the medical ethics and medical ethicists of the twentieth century than it does about those of the fifth century BC.[70] It is a paradox that the Hippocratic *Oath*, which, on my interpretation, gained in authority precisely because of its ethical compatibility with Christianity, should now so often be cited to resolve moral medical dilemmas which are largely the result of the decline of that Christian moral consensus that gave it its authority.[71]

Notes

1. Ludwig Edelstein, 'The professional ethics of the Greek physician', *Bulletin of the History of Medicine*, xxx (1956), 391–419 = *Ancient Medicine* (Baltimore: Johns Hopkins Press, 1967), 319–48. Cf. also his 'The Hippocratic Oath', *Supplement to the Bulletin of the History of Medicine*, i (1943) = *Ancient medicine*, 3–63. A succinct survey is given by Danielle Gourevitch, *Le triangle hippocratique dans le monde gréco-romain. Le malade, sa maladie, et son médecin* (Rome: Ecole française, 1984), 251–88. P. Carrick, *Medical ethics in Antiquity: philosophical perspectives on abortion and euthanasia* (Dordrecht: Reidel, 1985), adds nothing to Edelstein save error. This essay was written before the publication of Owsei Temkin, *Hippocrates in a World of Pagans and Christians* (Baltimore: Johns Hopkins University Press, 1991), a brilliant survey, which covers many of the points made here, albeit from a slightly different perspective. I have made only occasional reference to this book, which should be regarded (and read) as complementary to this essay.
2. I would set the *Law* and the *Oath* in the period 410–350 BC; the *Physician* perhaps a generation or so later; *Precepts* and *Decorum*, from their language and their social context, are unlikely to predate 200 BC, and could well have been composed in the last century BC A somewhat later dating presents problems, but is not entirely excluded. Although the *Oath* and, occasionally, the *Law* are included in English translations of Hippocratic writings, the other texts are usually not. However, all are to be found in the Loeb Library series; *Oath* and *Precepts*, vol. 1; the rest in vol 2 (where only ch. 1 of the *Physician* is printed).
3. Contrast *Oath*, line 10, with *Precepts*, chs 8 and 12.
4. *Precepts*, ch. 1, which begins with a reminiscence of *Aphorisms* 1.1; for the vocabulary, see Jones' introduction to his Loeb edition and translation, vol 1 (London: Heinemann, 1957) 305–11. *Decorum*, chs 1, 4.

5. *Law*, chs. 2–3, reflecting the well-known debate in Greek philosophy over the relationship between nature *(physis)* and custom (*nomos* - the word here translated as 'law').
6. Although acknowledging a strong interchange in the fifth and fourth centuries between medicine and philosophy, few scholars now would accept Edelstein's contention that this component in the *Oath* is Pythagorean. Cf. for the question of Pythagoreanism, Charles Lichtenthaeler, *Der Eid des Hippokrates* (Cologne: Deutscher Ärzte-Verlag, 1984), 279–92. Charles Singer, 'An early parallel to the Hippocratic Oath', *Gesnerus*, viii (1951), 177–80, drew attention to similar words and sentiments in religious regulations from the shrine of Agdistis in Lydia. Gourevitch, *Le triangle hippocratique*, 260–2, counselling against any direct relationship between the *Oath* and these regulations, adduces other similar examples from religious laws, notably from Pergamum. The question of Pythagorean or religious influence is independent of that of authorship, where, *pace* Lichtenthaeler, the probability still seems to me against the historical Hippocrates as the author of the *Oath*.
7. Cf. above, note 4, for parallels between the religious language of the *Oath* and those of *leges sacrae*.
8. For the *pholeon* at Velia, see now M. Fabbri, A. Trotta, *Una scuola-collegio di età augustea* (Rome: Bretschneider, 1989), who give a full bibliography of discussions of the rare word *pholeon*. A series of inscriptions and statues commemorates doctors who were also *pholarchoi;* all bear the (family ? or cult ?) name *Oulis*, and the whole association looks back to Parmenides *Ouliades*, the *physikos*, fl. 480 BC
9. Indeed, the *Oath* is unusual in its implication that an appropriate moral *attitude* must precede and determine good medical practice; for most writers in antiquity, sound medical *practice* inevitably produces a moral attitude, and hence discussions of medical ethics are couched in terms of appropriate action. I owe this point to Professor Robert Baker.
10. Edelstein interpreted the second noun to refer only to the patient, but see now Temkin, *Hippocrates*, 30–1.
11. The author of the Hippocratic tract *On the art* spent a great deal of time in rebutting the suggestion that a healer was an unnecessary and expensive luxury, for diseases either cured themselves or could be treated by simple self-help, see the *Art*, chs 8–9. For a general survey of attitudes, see D. W. Amundsen, 'Images of physicians in classical times', *Journal of Popular Culture*, viii (1977), 301–15; and my *From Democedes to Harvey* (London: Variorum, 1988), ch. VIII.
12. L. Gil, I. R. Alfageme, 'La figura del médico en la comedia Atica', *Cuadernos de Filologia Clásica*, iii (1972), 35–91. Plato at times took medicine as a model for his science, and in his philosophy knowledge of what is (morally) good inevitably results in moral actions. At *Republic* III, 406–7, Plato attacks Herodicus (and Hippocratic

doctors?) for keeping alive by medical means those who are no longer of any use to themselves or society. It is not entirely clear how far Plato's opinion represents a lay challenge to a medical moral belief, rather than an individual reaction to an individual theory.

13. Galen, *On prognosis* 4; XIV 622–4 K.
14. See above all, Galen, *On examining the best physicians,* A. Z. Iskandar (ed.) (Berlin: Akademie Verlag, 1988), with my article, 'The patient's choice: a new treatise by Galen', *Classical Quarterly,* xl (1990), 236–57.
15. *Digest* 50,9,1; and he could presumably also be re-examined and refused immunity, *ibid,*. 59,4,11,3 (the source of 27,1,6,6), on similar grounds. It should perhaps be noted that in the last two passages *'res publica'* does not indicate 'the state', but, as another work of Ulpian which mentioned civic doctors, *De officio curatoris rei publicae (On the duty of a financial overseer of the community),* shows, should be translated as 'community'.
16. *Tituli Asiae Minoris* II.2.663, Cadyanda. Similar phraseology is common on other honorific inscriptions. A list is given by L. Cohn-Haft, *The public physicians of Ancient Greece* (Northampton, Mass.: Smith College Studies in History, xlii (1956)), 77–85, but he does not pursue the question of the language of the decrees.
17. W. Dittenberger, *Sylloge inscriptionum graecarum,* ed. 3, n. 807, Magnesia ad Maeandrum. The last Greek word corresponds to the Latin *'mores'.*
18. The point is seen by Gourevitch, *Le triangle hippocratique,* 414–37, but is obscured by her failure to separate honorary decrees from tombstones and other private inscriptions. Similarly, her evidence for doctors as good parents, friends, masters, etc., is, in her discussion, only relevant indirectly to the appropriate moral standing of the physician. A study of both *Precepts* and *Decorum* in the light of what is now known of medical practice in the Hellenistic and Roman periods would be valuable. Cf. also for attempts to differentiate between medical and popular ethics, F. Kudlien, 'Medical ethics and popular ethics in Greece and Rome', *Clio Medica,* v (1970), 91–121.
19. It is worth noting that in the literature on the duties of a judge, governor, doctor, etc., associated by Edelstein with the Stoic Panaetius, fl. 140 BC, the moral element does not arise within the activities of the individual but corresponds to the moral norm of the surrounding society or sect (Stoic or Epicurean), and thus fluctuates according to the more general social changes in morality.
20. [Soranus], *Introductio,* Rose (ed.), 244 = *Erasistrati fragmenta,* Garofalo (ed.), fr. 31. Edelstein, *Ancient medicine,* 334, accepted the passage as genuine; Garofalo apparently rejects it; Gourevitch, *Le triangle hippocratique,* 268, suggests that only the first part of the sentence, which says that the best situation is one in which *'artes'* and *'mores'* are combined, is genuine, but not the hypothetical second section. If she is right, then a commonplace from Erasistratus has

been later developed to indicate a preference for morality over science. The morality of the less proficient healer will at least ensure that he performs as well as he can, and that the patient will not be financially cheated or otherwise abused.

21. F. Kudlien, *Der griechische Arzt im Zeitalter des Hellenismus* (Wiesbaden: Steiner Verlag, 1979), 98–103, discusses whether medical guilds sought to preserve the interests of the social group, and decides against it. An inscription from Ephesus, *Die Inschriften von Ephesos* 1386, records a decision (of the city or, more likely, of the doctors' guild) relating to fees, but its precise import can scarcely be reconstructed with certainty from the fragments of the stone.
22. See the discussion by V. Nutton in *From Democedes to Harvey*, ch. VIII, 30. About 40 BC the Roman triumvirs declared that all doctors, teachers, and 'sophists' were free from *eisphora* (special taxation) and from certain tolls, see D. Knibbe, 'Neue Inschriften aus Ephesos', *Jahreshefte des österreichischen archäologischen Institut*, liii (1981/2), 136–40, which may well imply that these tax privileges went back still further in the Hellenistic period in the East. But no text, as far as I am aware, lays down qualifications for recognition as a member of these groups. The pragmatic assumption, that a man was a doctor or teacher because he in some way or other healed or taught, was probably all that was necessary.
23. The legal status of the healer is nicely covered by F. Kudlien, *Die Stellung des Arztes in der römischen Gesellschaft* (Stuttgart: Steiner Verlag, 1986) but even he underestimates the variety of possible healers. See also V. Nutton, *From Democedes to Harvey*, chs VII–IX.
24. For surgeons, e.g. Celsus, *De medicina* 7, pr. 4; Oxyrhynchus papyrus 437 (= M. H. Marganne, *Inventaire analytique des Papyrus grecs de Médecine* (Geneva: Droz, 1981), no. 132); for the midwife, Soranus, *Gynaecology*, 1.2–3.
25. Scribonius Largus, *Compositiones*, pr. The fundamental study remains K. Deichgräber, *Professio medici, Zum Vorwort des Scribonius Largus* (Mainz; Akademie der Wissenschaften, 1950). Later studies are based on the new Teubner text by S. Sconocchia (Leipzig: Teubner, 1983), which alters the wording in a few places, but not significantly. The translation of the *Preface* by J. S. Hamilton, 'Scribonius Largus on the medical profession', *Bulletin of the History of Medicine*, lx (1986), 209–16, is distressingly unreliable, and the somewhat freer version of E. D. and A. A. Pellegrino, 'Humanism and ethics in Roman medicine', *Literature and Medicine*, vii (1988), 22–38, is even worse. For example, the crucial sentence that opens para. 2 (p. 1, lines 11–14 Sconocchia) is totally garbled in both these versions because their translators do not understand that 'medicinam spoliare .... usu medicamentorum' means 'to rob medicine of the use of drugs'. Such mistakes in simple grammar and syntax are, alas, only too common, with drastic consequences for the interpretation of the document.

26. Scribonius would certainly have been aware of the story that Hippocrates as a good Greek had refused to treat the King of Persia (cf. Plutarch, *Cato Maior*, ch. 23, where Cato is understood to claim that all Greek physicians had sworn a 'common oath' not to serve their enemies) and, in a Roman context, of the Romans' decision to reject as dishonourable the offer of Nicias, physician to King Pyrrhus of Ephesus, to murder his master on their behalf, Aulus Gellius, *Noctes Atticae* III.8.5, with Livy, *Historiae* XLII.47.6 (but both name and position of the plotter are open to doubt, cf. also Aelian, *Historia varia* XII.33, and Plutarch, *Pyrrhus*, 21.1, with the discussion of H. Münzer, in W. Pauly, G. Wissowa, *Realenzyclopädie*, Band VI Stuttgart: Metzler, 1909, 1935–6).
27. Text and translation are conveniently given by J. H. Oliver and P. L. Maas, 'An ancient poem on the duties of a physician', *Bulletin of the History of Medicine*, vii (1939), 315–23; and by Gourevitch, *Le triangle hippocratique*, 278–80 (with an up-to-date bibliography). Her layout of the poem obscures the restorations, and, 280, in talking of Sarapion's sexuality she makes overmuch of some very literary *flosculi*. Since the word for 'virtue', *arete*, can encompass both moral excellence and technical skill, the exact force of the word is uncertain, but, in the whole context of the passage, a purely ethical connotation is the most likely.
28. Two fundamental studies are O. Temkin, *Galenism. Rise and decline of a medical philosophy* (Ithaca: Cornell University Press, 1973); and Wesley D. Smith, *The Hippocratic Tradition* (Ithaca: Cornell University Press, 1979), which, despite its title, is largely about Galen's attitude to Hippocrates. Galen wrote three separate works on the *Timaeus*, a *Summary*, a *Commentary*, and *On medical statements in the Timaeus*. New fragments of the last have been found in a Greek manuscript in the Escorial, see now Carlos J. Larrain, *Galens Kommentar zu Platons Timaeos* (Stuttgart: Teubner, 1992).
29. Galen, I.53–63 Kühn (ed.); significant improvements to the Kühn text were made by I. v. Mueller, *Galeni scripta minora*, II (Leipzig: Teubner, 1891) 2–8; E. Wenkebach, 'Der hippokratische Arzt als das Ideal Galens', *Quellen und Studien zur Geschichte der Naturwissenschaften und Medizin*, iii (1932/3), 155–75; P. Bachmann, 'Galens Abhandlung darüber, dass der vorzügliche Arzt Philosoph sein muss', *Nachrichten der Akademie der Wissenschaften in Göttingen, phil.-hist. Klasse*, 1965. An English translation is given by Peter Brain, 'Galen on the ideal of the physician', *S. African Medical Journal*, lii (1977), 936–8. The date of the tract is very uncertain, since Galen gives no cross references to other works. Smith, *The Hippocratic Tradition*, 83, suggests composition during Galen's first stay in Rome, AD 162–6, but if the observation of Hans Diller, 'Zur Hippokratesauffassung des Galen', *Hermes*, lxviii (1933), 180, is correct, that Galen's quotations from *Airs, waters, and places*, I.59 K., come from his commentary, not from the text of

Hippocrates, then the date must be pushed considerably later, to the 180s or even beyond. But Galen's ability to reproduce the same thoughts in the same language over decades imposes hesitation.

30. Galen; XIV.660 K. The phrase reported by Galen, 'first among doctors and unique among philosophers' recalls the language of honorary decrees for champion athletes. Earlier in the book, XIV.614 K., Galen reports hostility in AD 163 'for the first time' directed at his medical skills and his 'dignified way of life'.
31. Lucian, *De saltatione.* Galen, we know, was acquainted with Lucian, but, since similar claims are made for architecture, poetry, and mathematics, as well as medicine, Lucian's satire need not be directed against him, cf. also B. P. Reardon, *Courants littéraires grecs* (Paris: Les Belles Lettres, 1971), 30–41.
32. I.55 K. Galen is not referring to their (literary) 'style' (so Smith, *The Hippocratic tradition,* 83) as such, but to their ability to express themselves clearly and accurately. Their double mistake consists in choosing the wrong concept and the wrong word.
33. Diller, 'Zur Hippokratesauffassung', 176–80, discusses Galen's sources. His disquiet at the presence of an allusion to *On places in man* (for which he provides an adequate explanation) would have been lessened by the (later) discovery of an Arabic text in which Galen also refers to this 'Hippocratic' work, see *Commentary on Epidemics II, CMG* V 10.1, 311.
34. He recorded the same stories, in greater detail, in his *Commentary on the Hippocratic Oath,* on which see further below, and, as we have already seen, some of them were known to Scribonius and Plutarch, if not to the Elder Cato. The significance of these stories in helping to fix the moral character of Hippocrates is well brought out by Temkin, *Hippocrates,* 39–78; and by Jody Rubin Pinault, *Hippocratic Lives and Legends* (Leiden: Brill, 1992).
35. Diller, 'Zur Auffassung', 172, noted the omission of *Precepts.* Neither *Oath, Decorum* nor *Precepts* features in Smith's list of texts in *The Hippocratic Tradition.*
36. See, above all, *On prognosis,* with my commentary on it, *CMG* V 8,1 (Berlin: Akademie Verlag, 1979).
37. Galen, *On diagnosing affections* 6; V.30 K., cf. his quotation of a verse from the poem at ch. 5: V.26 K. The same procedure is recommended by Seneca, *De ira* 3.36.3, and by Epictetus, 3.10.2. For Galen's religious beliefs, see F. Kudlien, 'Galen's religious belief', in V. Nutton, *Galen: problems and prospects* (London: The Wellcome Institute, 1979), 117–30; and Temkin, *Hippocrates,* 181–96. On a god as a protector and helpmeet, cf. Robin Lane Fox, *Pagans and Christians* (Harmondsworth: Penguin, 1988), 115–38.
38. F. Rosenthal, 'An ancient commentary on the Hippocratic Oath', *Bulletin of the History of Medicine,* xxx (1956), 52–87 (reprinted in his *Science and medicine in Islam* [Aldershot: Variorum, 1991]). For

doubts on its authenticity, cf. K. Deichgräber, 'Die ärztliche Standesethik des hippokratischen Eides', *Quellen und Studien zur Geschichte der Wissenschaften und der Medizin,* iii (1932), 97–8.

39. G. Strohmaier, 'Asklepios und das Ei: zur Ikonographie in einem arabisch erhaltenen Kommentar zum hippokratischen Eid', in Ruth Stiehl and Hans Erich Stier, *Beiträge zur alten Geschichte und deren Nachleben. Festschrift für Franz Altheim* (Berlin: de Gruyter, 1970), 143–53. Cf. also the parallels noted by me in 'The patient's choice', 254, answering an objection to authenticity raised by Kudlien, 'Galen's religious belief', 119. Pinault, *Hippocratic Lives,* 95–124, discusses the Arabic biographical tradition, and suggests that there was a lost intermediary between it and the Greek stories, but fails to realise that it was this Galenic commentary.
40. Since the commentary is said to have been only a single book in length, I calculate that we have approximately one quarter of the text.
41. Galen, *Commentary 2 on Epidemics I:* XVII A.148–9 K.
42. In the commentary on the *Oath,* fr. 2e: 67–76 Rosenthal, Galen uses the attributes of Asclepius of Pergamum to indicate the moral and intellectual qualities of the doctor when treating the sick. The restriction of ethics implied here does not seem to me fortuitous. Temkin, *Hippocrates,* says very little about this commentary.
43. Hippocrates, *Epidemics VI.*4.7; Galen, *Commentary IV on Epidemics VI,* 8–10: XVII B. 135–152 K., with the much improved text at *CMG* V 10.2.2, 199–207. These pages are the subject of a brilliant study by Karl Deichgräber, 'Medicus gratiosus', *Akademie der Wissenschaften und der Literatur, Mainz, Abhandlungen der geistes- und sozialwissenschaftlichen Klasse* (1970), 195–309.
44. Edelstein, *Ancient medicine, passim*; Gourevitch, *Le triangle hippocratique,* 169–216.
45. For details, see above, note 14.
46. An interesting comment on Galen's moral priorities. Ethical considerations are subordinated to the needs of effective practice.
47. *On examining physicians,* 9.3; the Arabic says that the man of intelligence and book-learning is superior to the man who has neither intelligence nor experience, but the underlying Greek may have given a slightly different sense. For the possibilities, cf. my 'The patient's choice', 248, n. 53.
48. For a relief of a doctor in front of his book cabinet, see J. Scarborough, *Roman Medicine* (London: Thames and Hudson, 1969), pl. 12 (but wrongly dated to 'late hellenistic period' instead of to *c.* AD 300).
49. For the use of *On examining physicians* in later literature, see Iskandar's introduction, 20–5. He unfortunately misses an important reference in al-Shayzari (fl. 1190), *Nihayat al-rutba fi talab al-hisba* (Cairo, 1946), 100, cited by G. Karmi, 'State control of the physicians in the Middle Ages: an Islamic model', in A. W. Russell,

The town and state physician (Wolfenbüttel: Herzog-August-Bibliothek, 1981), 75. Al-Shayzari declares that in his day there was almost no one (no *muhtasib*?) who adhered to the conditions laid down by Galen in *On examining physicians*. For the role of the *muhtasib*, see Karmi, 73–84, and M. W. Dols, *Medieval islamic medicine* (Berkeley: University of California Press, 1984), 33–4. By far the best introduction to medical ethics in Islam is given by J. C. Bürgel, 'Die Bildung des Arztes: eine arabische Schrift zum ärztlichen Leben aus dem 9. Jahrhundert', *Sudhoffs Archiv*, l (1966), 337–60. A. A. Naji, 'Medical ethics and the Islamic tradition', *Journal of Medicine and Philosophy*, xiii (1988), 257–75, renders some of Bürgel's conclusions accessible in English, but is otherwise thin.

50. Dols, *ibid.*, 55–66. He was not alone in laying great stress on the *Oath*, *ibid.*, 35, but his decision to write commentaries on the *Law* and on the so-called *Testament of Hippocrates* was very unusual. On the Islamic physician in general, see Franz Rosenthal, 'The physician in medieval Muslim society', *Bulletin of the History of Medicine*, lii (1978), 475–91 (reprinted in his *Science and medicine in Islam*).
51. J. C. Bürgel, *Untersuchungen zum ärztlichen Leben und Denken im arabischen Mittelalter* (Diss., Göttingen, 1970), 261–6, esp. 261, rightly noting the difficulty of reconciling the prescriptive deontological literature with the facts of practice; Karmi, 'State control', 75. For the wider context of Hippocratism in Arabic cf. also Manfred Ullmann, *Die Medizin im Islam* (Leiden: Brill, 1970), 32–3; A. Dietrich, *Ippocrate presso gli arabi* (Rome: Accademia nazionale dei Lincei, 1987), esp. 11–16; and Ursula Weisser, 'Das Corpus Hippocraticum in der arabischen Medizin', in G. Baader, R. Winau, (eds), *Die Hippokratischen Epidemien, Sudhoffs Archiv, Beiheft* 27 (Stuttgart: Steiner, 1990), 377–408, esp. 399–406. Even if a survey of the literary remains suggests a normative value for the *Oath*, exactly what this was is unclear. As far as I am aware, there are no discussions setting up the *Oath* as an ethic for doctors against the prevailing moral injunctions of the *Koran*, and I suspect that it gained in importance precisely because its moral guidelines could be easily subordinated to those of Islam.
52. Cf. the interpretation given by Ibn Abi Usaibi'a, cited by Rosenthal, 'An ancient commentary', 81.
53. Jerome, *Ep.* 52.15. For the problem of interpretation and for late antique Hippocratism, see Fridolf Kudlien, *Reallexikon für Antike und Christentum*, fasc. 115 (1989), s.v. Hippokrates, 466–80; and Temkin, *Hippocrates*.
54. Gregory Naz., *Or.* 7.10.
55. It is tempting to associate with Alexandria the commentary on the *Aphorisms* ascribed to Oribasius and preserved in Latin, ed. Basle, 1535, fol. 7, which claims that the *Oath* was the first work written by Hippocrates and administered by him to all intending medical

students. The date and place of this translation are unknown, perhaps Ravenna in the sixth century. A similar time and place may be suggested for the *Introduction* ascribed to Soranus, which seems to allude to several other deontological texts as well as the *Oath,* see Gourevitch, *Le triangle hippocratique,* 269–71.

56. Papyrus Oxyrhynchus 2547 = Marganne, no. 138. This papyrus entered the collections of the Wellcome Institute Library in 1968.
57. W. H. S. Jones, *The doctor's Oath,* (Cambridge: Cambridge University Press, 1924), 18–27. Note also the changes to the preamble of the Arabic version of the *Oath, ibid.,* 31.
58. A related example is the Hebrew 'covenant which Asaph .... and Yohanan .... made with their pupils', which is based in part on the Hippocratic *Oath,* albeit greatly modified, see the summary of the paper by S. Newmyer, 'The oath of Asaph and its Hippocratic original', *Newsletter of the Society for Ancient Medicine and Pharmacy,* xvii (1989), 10. See also Elinor Lieber, 'Asaf's *Book of medicines:* a Hebrew encyclopedia of Greek and Jewish medicine, possibly compiled in Byzantium on an Indian model', *Dumbarton Oaks Papers,* xxx (1984), 233–49, esp. n. 33, which gives the earlier literature. Although Dr Lieber rightly draws attention to the whole context of the *Oath,* I find few of her speculations convincing.
59. See the introduction to my edition, Berlin, 1979.
60. See, for the Latin Hippocrates, Pearl Kibre, *Hippocrates Latinus* (New York: Fordham University Press, 1985).
61. L. C. MacKinney, 'Medical ethics and etiquette in the Early Middle Ages: the persistence of Hippocratic ideals', *Bulletin of the History of Medicine,* vi (1952), 1–31. Kibre, *Hippocrates,* 198, 232–3, lists the manuscripts of *Praecepta* and of *De visitando infirmum,* both ascribed to Hippocrates.
62. MacKinney, 'Medical ethics', 13–5, with, 13, a photo of most of the relevant sections in Chartres 62, a manuscript that suffered severe damage in the last war.
63. *Ibid.,* 24, cf. also H. Sigerist, 'Early mediaeval medical texts in manuscripts of Montpellier', *Bulletin of the History of Medicine,* x (1941), 31–2; for the ascriptions to Hippocrates, see Kibre, *Hippocrates latinus,* 198, 233. A later tract on the same topic, usually anonymous, *ibid.,* 233, is Salernitan in origin and has links with Galen, see the apparatus to S. De Renzi, *Collectio Salernitana,* vol 2 (Naples: Filatre-Sebezio, 1853), 74–80.
64. MacKinney, 'Medical ethics', 23; Kibre, *Hippocrates latinus,* 91–3, 148. Kibre cavalierly deals with the various short ethical texts translated by MacKinney as if they were part of the same work, and, amazingly, declares that they 'coincide with the first two or three paragraphs of the Hippocratic *De arte*'. The briefest of glances at this tract, now available in a superb edition by J. Jouanna (Paris: Les Belles Lettres, 1988), shows the folly of this remark.

65. Deichgräber, *Medicus gratiosus*, 88–107, is fundamental, and my translation is based on the Greek text given on 97. An English version of the *Testament* is provided by Jones, *The doctor's oath*, 59–60, and by MacKinney, 'Medical ethics', 16–19, Document K., but his arrangement is confusing and shows no knowledge of the non-Latin variants. On the *Testament* in Arabic, see Bürgel, *Untersuchungen*, 99–113, and Deichgräber, *Medicus gratiosus*, 108–13, who also discusses a reworking of this treatise by Rhazes (d. 925). Kibre, *Hippocrates*, has no entry for this work, although she cites one manuscript of it, 92, as coming from *De arte*, and another 198, under the heading *Precepta*. (Her third entry under this heading is a manuscript of *De visitando infirmum*).
66. The section is not to be found in the redaction printed by Deichgräber, *Medicus gratiosus*, 97, or in the Arabic, given on 91, but occurs in that printed on 100, and in the Latin. If the Ambrosian manuscript represents the earliest stage, we have a good example of a modification of an ethical text to accommodate new external concerns, i.e. the changes in educational methods. One may speculate on the direction of the transmission, especially if the texts circulated in a bilingual community as in S. Italy or in 6th-century Ravenna.
67. I am not as confident as MacKinney, 'Medical ethics', 30, of the lack of Galenic influence, although his point about the parallels with *Precepts* and *Decorum* still stands.
68. I am using the term 'Hippocratic' to refer to the whole complex of traditional beliefs about the duties of the physician as listed by MacKinney. This does not imply either a direct descent from Hippocrates or from the *Oath*.
69. See W. Nolte, *Der hippokratische Eid und der Abschlusseide der früheren und jetzigen deutschsprachigen Hochschulen*, (Diss., Bochum: 1981), 92–3. This is not to say that some traces of the *Oath* cannot be found earlier, e.g. at Montpellier, see Jones, *The Doctor's Oath*, 60.
70. Note the use made of it by Robert Veatch, *A theory of medical ethics*, (New York, Basic Books, 1981).
71. It is no coincidence then that it is often cited by those who are resisting change on religious grounds, whether Christian, Jewish or Muslim, and that the sections on teaching and surgery, which offer advice contrary to the modern medical consensus, are never cited.

2

Medical Ethics in Transition in the Latin Medicine of the Thirteenth and Fourteenth Centuries: New Perspectives on the Physician-Patient Relationship and the Doctor's Fee

Luis García-Ballester

In this chapter, I would like to concentrate on the significant role played in some elements of the physician-patient relationship – with obvious ethical repercussions – by the introduction of intellectual novelties in a particularly crucial period in the development of the university schools, namely, the period between the late thirteenth century and the early fourteenth century. It is a period, and a subject, especially in territories of present-day Spain such as the Crown of Aragon,[1] that have not yet been fully investigated. It is a period in which the true foundations of the faculties of medicine were being established, a period in which Aristotle's natural philosophy and Galen's medicine were adopted by the schools of medicine, and a period in which the intellectual history of scholastic Galenism was established.[2] To these novelties should be added the rediscovery of Roman law texts in the law schools, especially that of Bologna and those law schools influenced by it, from the first third of the thirteenth century onwards.[3]

The 'New Galen', an Intellectual Movement with Deep Repercussions on Scholastic Medicine and Surgery.

During the 1280s and the following decades, an intellectual movement with significant consequences took place in the university medical circles of Montpellier, Bologna and Paris.[4] This movement not only broadened horizons and aroused scientific curiosity among the community of university physicians and surgeons, but also enabled them to re-interpret texts and concepts (for example, fever, *complexio,* quantitative grade, among others) that were already well-known, and led them to make the process of diagnosis increasingly technical. The doctor-patient relationship itself was affected by this movement, including the problem of doctor's fee. What four centuries later became known as problems dealing with medical ethics (not medical etiquette) could have originated in part during these medieval centuries. The protagonists of this significant development – among whom were Arnau de Vilanova, Bernard de Gordon, Henri de Mondeville, Jean de Saint-Amand, Pietro d'Abano, Taddeo Alderotti and Bartolómeo de Varignana – undertook such a process through three types of activity. In the first place, within the space of a few years, they introduced a considerable number of new medical works (mostly by Galen, but also by other authors such as Averroes), which gave their commentaries and systematic works an attractive complexity when compared with those of earlier writers. Secondly, they succeeded in institutionalizing this movement by means of direct participation in the reform of medical syllabuses. Thirdly, they encouraged the diffusion of this intellectual movement beyond the walls of the faculties of medicine with the intention of making it socially accepted. In order to achieve this last aim, they endeavoured to win over as large a number as possible of non-university physicians and/or surgeons.[5] At the same time, they tried to influence those persons (kings, popes, civil and ecclesiastical nobles, members of the bourgeoisie) and social groupings (particularly municipalities) with a capacity to encourage social changes that might favour the greater visibility and diffusion of those university professionals who were the products of this intellectual movement.[6]

It seems reasonable to state that the massive introduction of such important works of Galen's (among which stand out, *De virtutibus naturalibus, De interioribus,* the collection of pathological writings grouped under the title of *De morbo et accidenti, De complexionibus, De malicia complexionis diverse, De crisi, De creticis,* various works on the pulse, *De medicinis simplicibus,* and *De ingenio sanitatis*) into a medical 'curriculum' that had hitherto been limited to the description of and commentary on the various writings collected under the heading *Articella,* brought about, as a consequence, a far more detailed knowledge of the Galenic system than that in the possession of those physicians who lived before these developments. If the incorporation in full of Avicenna's *Canon* and the works of other Arab physicians such as Razes, Alkindi or Averroes is added to this, we possess all the intellectual elements that enabled the master physicians in the above mentioned medical circles, and those of the Latin European countries who were in contact with them, to reconsider old questions and to set forth audacious reflections and solutions that would broaden the intellectual and practical horizons both of the academic community and also of the medical community subject to its direct or indirect influence.[7]

This medical community came to include, moreover, a new type of surgeon who would find within this movement one of the elements that distinguished this new attitude from that of those who insisted on keeping surgery at a purely empirical level and on reducing the process of training to a mere oral or family tradition, as was denounced by university surgeons in the first decade of the fourteenth century.[8] The surgery ('manual work') that these learned masters talk of is not that practised by empirics, whether they acclaim themselves to be barbers or surgeons, but the form that is practised by a new surgeon who aspires to base his surgical technique (*ars*) on a 'medical science', in which, as we shall see, the 'new Galen' played a decisive role.[9] It was not by chance that Henri de Mondeville began his treatise on surgery by making reference to book V of Galen's *De morbo et accidenti.*[10] When the physicians and surgeons who belonged to the university circles that we are describing read the works of Galen, they found in them not only a wealth of doctrine, methods and techniques for curing, but also an intellectual stimulus upon which a new attitude might be developed. For example, in the work cited by Henri de Mondeville (*De morbo et accidenti*, book V, chapter 3), Galen states:

> ... if anyone wishes to understand the truth of a problem, let him read our work and pay attention to the natural world; if he does not follow our advice, never will he achieve perfect understanding of the problem.[11]

Such words were certainly attractive for a surgeon such as Henri de Mondeville, who took particular care to make it clear that his ambition would be to manage to unite in his work 'his (personal) experience and the doctrine of all his masters'.[12] In fact, the new surgeon resulting from the intellectual movement that has been summarised in the expression the 'new Galen' distinguished himself from other surgeons in two fundamental ways: (1) by knowing why he was doing what he was doing; and (2) by knowing how to do what he did well. The first part could only be achieved by means of 'medical science' or the so-called 'principles of medicine' based on Galenism; the second part could be accomplished through practice. For this reason, an unqualified, but experienced surgeon could carry out an operation very well, perhaps even better than a surgeon who had made an effort to gain knowledge of these principles of medical science; nevertheless, the former would never become a true surgeon.[13]

Intellectual appreciation of the 'new Galen' required that the university physician or surgeon should have a detailed knowledge of the Aristotelian natural philosophical corpus. This would provide him with the methodological guidelines, the terminology and the biological and social doctrines without which it was impossible to understand the confusing and complex world of Galen's writings, even with the aid of such doctrinally highly structured books as the *Canon* or the *Viaticum.* As is well known, in the course of the period between 1240 and 1275, the collection of Aristotelian *libri naturales,* as well as other works of Aristotle dealing with personal or social behaviour, like the *Politics,* became firmly established in the schools of arts.[14]

The Doctor-patient Relationship

However, not only was Galenism – and Aristotelianism – considered in greater depth with a resulting broadening of intellectual horizons, but, in addition, the *ars medica* or *chirurgica* thus established was perceived by university physicians and surgeons as an activity which was capable of providing solutions to medical and/or surgical daily problems. The activity of empirics entailed a real risk for society. Guillem Correger, a Catalan surgeon and a contemporary of Henri de Mondeville, did not hesitate to point out the social risk that empiricism involved, and the negative consequences of its application: 'the ignorance of these surgeons is harmful and results in the death of those who avail themselves of their remedies in order to cure their injuries and other illnesses'.[15] We find similar words by Henri de Mondeville. The latter, addressing his monarch (Philip IV of France), commented how relevant it was to carry the intellectual movement, whose socio-professional results we are commenting on, beyond the limits of the academic world. He pointed out that to pursue the liberal arts and the contents of university medicine 'may be beneficial for those surgeons who are not familiar with the liberal arts ... as well as for the health of their patients'.[16]

The new medical science which was developed from the late thirteenth century onwards imposed upon physicians and surgeons new intellectual and technical demands which also spread to the relationship between the practitioner and his patient. Medical care was affected by the intrinsic complexity of these doctrinal contents, which required the physician to make the process of diagnosis increasingly technical (*secundum artem medicam*). The increasing complexity of medical knowledge meant that a simple spontaneous relationship with the patient was no longer sufficient. Medical care, in other words, the whole series of activities which made up the process of diagnosis and cure, was also influenced by the intellectual developments that affected the university medical circles of Paris, Montpellier and Bologna so deeply, as Jean de Saint-Amand recorded, around 1285: 'scholars do not sleep, so feverishly are they searching in Galen's works...; they are tired and thirsty because of the effort that unravelling these writings involves'.[17] In this way, medical care came to be submitted to a series of hitherto unknown demands, that the new physicians of quality were supposed to fulfil. These demands, of a technical nature, were reinforced in social terms by the Church itself, which converted them into an integral part of a responsible doctor-patient relationship. Blameworthy ignorance of these demands on the part of the physician could make him fall into a state of moral sin; not respecting these same technical norms in the process of diagnosis might place his salvation in danger.[18]

We should not think that this intervention by the Church meant that whether medical attention was good or bad was a consequence of ecclesiastical endorsement or condemnation. Far from it. The Church limited its role to reinforcing an activity whose morality was derived from intellectual and technical reasons.[19] Let us consider then, to what extent the doctor-patient relationship became more technical, and how the doctor's fee was linked to it.

The Intellectual Complexity of the Doctor-patient Relationship

At a certain point in his commentary on the first of Hippocrates' aphorisms, Arnau de Vilanova asks himself before his pupils what one must do in order to become a good physician. His reply does not deviate from the then current western medical tradition, the number of prerequisites being limited to four:[20] in the first place, intellectual contact must be maintained with medical tradition, by means of reading and debate, that is to say, the medical apprenticeship must be within the university or incorporate its intellectual tools; secondly, one must look out for any type of development or experiment concerning treatment, wherever it may come from (even from popular beliefs), although without losing sight of the fact that the final criterion should be our sense of reason, as formed in accordance with the tools learned in the liberal arts;[21] thirdly, the physician should be able to express a series of judgements in which he tries out his professional qualities;[22] finally, he should know how to communicate his experience with patients to others, and even express it in writing.[23]

When Arnau mentioned the third of the prerequisites – the need of the physician to express a series of judgements in the performance of this true medical activity – he raised two sorts of problems: on the one hand, how could the physician choose from among the already substantial mass of medical writings with which he was supposed to be familiar, many of which were only available in somewhat unsatisfactory translations and which, at the same time, were subject to the inevitable intermediary influence of the oral commentaries of academic activity (*prolationes*), and which, then, were easy to distort?[24] On the other hand, how could the practitioners organize intellectually and technically (*secundum artem medicam*) the doctor-patient relationship?[25]

Even though it was generally accepted that the necessary point of reference for problems concerning natural philosophy was Aristotle, and that for physicians the surest guides were the writings of Hippocrates and Galen,[26] on many occasions the question was by no means so straightforward. What is to happen when medical authorities contradict each other or when there is no answer in these works to the problem under consideration, or when what our experience demonstrates does not correspond to what our eyes read or to accepted teachings? The criteria that Arnau explains to his students, which are illustrated with a large number of examples, can be cut down to one alone: to read attentively Galen's works, which were at that very moment circulating in abundance in university circles. He himself could not help becoming excited when he explained that in the previous year (we are talking about 1301), he had discovered a new consideration of the semiology of pain when he had to translate from Arabic into Latin, or to verify with the Arabic version, the first two books of Galen's *De interioribus*, which were absolutely incomprehensible in the Latin version that was circulating at that date.[27]

In the replies – which scarcely take up ten pages of the printed copy – that he gives to the problems that have been mentioned above about how to become a good physician, he displays before his pupils more than twenty works by Galen.[28] It was precisely the series of problems that the doctor-patient relationship posed at the beginning of the fourteenth century that found no organized reply in the medical writings that the university physicians had available (the writings of Hippocrates, Galen, the Arabic authors, or those of Salernitan tradition). It is true that many of the difficulties connected with diagnosis were touched upon by Galen, but this material was scattered in works which were particularly difficult to gain access to or to understand. This material needed to be given form or to be organized, at the same time as it was enriched. This process of transforming Galen was carried out according to the intellectual and social circumstances of each commentator who, in fact, 'manipulated' the contents of available Galenic works and put many 'Galens' in circulation.[29] And this is exactly what Arnau de Vilanova or Henri de Mondeville did

This was the context in which Arnau considered the second of the problems mentioned above: the question of the doctor-patient relationship. That is to say, the relationship that the physician has with the patient's body as long as the latter was the object of health. The above-mentioned relationship (that is to say, all the judgements that the physician was obliged to make while it lasted) had to be subjected to a technical or rational scheme, which was to be none other than that of the *res naturales, non naturales* and *contra naturam*,[30] to which a fourth factor, the *externa accidentia* was added.[31] We shall see the importance that this fourth factor was to possess. Henri de Mondeville, in the long introduction to the second book of his *Cirurgia* which received also the name of *Tractatus de contingentibus*, was to apply the same organizational scheme, although he gave the name of *res extraneae et diversae* to the fourth factor.[32]

However, this scheme – which was familiar to university physicians throughout the thirteenth century and which reached them by means of the *Articella* (to be precise Johannicius' *Isagoge*)[33] – was applied to the physician-patient relationship and endowed it with all the rich doctrinal contents derived from the complex knowledge of Galen that these physicians possessed in the opening years of the fourteenth century. What is more, the physician had to subject himself to these standards or procedures if he wanted to make evident all the efficacy that technically-acquired medicine was capable of performing. It was not enough to win the confidence of the patient – however important that might be[34] – nor was the mere examination of urine sufficient,[35] although perhaps, on occasions, the physicians had no alternative to doing this 'to give the impression that he is doing something'.[36] The physician who wished 'to improve in medicine' (*in medicina perficere*)[37] and to obtain the maximum benefit possible from therapeutic cures[38] should subject his relationship with the patient – that is to say the whole complex of diagnosis, prognosis and treatment – to the fourfold organizational scheme mentioned above.

Both Arnau de Vilanova and Henri de Mondeville, but especially the latter, went further: everything connected with the conduct of the physician – from strictly technical matters (for example, the exact identification of the patient's *complexio,* how to take the pulse correctly or the structure that the *anamnesis* or the enquiries concerning the patient's symptoms should have) to the question of fees or the problems of etiquette (what was technically known by the name of *res* or *accidentia extraneae* or *exteriores*) – was derived from this strictly technical organizational scheme.[39] For this reason, I put forward the opinion that what later became known as medical ethics had this technical, intellectual origin. The specific morality of the practitioner derived, therefore, from his being a healer technically trained, and was essential for his status as an expert in medicine. It was an aspect that attained a well-structured, mature form of expression for the first time in medieval western medicine – and which began to be taught as such at schools and faculties of medicine and surgery – at the very beginning of the fourteenth century.

We must not forget that the whole set of elements included in the physician-patient relationship, which define the activity of the practitioner and his behaviour as a professional, was set out by Arnau de Vilanova in a commentary (a typical literary genre of scholastic medicine) in the presence of his students; in the same way, everything leads apparently to the fact that the section of Henri de Mondeville's *Cirurgia,* was part of the lectures he gave at the surgery schools in Paris.[40] Naturally, what enabled the appraisal of technique and medical science to have social impact was something more than merely its intellectual content. In fact, I consider that the increasingly technical nature of medical diagnosis and of the doctor-patient relationship was yet another consequence – among other factors – of the reception of the 'new Galen', which filled the old scheme of Johannicius' *Isagoge* with new contents; this scheme was enriched with a wide range of fundamentally professional matters, which were provided with a definite form in the late thirteenth and the early fourteenth centuries. This 'something else' was to be included by these university physicians within the fourth element of the structural scheme, and also within the other three elements thanks to a new re-interpretation of their contents; so that all four elements are interconnected.

These university physicians were fully aware that the technical dimension of the doctor-patient relationship did not exhaust the contents of this same relationship. This relationship was something more than one between two abstract individuals and something more than an intellectual problem. Proof of this can be found in the frequent allusions made by both Arnau and Henri to the living, everyday world of clinical practice. What is more, I believe that the commentary on the first of Hippocrates' aphorisms is the medical text in which Arnau provides the lengthiest list of true case histories taken directly or indirectly from his own professional experience, or from practitioners closely bound to him.[41] The overall approach to the physician-patient relationship, as detailed by these writers, is impregnated with social aspects, which condition the technical structure of this relationship: fear of failure, problems derived from fame, the lack of comprehension on the part of the laity, the social structure of the spheres in which the physicians moved, problems concerning fees and the contractual relationship between the physician and his patient, and the complex world of inter-professional relationships at the patient's bedside, the problem of poverty, the problem of fashion within the world of medicine and treatment, and the already-mentioned problems of etiquette; not to mention such personal difficulties as age, the type of professional activity or the different sexes of patients. In my opinion, what increases the interest of what we are saying is that all these social connotations are included by both Arnau de Vilanova and Henri de Mondeville in the fourfold organizational scheme of the physician-patient relationship. They are not problems 'added to' but 'derived from' the technical nature of this relationship; this technical nature is evident in the four-part scheme which they used to provide it with intellectual structure.

Arnau de Vilanova dedicated all the last part of his commentary to what he called *de consideratione extrinsecorum accidentium.*[42] Henri de Mondeville also included in this section – *res extraneae et diversae* – what are, without any shadow of doubt, the most fascinating and original contents in his approach: this information enables us to probe in greater depth into the nature of everyday relationships with patients as conducted by these university physicians at the beginning of the fourteenth century.[43] This scheme was nowhere near as simple as the one that appeared in his straightforward explanation of Johannicius' *Isagoge.* It was a scheme which became increasingly complicated with the different contributions that gradually enriched university medical teaching in the course of the thirteenth century. In actual fact, Arnau's most ambitious medical work – his *Speculum medicine* – was to have the same format as its conceptual framework.[44]

As has already been emphasized, the most significant intellectual contribution to the content of medical science was what I have called the 'new Galen'. But we should not forget Avicenna's *Canon,* of growing importance from the 1190s onwards,[45] nor other Arabic treatises such as Averroes' *Colliget*[46] and the collection of commentaries on the *Articella*,[47] or the rich collection of new surgical treatises (for example, that of Teodorico Borgognoni *c.* 1280).[48]

With all this mental baggage, the doctor-patient relationship was no longer something purely intuitive, or the result of practice alone. In order to satisfy the new demands, the pre-Salernitan and Salernitan writings, which enjoyed wide circulation throughout the thirteenth and fourteenth centuries, were not sufficient. As is well known,[49] this kind of brief medical writings did not go beyond some simple and direct advice (it is, of course, true that it is possible to observe in them an increasing complexity) on how to take the pulse, to examine the urine, to gain the patient's trust, or how to manage the delicate subjects of the relationship with other colleagues and of collecting fees. The new doctor-patient relationship, on the contrary, demanded a process of technical education and implied a complex intellectual background. As Henri de Mondeville said, 'It is talent, technique (*ars*) and practice that will enable us to establish an accurate diagnosis'.[50] Arnau took pains to warn his pupils, physicians-to-be, of this:

> The problems involved in the training of the physician, those connected with the obedience of the patient, and the characteristics that those who surround the patient and attend him should possess, and everything that is connected with the external circumstances that bear upon the physician and the patient ... are not self-evident, and neither do they become apparent to us without any effort on our part; once again, they are the result of intellectual effort and reflection. Not everybody finds it easy to know what a physican has to do and to bear in mind in order to accomplish his task ... Moreover, I have not read what I am about to explain to you either in the works of Hippocrates or in those of any of his commentators.[51]

The Doctor's Fee.

Let us now consider one of the aspects of the doctor-patient relationship that related to the doctor's fee.[52] Even a matter such as that of the salary of the physician or the surgeon, or any of the other healers who took part in the process of curing, was considered to be derived from the medical or the technical structure of the doctor-patient relationship, so deeply affected by the so-called 'new Galen' and the previous reception of Aristotle. As will be seen, practical administrative procedures derived from the application of some passages of Roman law, which deal specifically with the civic salary to be given to doctors, affected this aspect of the doctor-patient relationship.[53] This does not mean that the question was not contemplated within the framework of the social, intellectual, legal and moral values that dominated thirteenth and fourteenth-century urban society in Latin western Christendom.

Throughout the thirteenth century and in the early fourteenth century, particularly in southern Europe, a social grouping which made trade and commercial exchange the most significant factor for social progress had developed and become predominant in European cities. This fact gave those cities controlled by such groupings a clear atmosphere of initiative. Such a development was not merely a way of doing things, but also a new philosophy which imbued human relations. This ideology was well expressed in the justifications that municipal councils of cities such as Valencia – from which the clergy were excluded and on which the nobility formed but a minority in terms of representation – felt obliged to attach to certain measures to encourage trade: 'the art of commerce and its operations are the best methods to make a land wealthy'; 'wherever trade is prevented or restrained all is poverty'; 'the lands where trade is encouraged are rich and prosperous, the others are poor and wretched'.[54] Not only was trade considered a means for personal enrichment, but also for the general well-being, the interests of the dominant social grouping becoming confused with those of society in general. The doctor-patient relationship was adapted to this norm of behaviour. It was converted into an item of barter, as it was subject to the contractural relationship between the physician and his patient; although, as we shall see, medicine was not considered to be a commodity as such, but a service rendered and one which was paid for. Moreover, the fact that the physician or surgeon was in possession of academic training had a direct repercussion on the amount involved in the contract. That is to say, medicine adapted the activity of its professionals to the commercial customs of the bourgeois groups that governed thirteenth or fourteenth-centuries cities. As a consequence, medicine was not only a source of health, but also of wealth, for those who practised it.

The renowned passage in the first book of Plato's *Republic* (340c ff.), in which he considers the question of whether human self-interest lies behind all human undertakings, and whether the physician – as Socrates maintained – should not be a healer rather than a money-maker (341c), is well-known.[55] Economic profit was not an intrinsic part of medicine, although it could not be completely separated from the art of producing health. If there were no financial gain for the physician, he would make no effort to be concerned about the health of others (346e–347a).[56] Aristotle was to maintain the same point of view (*Politics,* 1258a 10 ff.), but added an interesting consideration: from the point of view of economic theory, medicine would belong to the so-called art of acquisition, which was related to exchange or barter, with the result that it became a form of 'labour for hire' (*misthamía,* 1258b 25).[57]

As we know, Aristotle's writings were of particular interest to the scholars who exercised their intellectual activity in the faculties of arts in the mid thirteenth century.[58] Aristotle's *Politics* was a work which did not escape commentaries of the natural philosophers (between them Albert the Great and Thomas Aquinas), especially the opinions of the Greek natural philosopher on the economic side of the medical activity.

Although the aim of medicine, in the opinion of Albert the Great (d. 1280) in his commentary on the above mentioned work by Aristotle (*c.* 1261),[59] is to maintain health and recover it when lost, the social circumstances in which medicine was practised in the mid thirteenth century implied that those who practised made money.[60] A few years later, in 1272, Thomas Aquinas, in a commentary not void of criticism makes matters more precise, stating that medicine, with regard to gaining money through its practice, is *neutra,* but that in fact, the power of money is such that it has been converted into an *ars ad pecuniam.*[61] As we shall see presently, in the second decade of the fourteenth century, a university physician and surgeon, such as Henri de Mondeville, would include the salary as an intrinsic element of the doctor-patient relationship.

Among the three ways of acquiring money which Albert the Great identified in urban European society in the second half of the thirteenth century – merchandise (*mercatura*), usury (*usuraria*) and services (*ministrativa*) – medicine belonged to the latter.[62] Thomas Aquinas classified medical practice as mercenary (*mercenaria*) as far as one hires one's services in exchange for money, even though the 'useful' nature of the activity places it in a special category.[63] As such, the physician offers his technical knowledge in exchange for money. To charge for medical service would be just as much a part of the medical function as being technically well qualified. The salary of the physician or the surgeon was not something added to the doctor-patient relationship, but something inseparable from it. To practise free of charge would only be justified in the case of the poor, as an act of charity (*pro amore Deo*), but not as a general practice for the entire population. The nature of the 'service' of medical practice justified him charging for medical service, when this service was for those who could afford to pay. In this way Arnau de Vilanova reminds us that the physician achieves the two most important things for a medieval Christian of the urban bourgeoise: to secure eternal salvation (with the practice of charity) and to earn money from one's work.[64] The same type of reasoning was behind Henri de Mondeville's opinion, who translated this mode of thought into medical terms. The conflicts among the evangelical mandate of charity ('who is poor?' and 'who decides this?'), the supposed 'neutrality' of medicine in relation to health-money, and a pecuniary conception (*pecuniativa*) of medical activity, should have been constant in the period under consideration, if we take into acccount that all of this was collected in the form of *questiones* in the above mentioned commentaries of these university professors on Aristotle's *Politics.*

Together with these commentaries on Aristotle, we should not forget another type of evidence, also from university circles, which is connected with the reintroduction of Roman law in Latin medieval Europe. These are the commentaries that professors of Bologna's law school made on the newly rediscovered Roman law texts, the *Digest* and Justinian's *Code.* As Nutton points out,[65] some passages of the Roman legal texts deal with rights and privileges of doctors, and were commented upon in the early thirteenth century by members of the law school. These commentaries reveal that the idea of a *salarium* contracted between the doctor and a private patient or a public institution (such as a municipal council), began to be familiar in university circles at this time.[66] This fact coincides with the years in which we have the first documentary evidence of a doctor hired by a city in the Po Valley to attend to its citizens, from 1211–14 (Reggio, Bologna). The end of the thirteenth century and the fourteenth century witnesses the spread of public doctors to several major and smaller cities and even small towns throughout Italy.[67] Roman law spread in Languedoc (Montpellier), territories of the old Septimania (Toulouse), and continental territories of the Kingdom of Majorca (Cerdanya and Roussillon, just north and south of the eastern Pyrenees), in the second half of the thirteenth century.[68] When these last territories were joined to the Crown of Aragon in 1344–5, the massive presence of jurists from Roussillon in the court of the King Peter III (1336–87) contributed to the diffusion of Roman law in the Crown of Aragon and to its acceptance by the king and local governments.[69] The new university of Lérida (western Catalonia), created in 1300, adopted Bologna as a model, and the law school of Lérida was its most important centre and a place of reception and diffusion of Roman law in the Crown of Aragon, which maintained a strong relationship with 'the mother house' (Bologna), and the new Studia (Toulouse, Montpellier, Avignon).[70] All this could provide a stimulus to the social acceptance of the concept of *salarium* (a concept from Roman law) and, as we will see, to the employment of doctors by local governments. *Salarium seu pensio* would be the words used in the contracts found in the Crown of Aragon from the late thirteenth century onwards to indicate the money and other benefits that doctor (physician or surgeon) received as remuneration for his hired practice. In this sense, it does not appear to be a coincidence that the first documentary evidence of contracts with civic doctors belongs to cities and towns of Cerdanya (Puigcerdà) and the northeast coast of Catalonia (Castelló d'Ampuries), which had close relationships to Roussillon, Languedoc, Provence and the North of Italy.

Henri de Mondeville, who studied in North Italy and Montpellier,[71] derived the contractural nature of medical activity from the medical structure of the doctor-patient relationship itself. Effectively, one of the elements of this relationship belonging to the fifth *res non naturalis* (movements or accidents of the soul, *accidentia anime*) is the mutual confidence that should exist between doctor and patient. Without such confidence the efficacy of the curative action would be greatly undermined. 'Without confidence rarely will the treatment have any effect.'[72] In fact, the physician's or surgeon's confidence in his patient was demonstrated by two conditions of equal significance: the first one was that the patient should carry out what had been prescribed by the healer; the second that the patient should pay the remuneration agreed upon. The fee would be for the doctor the objective and tangible expression of his relationship with the patient and that of the patient with the doctor, while, at the same time, it would be a guarantee of continuity in treatment. To a certain extent, then, there is no point in raising the question that so occupied Plato in the *Republic*. Henri de Mondeville could not avoid being a citizen of his own times, and his text clearly reflects the particular social and moral values prevailing in the society in which he practised. For this reason he commented: 'The patient mistrusts whatever is given free of charge. He does not believe that he will be given something of value for nothing,'[73] and he cites some rather cynical lines which are especially illuminating for the common attitude towards the healer-patient relationship in this period of the Middle Ages: 'the cure costing large sums is held to be useful by many! If it is given free of charge, it serves no purpose.'[74]

Or this other popular proverb of his period: 'when we receive things, we should give things, and words when words are offered'.[75]

However, this same contractual relationship also involved a series of obligations for the physician, which society came to subject to legal norms. The patient could count on legal means to defend himself from increasingly aggressive treatment and from an increasingly more complex network of practitioners and medical care (physicians, physician-surgeons, surgeons, barbers, apothecaries), who were becoming more and more expensive. These practitioners displayed a high degree of adaptability to the laws of the already sensitive market, to the laws of supply and demand, and in addition to the practical administrative laws which were inspired by Roman law. Likewise, the explanation by university physicians of what the physician-patient relationship should be like supplied interesting material to lay society, which allowed its members the possibility of checking whether daily practice really corresponded to what was explained by physicians to their students or not.[76]

Medicine was to be something other than individual practice, and the responsibility of the qualified healer had to go beyond that of the strict relationship between two individuals. Scholastic medicine had the expertise and the good fortune to know how to demonstrate its efficiency in the field of the preservation and promotion of health, or how to recover it when it has been lost. The ruling classes saw it in this way and clearly supported it, thereby instigating a whole series of measures for its promotion. This became a task involving those who governed society, basically the royal and municipal powers, who did not renounce real control over the physician-patient relationship.[77] In this way, a form of relationship between the civil authorities, on the one hand, and medicine and physicians, on the other, was inaugurated in the Latin West. This relationship was made up of at least three intellectual elements from the new scholasticism: rediscovered Roman law, Aristotelian natural philosophy, and the new Galen.

The physician came to have a series of social responsibilities, something that did not exist in medicine in Antiquity.[78] In compensation, the physician's norms of conduct were supported and legitimized by the same civil power and by the medieval system of professional organization: the university system and the guild system. Moreover, health came to be seen as something good in itself, something positive for the community; something, therefore, which had to be protected and encouraged. At the same time, health acquired political and moral characteristics. Preservation of health became a moral obligation of the public authority (whether wielded by royal or municipal powers). And all of this was perceived by normal citizens. The political authority regarded the physician or the surgeon who had been trained in medical science to be an element that contributed to the better health of the *res publica,* and also considered that the physician's action not only defended but also extended the demand for health, so obvious among the civil population of Mediterranean Europe[79] in the thirteenth and fourteenth centuries. The whole of this social aspect, which went beyond the strict personal relationship between the physician and his patient, acquired social validity in the period under consideration. Throughout antiquity, medicine remained free from supervision by civil authorities.[80] A situation which, we might say changed radically in the thirteenth and fourteenth centuries when civil society, the university system and the professional associations began to control the medical profession efficiently and to enforce rules of conduct.[81]

From the first third of the thirteenth century onwards and throughout the fourteenth century, we already have documentary evidence in Italy[82] and the south of France,[83] as well as in the Crown of Aragon, that for the ordinary people, in small as well as large cities and even small towns, sickness was understood in rational terms, and its treatment and possible cure left in the hands of physicians and surgeons by the town councillors, who contracted them to do this work.[84] The concern of the municipal councils for medical assistance was manifested in the conditions they demanded from the medical practitioners. These conditions were stipulated in public contracts, more or less in detail, before a public notary and constituted a form of recognition of the social responsibilities of the physician, something rather peculiar also to the late medieval European world. I shall not attempt to analyse at this point all the characteristics and variants which were laid down in these contracts throughout the thirteenth and fourteenth centuries, but rather to study the commitment undertaken by physicians in these contracts related to the paid or free assistance to patients as citizens of towns that had contracted the doctor's assistance. For this, I will use evidence from small cities in north-east Catalonia and the valleys of the Pyrenees.

Some of the earliest evidence that we possess relates to the year 1292–3, and belongs to the town of Puigcerdà,[85] the most important town (6,000 inhabitants or so, in 1345)[86] of the Cerdanya valley in the Catalan Pyrenees. Nevertheless, the most interesting contract for our purpose was that signed in 1307 between Magister Bernardus de Crenis (Cremis), *fisicus*, and the municipal council of Castelló d'Ampuries, capital of a prosperous region in north-eastern Catalonia,[87] where we have documentary evidence of private contracts from 1288 onwards.[88] The above mentioned character of social responsibility was compatible with the gospel of brotherly love, which took account only of the relationship between the individual doctor and the individual patient, when the latter was poor. Among physicians and surgeons – particularly those trained in a university and living in societies of the western Mediterranean, where technical knowledge became a matter of barter – the conviction was increasing that medical practice had an economic dimension to be resolved between the practitioner and the patient as individuals, provided that the latter had means;[89] an economic dimension that – it could not be ignored – formed an integral part of the doctor-patient relationship itself. There existed therefore, three aspects, often contradictory, which had to be harmonized: (1) the evangelical commandment of charity; (2) the fee for medical practice according to the patient's means and to the practitioner's skill; and (3) the responsibility of the municipal authorities for the health of its citizens, who, in this respect, came up against, as we shall see, the demand for free treatment from the physicians and surgeons.

We have already mentioned that this last responsibility manifested itself in contracts with the doctors and surgeons. According to these contracts, the doctor was obliged to examine the patient's urine; to attend them a minimum number of times when informed of their disease; to point out the efficacy or otherwise of phlebotomy, or of another form of therapy by means of diet or drugs without sharing with the apothecary any benefit from the drugs prescribed; and to inspire confidence by his mere presence by forbidding him to absent himself from the community. And to do all of this without charging his patients. It was this last condition which was always present in all contracts written up throughout the fourteenth century, at least in the town of Castelló d'Ampuries.[90] The only salary received by the doctor from the municipal authorities was in the form of three monthly or six monthly payments plus certain exemptions from municipal taxes. This formula gave a contractual character to the commandment of charity: everyone, including the poor, received medical assistance.[91] Christians, as well as Jewish doctors, were hired. Municipalities wanted to strike 'a balance between the doctor's desire for money and the city's obligation towards its poorer citizens'.[92] However, many of the contracts agreed in the Crown of Aragon throughout the fourteenth century do not distinguish between well-to-do and poor citizens. As we shall see later, it was to be a source of disputes between hired doctors and local governments.

What gave rise to this concern on the part of the municipal authorities for the preservation of health and the cure of diseases? I believe, in agreement with Nutton,[93] that behind these contracts, in which a series of socio-medical obligations on the part of the practitioner is laid down by the municipal authorities, there lies, among other factors, the result of the reception of Roman law. The contract itself and the notarial intervention are consequences of its acceptance.[94] But I also think that there is another type of evidence which provides an additional reason to explain the attitude of the municipal councils, at least from the last third of thirteenth century onwards. This is the doctrine resulting from commentaries on concrete works by Aristotle, such as *Politics,* which, as I already mentioned, were widespread throughout European university circles in the schools of arts in the mid thirteenth century. In this work, the theme of the responsibility of the authorities for the problem of the health and illness of the citizens was dealt with. When Henri de Mondeville wrote in 1306 the dedication of his *Cirurgia,* he made reference to this responsibility and in this context he cited Aristotle's work on *Politics.*[95] I do not think that the intense process of Aristotelization to which Latin Europe was subjected from the fourth decade of the thirteenth century onwards[96] was foreign in character to payment for medical practice which was clearly seen in the northern territories of the Crown of Aragon during the early years of the fourteenth century, nor alien in character to the form in which the municipality contracts were drawn up with the practitioners (physicians or surgeons). At least, I believe, it must be considered as another part of its intellectual background apart from other social and economic factors, such as the intense process of urbanization in western Europe, and the growth in commercial activity, already mentioned.

Albertus the Great's commentaries on Aristotle's *Politics,* in the mid thirteenth century (1260s), and the subsequent commentaries by Thomas Aquinas in 1272, impressed upon university circles and, as a result, on society in general that 'the urban authorities should be particularly concerned about the health (of the body) of their citizens'.[97] The government of society should also understand the problems of health and illness.[98] An important detail was added: these problems were to be resolved by the doctor technically, the preservation of health as well as the treatment and cure of diseases. In Albert the Great's opinion, the already technical character – based on Galenism – of the medicine of his period,[99] brought him to the belief that, if the civil authorities were obliged to provide a doctor for the community, it was the exclusive responsibility of the physician not only to use his technical training which enabled him to carry out his practice as such, but also to make the series of decisions that resulted directly from his technical work; namely, to identify the cause of disease, and its mechanisms of production, as well as to know the function of drugs and their correct application in curing.[100]

There remained at least two latent problems not directly touched upon by Aristotle's commentators. First of all, how were the civil authorities – the nobility in the case of the feudal dominions, the king in his realms, or municipalities – to be sure that the practitioner (physician or surgeon) was well qualified? Secondly there was the the problem of the doctor's fee, or more precisely, the economic factor of the doctor-patient relationship. One solution to the first of these problems was the control of medical practitioners by means of an examination;[101] another way seemed to be found in recognizing the qualifications of the physicians and surgeons issuing from the new scholastic faculties of medicine. In fact, the institutions of the new university demonstrated that the conversion of medicine into a *scientia* was perceived to be effective, highly commendable and socially useful.[102] The civil authorities established a link between health (*spes salutis*) and presence of well trained physicians, surgeons and apothecaries.[103] However, the limited number of professionals supplied by the medical faculties in the thirteenth and fourteenth centuries, made it possible for only a part of the population to receive medical care by them. The fact was that many civil authorities – even from small communities – sought university-qualified practitioners to solve the problems of medical care, guided by their evident prestige.[104] A very early piece of evidence, in the territories of present-day Spain, of the high esteem of municipal councils for university medical studies, was that in the contract between the town of Castelló (north of Catalonia) and the physician

Bernat of Borriacho (29 November, 1307), the latter was allowed to spend three winters at the University of Montpellier *'causa recipiendi suum magisterium'*.[105] The high esteem exhibited by civil society for the university degree was maintained throughout the fourteenth century despite the great mortalities. In 1394 the *consules* of the same town paid Johannes Maguessa, physician of the city, a great sum of money (50 gold florins) for the expenses of obtaining his *magister in medicina* degree.[106] In spite of the existence of university-qualified doctors, and perhaps because of the lack of these, the civil communities established methods of controlling the skill of medical practitioners, whether university trained or not, whether Christian, Muslim or Jew. Health was under municipal, and also royal, control, at least by law.[107]

The problem of salary, and of the economic factor in relation to the patient, at the outset, did not appear to present any problem. A contract where the doctor's fee was clearly laid down (annual, biannual, quinquennial, decennial, or life-long) sufficed. And this whether the contract was made by the medical practitioner with several individuals or families, or if made with a civil or ecclesiastical community.[108] But the ambiguity in Albert the Great's own commentary on Aristotle when he declared the technical autonomy of the physician (an ambiguity maintained in the commentaries of Thomas Aquinas on the same work by Aristotle), along with the evident accumulation of money by individuals who belonged to social groups that had prospered under the commercial activity of the great and small cities in Mediterranean Europe, introduced exceptions to the evangelical commandment of charity and to the contractual demand for economic equality for all (free medical service for all citizens of the municipality). Without ruling out, of course, the greed of certain physicians and surgeons.

Practitioners did not encounter any problem in making this compatible with the practice of free medical attention given to the poor. The latter concept – that of poverty – is very difficult to define, especially if payment for the visit of the doctor, or the amount of the doctor's fees, depended on it. Henri of Mondeville, for example, took particular care to establish a scale for the poor, according to which one could range from free care to small sums.[109] This principle had to be made compatible with the evangelical commandment of charity, characteristic of a Christian society, and with that of an incipient system of organization within medical care on the part of these same municipal corporations, a principle which became increasingly strengthened as the fourteenth century advanced.[110] We are not referring to the creation and maintenance of hospitals, which were directed more to the destitute than to those sick who were the recipients of medical attention, but instead to the contracting of individuals qualified in the field of medicine who were responsible for the medical care of the population (both human beings and animals) on behalf of the town councils (physicians, surgeons, barbers and even veterinary surgeons). I have had the opportunity to check that such practices existed in towns of all sizes in Catalonia, Aragon, Valencia and Majorca throughout the fourteenth century and, naturally, the custom was not without its own difficulties.

Fortunately the archives of Catalonia give us an insight into a conflict on this very problem, between the university physician Gilbertus de Alamaneis (*fl.* 1350), a graduate of Padua, and the municipal council of the already mentioned city of Castelló d'Ampuries.[111] A few months after the Black Death (prd. kal. febr. 1349 = 31 January, 1350), the municipal authorities and the chief adviser to the important Count of Ampurias (son of the King of Aragon and Lord of the region), met to make a decision on the grave sanitary condition of the town and country due to the 'dire shortage of doctors' (*summa indigentia medicorum*), a problem which had developed in this part of Catalonia from the beginning of the century (at least from 1307).[112] They decided to set out for Avignon and to contract a university physician. From there, they brought the aforementioned Gilbertus, *magister in artibus et in medicina* from the prestigious university of Padua. The doctor signed two contracts. One with the Count of Ampurias, to attend him and his servants, and members of his court; another with the municipality. In the first one, through the payment of 1,400 sous Barchinone (70 pounds) per annum, plus barley to feed two horses, medical assistance was guaranteed *iuxta artem et scientiam medicine,* to the Count, his wife and children, whom he would accompany on their journeys. As regards his courtiers and servants, there was to be a distinction: those who could afford were to be charged a fee; on the other hand those who were poor would be attended to 'for God's sake'. In the contract with the municipality, the physician, by an annual charge of 1,000 sous malgorenses (50 pounds), payable in three instalments, he undertook to: to establish his and his family's residence in the town; to examine the town's sick prescribing what was most appropriate; to make home visits, when requested, at least twice, despite the nature of the disease; under no circumstances to demand fees for this. At the end of a year, the municipality renounced the contract, because that physician demanded *magna et inmoderata salaria* for visiting his patients. This was considered *peccatum maximum* by the members of the city council, and provoking *maximum dampnum, perjudicium et scandalum.*[113] The physician denied the charges, citing the terms of contract signed by the Lord of the region. Despite this, and the intercession of the Countess, the physician had to leave, being substituted by another university doctor, Bartholomeus de Tribus Bonis, *magister in artibus et medicina,* coming from Toulouse, who signed a new contract.[114] Unfortunately, this contract with the new physician has not been preserved.

It is interesting for us to note how the attitude of the physician of Padua was considered by the members of the municipal council as a 'great sin' (*peccatum maximum*), and this in a civil context, neither religious nor ecclesiastical. The social consequences of this civil offence took on a civil character too, in the form of negligence of health, decrease in medical attention for the citizens, and the loss of confidence which should have existed between patients and their doctor (*maximum dampnum, perjudicium et scandalum*). This medical attention which the citizens wanted – and looked for – was one to be undertaken by a physician with the highest university degree from Padua, one of the most prestigious schools of medicine in Europe at this time, which led, together with Montpellier and Paris at least, the medical intellectual movement of the 'new Galen'. We should not forget that Bologna and the cities of the Po Valley were the first to incorporate Roman law in the first third of the thirteenth century, whilst the territories of the French Midi of today, and Catalonia introduced it about the middle of the century,[115] and that the doctors coming from there were specially familiarized with the problems involved with contractual relationships.

The attitude of the physician of Padua was shared by some Jewish physicians, as stated by Leon Joseph of Carcassone (*c.* 1350-*c.* 1418), a Jewish doctor who practised medicine in Languedoc and Roussillon (Perpignan). He wrote: 'The majority of those who practice the art of medicine among my people ..., say that a learned physician is he who asks for a large sum of money and does not heal free of charge'.[116] To gather a fortune by medical practice would be the best way of showing professional success.

The problem of salary which we have posed is just an example of the complicated framework that the question of the doctor-patient relationship gradually developed in the course of the fourteenth century; in addition, it shows how medical, intellectual, social and ethical matters overlapped in this period.

Notes

1. In the period which we are considering, the kings of Aragon in north-eastern Spain governed three countries that were linked only by the rule of their common monarch: the principality of Catalonia, the kingdom of Aragon, and the kingdom of Valencia. To these was added in 1344–5 the kingdom of Mallorca, which was formed by Balearic Islands and continental territories, such as Cerdanya (the eastern Pyrenees) and Roussillon, whose capital was Perpignan. See T.N. Bisson, *The Medieval Crown of Aragon* (Oxford: Oxford University Press, 1986).
2. A good brief survey is N.G.Siraisi, *Medieval and Early Renaissance Medicine. An Introduction to Knowledge and Practice* (Chicago and London: University of Chicago Press, 1990).
3. See the lucid chapter by V. Nutton, 'Continuity or Rediscovery. The City Physician in Classical Antiquity and Mediaeval Italy', in A.W. Russell (ed.), *The Town and State Physician in Europe from the Middle Ages to the Enlightenment* (Wolfenbüttel: Herzog August Bibliothek,1981, 9–46, repr. in V.Nutton, *From Democedes to Harvey: Studies in the History of Medicine* (London: Variorum ,1988). On the relationships between Bologna and the thirteenth/fourteenth centuries, universities of the present-day French Midi and Catalonia, see A. Gouron, 'The training of southern French lawyers during the thirteenth and fourteenth centuries', in *Post Scripta, Essays...in honor of Gaines Post* (Rome: 1972), 219–27 (Studia Gratiana, XV), repr. in A. Gouron, *La science du droit dans le Midi de la France au Moyen Age* (London: Variorum Reprints,1984).
4. See N.G. Siraisi, *Taddeo Alderotti and his pupils. Two generations of Italian medical learning* (Princeton, N.J.: Princeton University Press, 1981); L. García-Ballester, 'Arnau de Vilanova (c.1240–1311) y la reforma de los estudios médicos en Montpellier (1309): el Hipócrates latino y la introducción del nuevo Galeno', *Dynamis*, ii (1982), 97–158; D. Jacquart and Françoise Micheau, *La médecine arabe et l'occident médiéval* (Paris: Editions Maisonneuve et Larose, 1990),176–185.
5. Conviction about this led the new surgeons to adopt a clear, specific teaching purpose in their writings. In fact they imposed upon themselves the demand that they should spread the new doctrinal contents that supported surgical techniques among those who were unable to gain access to them because they lacked the necessary intellectual tools (they did not have Latin and lacked training in scholastic methodology as a result of not having studied the arts) and they took great pains to inform uneducated surgeons of the usefulness and expediency of their new attitude. See Julius L. Pagel (ed.), *Der Chirurgie des Heinrich von Mondeville* (Berlin: Verlag von August Hirschwald, 1892) (*Cirurgia*, ed. Pagel, thereafter), 11–12. I

also use in some passages E. Nicaise (ed. and transl.), *Chirurgie de Maitre Henri de Mondeville* (Paris: F. Alcan Editeurs,1893) (*Cirurgie*, ed. Nicaise, thereafter). Guillem Correger, a Catalan surgeon contemporary of Henri de Mondeville, shared this attitude with him, and translated *c.* 1306 the *Cirurgia* of Teodorico Borgognoni into Catalan. Addressing also his monarch (James II), wrote: 'My lord ... on seeing that all (the surgeons) of my land were acting more through routine than through knowledge of the cause ... and seeing that they did not have access to the best works of surgery, written in Latin ... I took the liberty of translating this work to avoid errors which were the consequence of ignorance' (Translator's foreword, MS Paris, Bibl. Nat., fons espagnol, 212, fol. 1ra). The efficacy of his project is demonstrated by the fact that the presence of copies of the Catalan version of Teodorico Borgognoni's *Cirurgia* has been detected in the libraries of several fourteenth-century physicians and surgeons in towns of the Crown of Aragon.

6. On the influence of Arnau de Vilanova on the rich Valencian merchant Bernat dez Clapers, see A. Rubio, 'Un hospital medieval según su fundador: el testamento de Bernat dez Clapers (Valencia, 1311)', *Dynamis*, iii (1983),373–87. See also, L. García-Ballester, M. McVaugh and A. Rubio, *Medical licensing and learning in fourteenth-century Valencia* (Philadelphia: The American Philosophical Society, 1989) (trans. Amer. Phil. Soc., 79, part 6).
7. L. García-Ballester, Introduction to *Commentum s. tractatum Galieni de malicia complexionis diverse*, in *Arnaldi de Vilanova Opera Medica Omnia*, vol XV (Barcelona: Universidad de Barcelona, 1985), 22–37.
8. On the new university surgeon of this period, see Jole Agrimi and Chiara Crisciani, 'The science and practice of medicine in the thirteenth century according to Guglielmo de Saliceto, Italian surgeon'; N.G. Siraisi, 'How to write a Latin book on surgery: organizing principles and authorial devices in Guglielmo da Saliceto and Dino del Garbo'; C.O'Boyle 'What was the effect of the new university medicine on the role of the surgeon?'; D.Jacquart, 'Medical practice in Paris in the first half of the fourteenth century'; and M. McVaugh, 'Royal surgeons and the value of medical learning: the Crown of Aragon, 1300–1350', in L. García-Ballester, R. French, J. Arrizabalaga, and A. Cunningham (eds), *Practical medicine from Salerno to the Black Death* (Cambridge: Cambridge University Press,1993).
9. To this was added the positive social evaluation of manual work, characteristic of an urban culture in which artisan classes and commercial endeavour played a significant part. Henri de Mondeville did not hesitate to remind his readers that God himself, when he moulded the clay with which he created Adam with his own hands, gave the greatest dignity imaginable to the potter's craft, and to any task performed with the hands in general, especially surgery, which

was not only work carried out with the hands, but involved the very material of the human body, and was the intellectual fruit of medical science. (*Cirurgia*, ed. Pagel, 79).

10. *Cirurgia*, ed. Pagel, 11.
11. 'Si vero rei veritatem cupit intelligere, particulam nostram ... legat et perscrutetur naturali, quod si neglexerit non potuerit hoc opus egregium intelligere perfecte', *Opera* (Venice: 1490), fol. 132rb.
12. *Cirurgia*, ed. Pagel, 10–11.
13. *Ibid.*, 11–12; 80–1.
14. On the role played by the Aristotle's *libri naturales* in the schools of arts of the mid thirteenth century, see J.A. Weisheipl, 'The Parisian faculty of arts in mid-thirteenth century: 1240–1270', *American Benedictine Review*, xxv (1974), 200–17.
15. Translator's foreword, *op. cit.*, note 5 above, fol. 1ra.
16. 'Sunt autem alii iliterati cyrurgici ... quod litterarum scientiam et artem cyrurgiae non noverunt confitentes illud modicum de scientia, quod ipsos possibile est habere, a cyrurgicis litteratis et medicis habuisse, quibus merito concedatur, quod sibi et suis patientibus in suis aegritudinibus hujusmodi doctrina nostra proficiat ad salutem', *Cirurgia*, ed. Pagel, 12. Empiricism was also an intellectual attitude which rejected medical practice based on Hippocratic or Galenic medical principles. We only know that it was a very active movement in the same university circles and at the same time where 'new Galen' rose. See García-Ballester, *op. cit.*, note 4 above, 107–09, and William Eamon and Gundolf Keil, 'Plebs amat empirica: Nicholas of Poland and His Critique of the Mediaeval Medical Establishment', *Sudhoffs Archiv*, lxxi (1987),180–96.
17. O. Paderstein (ed.), *Abbreviationes librorum Galieni seu Revocativum memorie (de morbo et accidenti, Megategni, de interioribus, de criticis diebus)* (Berlin: 1892), Prohemio, 10.
18. García-Ballester, McVaugh, and Rubio, *op. cit.*, note 6 above, 44.
19. *Ibid.*
20. 'Quatuor sunt ea que oportet agere quemlibet volentem notabiliter in medicina perficere, quorum primum est antiquorum tradita scrutando vel discutiendo perlegere, secundum caute experiri, tertium vero subtiliter iudicare, quartum experta certificata stilo brevi et ascribere'. *Repetitio Arnaldi de Vilanova super canonem 'Vita brevis'*, Michael McVaugh (ed.). *Arnaldi de Vilanova Opera Medica Omnia*, vol XIII (Barcelona, forthcoming).
21. 'Multa enim sapientes a vulgo recipiunt ... De modo enim operandi quam vulgus servat, considerandum est utrum sit consonus rationi vel non, quia si sit, procedit medicus secundum modum vulgi; si non, tunc procedatur iuxta regulam rationis. Que si manifeste repugnet rationi, detestabilis est et superstitiosus, sicut sanare fracturas absentium cum ligatione fissarum arborum'. *Ibid.*
22. 'Medicus habet iudicare non solum de his que docendo traduntur,

sed etiam de ceteris effectibus que apparent in sanabili corpore prout tale'. *Ibid.*

23. 'Ostensum est igitur breviter et quantum proposito pertinet qualiter medicus debeat inventa scribere sub stilo amphoristico'. *Ibid.*
24.. 'Publica enim et successiva relatio sepe deficit in una generatione et quod deterius est citissime variatur. Ex hoc iam patet secundum, quod modus conveniens acceptandi vel recipiendi auxilium quod ab antecessoribus preparatur est eorum scripturas diligenter intueri vel perscrutari'. *Ibid.*
25. Arnau de Vilanova dedicated the second part of his commentary to answering this question. *Ibid.*
26. 'Advertendum est utrum id quod traditur sive ponitur ab aliquo concordet cum sententiis, precipue Ypocratis et Galieni in medicina et Aristotelis in naturalibus'. *Ibid.*
27. 'de primo habere a Galieno in principio secundi *de interioribus*, ubi dicit quod diligenter considerandum est dictis Archigenis in differentiis indiciis et causis dolorum quas assiganat; et quia ille due particule *de interioribus* utilem continent doctrinam et valde necessariam medico, nec per communem translationem poterat intellectus elici Galieni proprie divina directione, reducte fuerunt anno preterito ad stilum latinorum, ita quod omnis studens potest in eis modo proficere; et notabiliter est defectus medicus qui caruerit scientia illarum particularum'. *Ibid.* See *Arnaldi de Vilanova Doctrina Galieni de interioribus*, R.J. Durling (ed.), in *Arnaldi de Vilanova Opera Medica Omnia*, vol XV (Barcelona: Universidad de Barcelona, 1985), 297–351.
28. *Op. cit.*, note 20 above.
29. See F. Salmon, 'The Many Galens of Medieval Commentators on Visual Theory', unpublished paper.
30. 'Bonitas autem...iudicii [medici] consistit in recta cognitione et consideratione rerum naturalium et non naturalium et contra naturam'. *Op. cit.*, note 20 above.
31. 'ea que de se nullo modo requiruntur ad opus [medicine] sed accidentaliter superveniunt ei et possent eius impedire processum'. *Ibid.*
32. 'circa morborum curationes assumit cyrurgicus quaedam ex rebus naturalibus, quaedam a non naturalibus rebus, alia a rebus contra naturam et alia a quibusdam rebus, quae videntur a rebus naturalibus et ceteris praedictis quamvis non sint extraneae et diversae', *Cirurgia*, ed. Pagel, 82. MS Paris, Bibl. Nat. latin. 13002. The explicit of this manuscript ('tractatus de contingentibus cum Dei auxilio hic finitur') is cited both by *Cirurgia*, ed. Pagel, 121, and *Cirurgia*, ed. Nicaise, 181.
33. See the edition by G.Maurach, 'Johannicius, Isagoge ad Techne Galieni', *Sudhoffs Archiv*, lxii (1978),148–74.
34. 'Confidentia de medico plus confert ad curam morbi quam medicus cum suis omnibus instrumentis', *Cirurgia*, ed. Pagel, 114.
35. 'medicus non potest cognoscere per urinam omnia..., scilicet causam morbi et accidens', *Ibid.*, 112.

36. 'Et non in omnibus dictis morbis medici inspiciunt ad urinas non propter necessitatem, sed ut videatur aliquid facere', *Ibid.*
37. *Repetitio Arnaldi de Vilanova super canonem 'Vita brevis'*, M. McVaugh (ed.), *op. cit.*, note 20 above, 15.663.
38. *Ibid.* 37.68–70.
39. Arnau de Vilanova exposed both opinions circulating throughout academic circles: 'Una opinio est quod ideo dicuntur accidentia extrinsecus vel extra quia cadunt extra limitem regulationum artis ... [alia opinio] supponit quod cadunt sub regulatione artificis, quoniam necessario pertinere dicit ad eius considerationem'. *Ibid.* He finally adopted the last one: 'pro tanto quisque sapiens medicus se debet in eis diligenter exercitare'. *Ibid.*
40. Introduction to *Cirurgia*, ed. Nicaise, xxv.
41. See the six case histories, *op. cit.*, note 20 above.
42. *Ibid.*
43. *Cirurgia*, ed. Pagel, 64–121; *Cirurgia*, ed. Nicaise, 95–181.
44. *Arnaldi de Vilanova Opera*, Lyon, 1504. fols. 1ra-45rb.
45. D. Jacquart, 'La reception du *Canon* d'Avicenne: comparaison entre Montpellier et Paris aux XIIIe et XIVe siècles', *Histoire de l'Ecole médicale de Montpellier, Actes du 110e Congrès national des sociétés savantes* (Paris: CNRS, 1985), 69–77.
46. The *Colliget* was translated into Latin in 1285. See, M. McVaugh, Introduction to his edition of *Aphorismi de gradibus, in Arnaldi de Vilanova Opera Medica Omnia*, Vol. II, Granada-Barcelona, Universidad de Barcelona, 1975),118.
47. On the formation of the collection of medical works known as *Articella*, from the twelfth century onward, see P.O. Kristeller, 'The school of Salerno: its development and its contribution to the history of learning', *Studies in Renaissance Thought and Letters* (Rome: Edizioni di Storia e Letteratura, 1956), 514ff. (repr. 1984); *Idem*, 'Bartholomaeus, Musandinus, Maurus of Salerno and other early commentators of the Articella with a tentative list of texts and manuscripts', *Italia Medioevale e Umanistica*, xix (1976),57–87.
48. *Cyrurgia Theodorici* (Venice: 1498).
49. For descriptions of manuscripts and the Latin texts, see S. de Renzi, *Collectio salernitana* (Naples:1852ff.), vols II, 73ss, V, 102ss., 333ss.; E.Hirschfeld, 'Deontologische Texte des frühen Mittelalters', *Archiv für Geschichte der Medizin*, xx (1928), 353–71; L.C. MacKinney, 'Medical ethics and etiquette in the early middle ages: the persistence of Hippocratic ideals', *Bull. Hist. Med.*, xxvi (1952), 1–31.
50. 'quod ingenium, ars et exercitium coadjuvant in contingentibus elicendis', *Cirurgia*, ed. Pagel, 121.
51. 'Recoligamus ergo genera istorum considerabilium que dicit necessitati ceteris medicis ad opus nostram perfectionem et videamus in generali que sunt observanda circa unumquodque illorum. Sunt ergo illa quatuor in genere: diligentia medici, obedientia infirmi,

ydoneitas ministrorum, et quartum congruitas extrinsecorum accidentium ... Sed certam est quod non sunt per se nota, quia nec offerunt se sensui nec etiam apprehenduntur ab intellectu nisi per discursum rationis et studiosam meditationem. Similiter patet quod non sunt omnibus nota etiam medico; non enim omnes prompte cognoscunt ea que medicus habet agere vel observare ad sui directionem in finem operis medicinalis ... Sed que sint hec considerabilia et ordinabilia in speciali non explicat Ypocras nec etiam eius expositores'. *Repetitio Arnaldi de Vilanova super canonem 'Vita brevis'*, M. McVaugh (ed.), note 20 above.

52. The economic side of the doctor-patient relationship has not been systematically studied in thirteenth and fourteenth century Europe. See, M.C. Wellborn, 'The long tradition: a study in fourteenth-century medical deontology', in J.L. Cate and E.N. Anderson (eds), *Medieval and Historiographical Essays in Honor of James Westfall Thompson* (Chicago: 1938), 344–57; E.A. Hammond, 'Incomes of medieval English doctors', *J. Hist. Med.*, xv (1960),154–69. C. Rawcliffe, 'The Profits of Practice: the Wealth and Status of Medical Men in Later Medieval England', *Social History of Medicine*, i (1988), 61–78. For a general outlook see, D.W. Amundsen, 'History of Medical Ethics. 2. Medieval Europe: Fourth to Sixteenth Century', in W.T. Reich (ed.), *Encyclopaedia of Bioethics*, vol 3 (New York-London: 1978), 938–951.
53. See Nutton, *op.cit.*, note 3 above, 27–8
54. Cited by Agustín Rubio-Vela, 'Ideologia burgesa i progrés material a la València del Trescents', *L'Espill*, ix (1981),11–38, at 24–8; *Idem*, Epistolari de la València medieval, (Valéncia, Universitat de Valäncia) 1985, 14–21, 133–4.
55. See, L. Edelstein, 'The professional ethics of the Greek physician', *Bull. Hist. Med.*, xxx (1956), 391–419, at p.397.
56. *Ibid.*, 397–389
57. *Ibid.*, 397–401 and 397, n.12
58. See note 14 above.
59. Albertus Magnus, *In octo lib. Politicorum Aristotelis commentarii, Opera Omnia*, P. Petrum Iammy (ed.), vol IV/2 (Lugduni: 1651). On the redaction date, see James A. Weisheipl, 'Albert's work on natural science (*libri naturales*) in probable chronological order', in J.A. Weisheipl (ed.), *Albertus Magnus and the Sciences* (Toronto: Pontifical Institute of Mediaeval Studies, 1980),565–577, on 575.
60. *In octo lib. Politicorum*, lib. 1, c. 6 (ed. Iammy, 37).
61. 'Medicinalis [ars] propter sanitatem, neutra tamen est propter pecuniam: sed quidem ... medicinalem convertunt ad acquirendum pecuniam, et ita faciunt...esse pecuniativam, idest acquisitivam pecuniae, ordinantes huiusmodi artes ad pecuniam, sicut ad finem ad quem oportet ordinari omnia alia'. Thomas Aquinas, *In octo libros Politicarum Aristotelis expositio*, P.R.M. Spiazzi (ed.), (Taurini-

Romae: 1966), li. I lect. viii no. 128, 40. On the date, see Introduction,xxiv–xxv.

62. *In octo lib. Politicorum,* lib. 1, c. 8 (ed. Iammy, IV/241).
63. *In octo lib. Politicorum,* lib. 1, lect. ix. no. 141 (ed. Spazzi,44).
64. 'tunc splendebit pericia medici et erunt omnia opera eius meritoria postquam ex caritate fiant; nam apud Deum merebitur gratiam et ab hominibus et emolumentum', *Repetitio Arnaldi de Vilanova super canonem 'Vita brevis',* M. McVaugh (ed.), note 20 above.
65. Nutton, *op. cit.*, note 3 above, 27 and the references cited there.
66. *Ibid.*, 28.
67. *Ibid.*,26 and 28–9.
68. Gouron, *op. cit.*, note 3 above, 220–6.
69. J. Reglá, 'La Corona de Aragón y Navarra en la segunda mitad del siglo XIV', in R. Menéndez-Pidal (ed.), *Historia de España,* Vol. XIV (Madrid: Espasa-Calpe Ed., 1966), 379–605.
70. J. Vincke, *Die Hochschulpolitik der aragonischen Krone in Mittelalter* (Braunsberg: Staatliche Akademie zu Braunsberg, 1942); *Idem,* 'Los familiares de la corona aragonesa alrededor del año 1300', *Anuario de Estudios Medievales,* i (1964), 333–51; Gouron, *op. cit.*, note 3 above, 224–5. On the relationship of medical practice and the diffusion of Roman law in the Crown of Aragon, see L. García-Ballester, *Historia social de la medicina en la España de los siglos XIII al XVI* (Madrid: Akal Editor, 1976), 46, note 110.
71. D. Jacquart, *Supplément* to E. Wickersheimer, *Dictionnaire biographique des médecins en France au Moyen Age* (Genève: Librairie Droz, 1979), 117–8.
72. *Cirurgia,* ed. Pagel 114, see note 34 above, where he cites Avicenna's commentary on book VI of Aristotle's *Naturalia.*
73. 'Et vere nihil confert, aut parum patienti, quia minus confidit ex quo mente concipit, quod vix datur gratis aliquod pretiosum, et similiter medicina data gratis nil confert cyrurgico penitus, immo nocet', *ibid.*, ed. Pagel, 98.
74. 'Empta solet care multos medicina juvare! Si detur gratis, nil confert utilitatis', *ibid.*
75. 'res dare pro rebus, pro verbis verna solemus!' *ibid.*
76. The number of copies of manuscripts from thirteenth to fifteenth centuries on medical etiquette belonging to the pre-Salernitan and Salernitan period, which have survived, is evidence of the popularity of this kind of medical literary genre. See note 49 above. Many times, the following words written by Arnau de Vilanova at the end of his commentary on the first of Hippocrates' aphorisms, were turned against the daily behaviour of the medical practitioners: 'Medicus debet esse in cognoscendo studiosus et in percipiendo cautus et ordinatus, in respondendo circumspectus et providus et in pronosticando ambiguus, in promitendo iustus ut non promittat sanitatem quia tunc usurparet divinum officium et faceret Deo iniuriam; sed promittat fidelitatem et

diligentiam in visitando et sit discretus et diligens, in sermone modestus, in affectione benevolus ... Extrinsecus autem accidentalia convenit esse ne corpus patientis inde ledatur aut animus perturbetur', M. McVaugh (ed.), see note 20 above.

77. See García-Ballester, McVaugh and Rubio, *op.cit.*, note 6 above, 10.
78. O. Temkin, 'Medicine and the problem of moral responsibility', *Bull. Hist. Med.*, xxiii, (1949) 1–20; 10
79. García-Ballester, McVaugh and Rubio, *op.cit.*, note 6 above, 3–4.
80. Edelstein, *op.cit.*, note 55 above, 417, n.49. Nutton has made this statement more precise: see op.cit., note 44 above,11–23
81. For this problem in the Crown of Aragón, especially in the Kingdom of Valencia, see García-Ballester, McVaugh, and Rubio, *op. cit.*, note 6 above.
82. Nutton, *op. cit.*, note 3 above, 24ff, and the references cited there.
83. See J. Shatzmiller, *Médecine et Justice en Provence Médiévale. Documents de Manosque, 1262–1348* (Aix-en-Provence: Université de Provence, 1989).
84. See Nutton, *op. cit.*, note 6 above, 24ff. Michael McVaugh and myself are working on this topic with materials the archives of the Crown of Aragon, from 1280–1400. The assertion on the rational understanding of the sickness does not exclude people from receiving medical care by empirical healers and using magic procedures.
85. The first documentary evidence we have belongs to a contract signed by Magister Bonet Cohen, medicus, a Jewish doctor (Arxiu Històric Comarcal de Puigcerdà, Notarial records:Pere Ferràn, Liber firmitatis, 1292–3, Nonas April 4, 1292 = 2 April, 1293). The next contract belongs to a Christian physician, Magister Raymundus de Vilalta, phisicus (*ibid.*, Ramón de Caborriu, Lib. firmitatis, 1298–9, Kal. August 14, 1298 = 19 July).
86. *Ibid.* Ramón Guillem de Lorà, *Lib. firmitatis,* 1345–6, August 10, 1345: 'Convocata et congregata universitate hominum ville Podioceritanie ...', and there follow the names of 1,270 citizens.
87. *Arxiu Històric de Girona* (AHG thereafter), Castelló d'Ampuries, Notarial records, Fragments, Box 4 no.1, Nonas Madii 5, 1307 = 3 May.
88. AHG, Castelló, Fragments 1–A, number 3, Kal. August 7, 1288 = 26 July. Michael McVaugh has reproduced 22 private contracts from this city in 1307–08, see 'Bernat de Berriacho (fl. 1301–43) and the ordinacio of bishop Poná de Gualba', *Arxiu de Textos Catalans Antics,* ix (1990), 253–4.
89. In this sense, see the long passages dedicated by Henri de Mondeville to this topic in his *Cirurgia,* among others: 'bene et cum salva conscientia potest cyrurgicus reportare a divite centum libras, sicut a mediocri quinquaginta et sicut a paupere ancam, anatem, gallinam, pullos, caseum sive ova. Sed si patiens fuerit verus pauper, nihil retineat de praedictis', ed. Pagel, 134.
90. See note 87 above (1307 May 3), and the contract between the city

council and the physician Gabriel Quintana 'licenciatus in artibus et bacallarius in medicina': 'Et visitabo etiam infirmos habitatoris dicte ville cum inde fuerit requisitus videlicet bis tantummodo in qualibet infirmitate sine pensione alicuius salarij', AHG, Castelló, reg. 345, s.f., 1371 June 16. The contract was renewed two years later (1373 October 6) on the same terms, *ibid.*

91. We could cite, as an example, the contents of the contract mentioned above between the municipal council of Castelló d'Ampuries and the physician Bernardus de Crenis (1307): 'Ut essent summa indigentia medici seu medicorum in villa Castilionis fuit tractatum et ordinatum per consules et alios probos homines ville Castilionis convocato consilio ut moris est ..., ordinaverunt inter se quod Magister Bernardus de Crenis, fisicus, staret et continuam residenciam faceret in dicta villa pro medico. Et quod pro pensione seu salario dare singulis annis comuni decem libram malgorenses eidem Magistro Bernardo, quarum medietas solveretur [eidem] consules dicte ville qui pro tempore fuerunt, in festo Sancti Michaelis quolibet anno et alia medieta solveretur eidem in festo Pasche quolibet anno..., et quod bene et legaliter pro posse suo videbit et judicabit omnes urinas que apportabuntur sibi per omnes habitatores dicte ville, et quod debit eis consilia tam flebotomiis quam eciam dietis et generaliter regimina et consilia, et quod bis illos infirmos visitabit (et de quibus fuerit requisitus). Et quod de hoc nichil accipiet ab eis nec ab alio ipsorum, immo libere et gratis predicta exhibebit pro posse suo... Promisit eciam dictus Magister Bernardus quod non haberet partem nec comunionem cum aliquo ypothecario super lucro ipsius ypothecarie', AHG, note 87 above.
92. Nutton, *op. cit.*, note 3 above, 27.
93. *Idem.*
94. J.Plescia, 'The rise of modern jurisprudence: Roman law, glossators and commentators', *Annals of the Archive of Ferran Valls i Taberner Library*, vi (1989),193–210.
95. 'insuper ad utilitatem communem, que secundum philosophum XI politicorum praeponenda est utilitate singulari', ed. Pagel, 10.
96. The Aristotelian model of asking about human nature and its environment was made fully available to the Middle Ages by Albert the Great, who was conscious of his programme of Aristotelization: 'Our intention', he said,'is to make all the aforesaid parts [from natural sciences, logic or mathematics to ethics, economics, politics and metaphysics] intelligible to the Latins', *Opera Omnia. Physica*, lib. I, tr. 1, c.1, P. Hossfeld, Aschendorff (ed.), 1987, 1, l.43–49. See, B. M. Ashley, 'St. Albert and the nature of natural science', in J.A. Weisheilp (ed.) *Albertus Magnus and the sciences* (Toronto:Pontifical Institute of Mediaeval Studies, 1980), 73–102, on p. 73; J. A. Weisheipl, 'The life and works of St. Albert the Great', *Ibid.*, 13–51, at p. 30; and W.A. Wallace, 'The Scientific Methodology of St. Albert

the Great', in G. Meyer and A. Zimmermann (eds), *Albertus Magnus Doctor Universalis,* 1280/1980 (Mainz: Matthias-Grünewald-Verlag, 1980), 385–407, at 387–88.

97. '[Conditor civitatis] primum quidem tanquam necessarium ad sanitatem, scilicet quod cives in ea sani permaneant', 'legislator qui curat de vita hominis, prius debet ordinare vitam secundum corpus quam secundum animam', Albertus Magnus, *In octo lib. Politicorum,* lib. VII, c.9 and 14 (ed. Iammy, IV/2, 433 and 459); 'primo dicit quoniam conditorem civitatis oportet esse solicitum multum de sanitate inhabitantium civitatem', Thomas of Aquinas, *In octo libros Politicorum,* lib. VII, lect. 3 (ed. Spiazzi, 377).
98. 'principis enim oeconomi est providere ut habeatur medicus in sanitate conservans familiam, et curans aegrotos, et hoc modo pertinet medicina ad oeconomum et principem', Albertus Magnus, *In octo lib. Politicorum,* lib. I, c.7 (ed. Iammy, IV/2, 37).
99. 'Unde sciendum, quod Augustino in his quae sunt de fide et moribus plus quam philosophis credendum, si dissentiunt. Sed si de medicina loquitur, plus ego crederem Galeno vel Hippocrati, et si de naturis rerum loquatur, credo Aristoteli plus vel alii experto in rerum naturis', *Super II Sententiarum,* d.13, C, a.2, *Opera omnia,* Paris, 1890–99, vol XXVII, 247, cited by Albert Zimmermann, 'Albertus Magnus und der lateinische Averroismus', in Meyer and Zimmermann (eds), *op. cit.,* note 96, 465–493, at p. 475, note 41.
100. 'sed medici [pertinet] cognoscere causas morborum et curarum, utrum purgativis et alterativis sit utendum in morbis, hoc est medici', *Ibid.* Thomas of Aquinas responding to a question said: 'Quare ars medicinalis nos est pars economicae, sicut pecuniativa? Et respondendum, quod ad dispensatorem domus et ad principem civitatis pertinet quodammodo considerare de sanitate, scilicet utendo consilio medicorum ad sanitatem subiectorum: alio autem modo non pertinet ad eos, sed ad medicos, considerando scilicet ex quibus rebus sanitas conservetur vel restituatur', *In octo libros Politicorum,* lib. I, lect. 8 no. 132 (ed. Spiazzi, 40).
101. For this procedure in the territories of the Crown of Aragon, especially the Kingdom of Valencia, see García-Ballester, McVaugh, and Rubio, *op. cit.,* note 6 above.
102. M. McVaugh and L. García-Ballester, 'The Medical Faculty at Early Fourteenth-Century Lérida', *History of Universities,* viii (1989),1–25.
103. 'Ut provisiones medicorum phisice et cirurgie et apothecariorum qui nostrum felix sequantur stoleum, ut per eorum providenciam et scienciam medicine Nos et nostri subditi preserventur a noxis et habere possimus absque periculo spem salutis', *Arxiu de la Corona d'Aragó,* C., reg. 1145, fol. 24v (1354, February 12).
104. The municipal council of the town of Castelló d'Ampuries sent a messager to Avignon in 31 January, 1350 (prid. kal. February 1349) to look for a university physician and to contract him (see, AHG,

Castelló d'Ampuries, reg. 2062, s.f., 1351 February 2). The same attitude was shared by the municipal council of Barcelona just after the Black Death (1348 kal. October = October 2): Magister Raymundus de Thesaraco, *magister in artibus et in medicina,* was hired by the city (see *Municipal Archive,* Barcelona, Consellers, Imposicions. 5. reg.1348–51, fols 5v–6).

105. 'Retinuit tamen sibi dictus magister Bernardus ... quod ipse possit studere tribus hiemibus apud Montempessulanum causa recipiendi suum magisterium, quem hiemem intelligit de festo omnium sanctorum usque ad festum carnisprivii [November to February]', AHG, Castelló, reg. 142, fol. 24v, 3 kal. December 1307 (= 29 November). Reproduced by M. McVaugh, *op. cit.*, note 88 above, 251–52.
106. AHG, Castelló, reg. 508, fol. 200, 24 December, 1394
107. García-Ballester, McVaugh, and Rubio, *op. cit.*, note 6 above.
108. For instance, the contracts between the bishop and chapter of canons and the physician for medical attention to their persons and families. We have many examples in the Crown of Aragon: e.g. in Vic (Catalonia), *Arxiu Curia Fumada, Liber primus vitae,* 1288–1345, fols. 39r–v, contract with Magister Johannes de Portugal, *fisicus,* Kal. June 16, 1312 = 17 May; another contract (fol. 49) with Magister Bernardus, *cirurgicus,* Idus July 8, 1315 = 8 July. The bishop of Valencia signed a contract with Magister Mironus de Corça, *magister in artibus et in medicina, Arxiu del Regne de València,* Notarial records, reg. 2923: Domingo Moliner, Nonas October 6, 1341 = 2 October.
109. *Cirurgia,* ed. Pagel,133 –4 (Nic. 196–202).
110. Michael McVaugh and myself are working on the characteristics of the network of medical attendance established throughout the fourteenth century in the territories of the Crown of Aragon.
111. AHG, Castelló d'Ampuries, No. 2062, s.f., from Nonas February, 1349 = 5 February, 1350 to Kal. Februar 16, 1351 = 17 January, 1352.
112. See note 91 above (ut essent summa indigentia medici seu medicorum in villa Castilionis), Nonas May 5, 1307 = 3 May. The most respectable doctor of the town, the university physician Mauratus Vitalis, *magister in medicina,* died in 1346 (AHG, Castelló, No. 215, s.f. between Kal. February 12, 1345 = 21 January, 1346 and Idus February 8, 1345 = 6 February, 1346). The city had at least two physicians, one surgeon, two barbers and three apothecaries. In Barcelona, the head of the municipal council recalled, in the contract with the university physician, the *medicorum penuria et deffectus* after the plague of 1348, see note 104 above.
113. 'Cum vos Magister Gilbertus d'Alamaneis fisicus habitator Castilionis promissistis et conveneritis bona fide venerabilibus Nicholao Micerij, Raimundi Strucij, Paulo Mathei et Guillelmo Blanchi consulibus anno proximo preterito ville Castilionis ... quod vos de omni vita facietis personalem et continuam residentiam in

dicta villa et judicabitis fideliter atque bene secundum noticiam vestram orinas habitatorum dicte ville que ad vos venient et aportabuntur et dabitis et prestabitis cuilibet postulanti consilium super flebotomijs dietis et aliis similibus que infirmis habitatoribus dicte ville fuerint utilia et necessaria super eorum infirmitatibus. Et visitabitis infirmos habitatores dicte ville cum inde fueritis requisitus videlicet bis in qualibet infirmitate sine aliquo salario.

Et vos dictus Magister Gilbertus ... cessaveritis et cesseris penitus facere servicium supradictum in totum nec etiam in partem aliquam nec vultis visitare infirmos neque eis dare consilium super eorum infirmitatibus ut promisistis et convenistis. Imo vultis habere a dictus infirmis de consilijs per vos eis dandis magna et inmoderata salaria contra promissionem et conventionem predictam.

Verum cum frangenti pacta et conventiones assimili videmus frangi debeant. Ideo nos ... consules nunc ville Castilionis ... denunciamus et dicimus vobis dicto Magistro Gilberto quod nos et nostri successores de certe non debemus nec dare intendimus vobis dictam pensionem nec aliquid aliud. Imo dictam pensionem vobis suspendimus ... cum esset peccatum maximum ... et ... esset in maximum dampnum perjudicium et scandalum dicte ville...dicti venerabiles consules petierunt sibi fieri publicum instrumentum. Quod fuit actum ... in villa Castilionis (iij Nonas febrerij anno Domini Mo CCCo Quinquagesimo)', AHG, Castelló, reg. 2062, s.f.

114. *Ibid.* The contract with Bartholomeus de Tribus Bonis was signed the 2 kal. febr. 1351
115. Nutton, *op. cit.*, note 3 above 26–27 and Gouron *op. cit.* note 3 above, 220–6.
116. Prologue to his Hebrew translation of Gérard de Solo's *Practica super nono Almansoris.* Hebrew text with English translation in L. García-Ballester, L. Ferre, and E. Feliu, 'Jewish appreciation of fourteenth-century scholastic medicine', *Osiris*, vi (1990),85–117 at 106–16, Appendix D.

3

The Medical Ethics of Gabriele de Zerbi

Roger French

Introduction: How Ethical were Medical Ethics?

In this and a subsequent chapter in this book, 'ethics' will be used in a particular sense. The current interest in medical ethics is an interest in ethical problems. It might seem unproblematic that medical ethics have a history, and that these problems can be studied in the past. We might, for example, take the problem of abortion, and look at it historically. But then we would find that there have been times and places in which abortion provided no ethical problems. Such a history would be the history of a practice, not of an ethical problem. In other words, modern medical ethics derives from the particular nature of modern medicine and the society in which it exists. So a history of medical ethics is a history of medicine and of society and of the problems that looked ethical to them, but not necessarily to us. Looked at in this way it soon becomes clear that ethics have a function, for the group that practises them, other than the internal, explicit injunctions that are normally seen as 'ethical' in some abstract way. Most of the Hippocratic ethical works can be read as defences of the medicine of one group when threatened by another. Asclepiads and groups making use of presocratic philosophy and the methods of the sophists can be identified in texts like *Ancient Medicine, Oath, Law,* and *Decorum,*[1] books that lay down rules for the proper practice of real medicine; that is, the medicine of the group to which the author belongs. Ethics comprise a system of rules that not only characterizes the group, but which in directing the behaviour of the group contributes to its success. Whatever the source of the rules and however they came to be written down (if they were) it is unlikely that that they originated with this explicit intention of benefiting the group. Rather, if the cumulative effect of such rules, whatever their nature and origins, was good for the group, it survived. Other groups, perhaps in direct competition, may have had ethics that did not have this effect.

Looked at in this way we can see that it is the group, not the individual member, that is the beneficiary of its ethics. The members may have to make sacrifices to remain in the group. They enter and leave it, but the group persists. In this account, too, we can see why ethical rules are largely moral rules: they are obeyed not because of a rational awareness of any penalties, which would be the case if the rules were rationally derived for the interests of the group, rather they are obeyed because of the deeper-than-rational moral loading that a successful group can put on its members.

The Hippocratic ethical works provided a resource for those who later came to think about medical ethics. They did so primarily because they were concerned with the internal regulation of a group of medical men and the reputation of the group of the whole. Thus the Arab Haly Abbas found it useful to assert, as did the Oath, that the beginner should honour his teachers as parents and treat his fellow students as brothers; should select whom to teach and do so without payment; should not supply abortifacients or the means of suicide; should respect his patients' secrets; should dress cleanly and should be suspicious of a smooth tongue. To these plainly Hippocratic injunctions he adds one that seems to derive from the Arabic doctor's environment of practice, namely to improve his learning by visiting hospitals and talking to the doctors there. Haly's views in turn acted as a resource for Gentile da Foligno, the man who did a great deal (before his death in the plague of 1348) to bring Arabic medicine into the West while the New Galenism (described by Garcia-Ballester) was being absorbed and developed from other sources. Gentile developed a 'way of the physicians' – *via medicorum* – that was 'ethical' partly because it was technically ideal, like the New Galenism, and partly because it drew upon the Hippocratic ethical works, no doubt by way of Haly Abbas.[2]

Learning, Ethics and Reputation

When they rewrote the statutes of the student *universitas* at Padua in 1468, one of their philosophy teachers was Gabriele de Zerbi. He had been there about a year. Many of the statutes are concerned with the political structure of the *universitas* and in particular who was allowed to vote. (Zerbi was named among those on whom the obligation to vote was not to be enforced.) As for the statutes that governed the teaching and practice of medicine, they pay particular attention, in very strong language, to two special points, the regular performance of human dissections and to the control of unlicensed practice.[3] We shall return to these statutes in finding reasons to explain how Zerbi's ethics came to have the shape they did. (We shall also see how Zerbi's well-known book on anatomy is closely linked to his ethics and the statutes.)

Seven years later Zerbi moved to Bologna[4] where he taught logic, philosophy and medicine for eight years. The subsequent ten years that he spent in Rome brings us to 1494, when he moved back to Padua as the *ordinarius* in medicine. In the following year he published his little book on advice to medical men, the *De Cautelis Medicorum,* 'advice to medical men'.[5] This calendar of events likewise contributes to our understanding of 'ethics' at Zerbi's particular place in time, as we shall see.

The *De Cautelis Medicorum* is a textbook of ethics in the sense that it consists partly of advice, devices and strategies that the doctor can employ to enhance his reputation. The advantage that follows from this is not only the benefit of the individual but also that of doctors as a group and of a certain kind. The 'ethical' doctor leaves behind a reputation that will encourage the patient and his family to call a doctor a second time, rather than one of the different kinds of unlicensed practitioners.

The image of the doctor that Zerbi wanted his colleagues to maintain was – to deal with one aspect first – that of the serious and reliable doctor. To gain and retain the confidence of the patient, the good doctor should not take part in festivities; should not sing or dance, or play a musical instrument; and he should not hunt or use weapons.[6] In other words, Zerbi thought that a frivolous doctor would not be trusted by the patient. And neither would a loose-living doctor, who consorted with evil men. The patient's confidence in his doctor would also be diminished, said Zerbi, if the patients knew that the doctor took part in public affairs and consequently did not devote himself entirely to medicine: the authority of the doctor would be diminished and his medicine useless.

It was important for Zerbi that the doctor came from the right social class. It was in the nature of the vulgar, he argued, that they could not command respect, and as doctors they could have no authority and were not associated with learning. The doctor should therefore emphasize the signs of his class. His house, said Zerbi,[7] should be large and obvious, so that everyone knows where it is (and can reach it rapidly in emergency). His clothes and behaviour should be distinctly non-plebian[8] (decent, but avoiding the over-dressing of the doctor who sought success by merely pleasing his patient). He should not go shopping for food and household necessities, for he would be noticed by the vulgar, which would cheapen him. The Good Doctor does not cultivate land (by which Zerbi no doubt means that the doctor should not be associated with the rustic class and should not spend time on non-medical activities).

The doctor's position in the middle of the social scale meant that special parts of Zerbi's ethics are devoted to behaviour at his upper and lower class boundaries. This is most directly stated in his account of how to deal with plebians. This is not difficult, he says, because every plebian is ignorant and vulgar. But there are pitfalls even for the refined and distant physician, for in their ignorance the common people break up what the doctor says into contraries.[9] What Zerbi leaves unsaid here is that a coarse but penetrating wit might well have punctured the pomposity of the university-trained physician. He is indeed more explicit when dealing with the situation where other medical attendants bring unlearned assistants into a case on which Zerbi's Good Doctor is already at work. Such men, says Zerbi, 'are not solemn', and if – as often happens, he adds – they have a way with words and are men of shrewd native judgement, then they deride the solemn and learned opinions of the Good Doctor.[10]

Outside the sickroom the ethical doctor was not in such medically and embarrassingly close contact with plebians, and could afford to be distantly polite. Never be familiar with plebians, advises Zerbi, for it is sure to breed contempt. The reputation of the physician would suffer as a result; that is to say, he would prove less attractive to the class with the power to pay his fees. Do not even talk to plebians if you can avoid it, advises Zerbi, and if you are obliged to, never dispute with them but agree where possible and talk of things common to all men.

On the other hand, the physician, as middle class, had to cultivate an ethic that smoothed the boundaries between him and the higher classes. The Good Doctor, advises Zerbi, is not pompous, and can address all classes in the same way, exchanging courtly greetings with knights.[11]

The reputation of the doctor depended on success. It was, therefore, ethically important not to take on hopeless cases. Zerbi says quite precisely[12] that cases involving children, pregnant women and diseases of the eyes are likely to damage the reputation of the doctor and should not be taken on. No doubt high infant mortality and the technical difficulty of eye diseases accounted for Zerbi's gloomy assessment of these two kinds of case. The problem of pregnant women was that powerful remedies might result in miscarriage, when the doctor would be in danger of being accused of procuring an abortion. To avoid this in cases where it became necessary to treat a pregnant woman, Zerbi advises the use of phlebotomy only in the presence of a colleague; and the use of weak medicines, the preparation of which is to be entrusted to the family. Zerbi is here able to use the Hippocratic Oath and its prohibitions against abortifacients and poisons. Like the Hippocratic doctor, the Zerbist did not cut for the stone: not only was it Hippocratically unethical but also unlikely to be successful, Zerbi says. (Zerbi had his followers, at least in anatomy. Berengario da Carpi disparagingly called them *Zerbistae.*)[13]

Ethics and Money

The ethical problems of the doctor's fees were complicated. The patient was buying health and wanted to strike a good bargain. But medicine was a highly technical business – and the doctor took care it should remain so – and the patient was never entirely sure of what procedures of the doctor were appropriate to the final result, health. He knew very well that what he paid the doctor depended on how long the cure took, and how many times the doctor called, and he must often have suspected that the doctor came too often and extended the cure for the sake of a bigger fee. To maintain the doctor's reputation, it is, therefore, ethically important, Zerbi says, to cure as quickly as possible, for a lengthy treatment generates a bad name, particularly among the vulgar. Become the authority of the sickroom, advises Zerbi: everyone will obey quickly in order to save money.[14] The image of the quick and efficient doctor was enhanced by his use of expensive and thus apparently effective remedies. 'Expensive medicines cure quickly' is one of Zerbi's aphorisms; if they are given free, he says, they do not help very much.

The ultimate claim the doctor made to counter the patient's fears that he was paying too much was that the doctor's aim was not money but health. Zerbi adds (not from the church but from the Arabic author Haly Abbas) that the physician knows that he will be rewarded by God. It was, nevertheless, uncommonly useful that the doctor should also be rewarded by the patient. So much so that Zerbi describes as divine the kind of patient who, seriously ill, prays and pays at the same time. In contrast they are diabolical who, restored to health, refuse to pay and avoid the doctor afterwards. To

Zerbi's despair, it was commonly held that cure of a disease was due to the astrological influence of Mars: an odious belief, says Zerbi, and unremunerative (because the patient could use it as an excuse to refuse payment to the doctor).

Zerbi's advice is, therefore, to take your fee at an early stage, unless your patient is magnificent, curial, a relation or a pauper. It is proper to accept what is offered, however small (Zerbi no doubt means from a pauper): be *mercenarius* about your *mercedes*. But do not turn away a patient from whom you think you may not get a fee. Take the case, for pity's sake, because it is a Christian thing to do, and because 'it generates a laudable reputation' says Zerbi. Such a reputation would be destroyed, he adds, by any obvious pursuit, particularly at law, of a patient reluctant to pay. Yet all too often the doctors of the late fifteenth century did just this, and Zerbi bewails the fact that the result is that 'it makes our art look ignoble'.[15] Do not sue your patient, but seek the intercession of a third party, such as a friend or relative of the patient, or an apothecary.

But it is best, says Zerbi, to secure payment by means of your technical knowledge of medicine. Remember that when the patient is in pain and the disease is strong, he will readily offer promises to the doctor (and the doctor in return should pledge his best help). But when the weakness has passed, the patient retains little memory of the devotion shown by the doctor. So act opportunely in securing your fee in acute cases; and in recurrent fevers you will be given renewed opportunities with the return of the critical days. Receive your fee, Zerbi concludes, with all the modesty you wish, and as if the soul, while noticing, appears not to notice; or as if while your soul in its liberality declines the fee, the hand in its dexterity is extended to receive it. In short, do not appear to be greedy.

Ethics and People

Treating ethics as a code of behaviour that characterizes and informs the actions of the group, we should expect to see ethical problems at the places where the group meets others. This is particularly so if the other groups are engaged in competitive activities. Surgeons and physicians shared a common university training in Italy and were not professional rivals in the way that they were in Northern Europe. It is for this reason that Zerbi's ethics contain no advice on how the physician should deal with surgeons. But he does have things to say on apothecaries, students, different kinds of patients and the assistants and bystanders in medical cases.

The doctor's ethical behaviour to apothecaries is mainly a question of choosing a good one, a 'faithful' person, in Zerbi's words.[16] The greatest danger to the doctor is in the power and quantity of the medicines he orders, particularly the opiates and purges. The strength of these medicine is such, says Zerbi, that mishandling them can cause death. The doctor should be personally present when these are being made up. He should not write down in a single prescription the whole of what a patient will need. Indeed, says Zerbi, it is a good *cautela* to write nothing down, in case anything goes wrong and angry friends and relatives of the patient go to the apothecary's shop to find out what the medicine was. A written prescription in such a case would be a ticket to disaster in terms of reputation, says Zerbi.

A section of Zerbi's advice[17] is devoted to the appropriate behaviour of the medical man when another doctor is also in attendance on the case. If the medical man finds himself with a case that might arguably end fatally, it is wise to call in one or more colleagues. Perhaps they can add to the first doctor's knowledge of remedies, and certainly a fatal outcome will bring less blame to a small group of consulting doctors than to an individual. Society does not withdraw its reward, says Zerbi in his aphoristic style, but singularity more often brings infamy.

Part of the function of this ethical manoeuvre is thus to avoid a bad reputation. The same is true of Zerbi's advice about choosing a colleague who is to act in these circumstances. First make sure that everything is prepared, so that the incoming doctor and the practitioner calling him should not suddenly appear to need something. The new colleague should be senior, sympathetic to the patient and, in first place, 'faithful'. It is important that the colleague thus chosen, says Zerbi, should be learned in the *scientia* of medicine, which will make full and private discussion of the case possible. In this case the best course of action, says Zerbi, is to issue a single, joint *consilium*. We can see from the context of Zerbi's advice that the advantage of this was, again, that responsibility was shared and criticism deflected. The danger in issuing two *consilia*, particularly if differing in advice, and especially if written, was that the learning of the practitioners, their very claim to monopolistic practice, would be called into question. We have already seen the dangers to the learned doctor's reputation when the bedside is surrounded by impudent but clever quacks.

In the converse case, that is when the doctor whom Zerbi is addressing is called to another doctor's case, then the function of

Zerbi's ethics is the same. Here, too, the imperative is to close professional ranks and maintain a common reputation of learning and behaviour. Ask the first doctor if he has seen the patient yet, advises Zerbi. If he has, then praise some of his remedies and propose collaboration. If the first doctor's pupil is at the bedside, continues Zerbi, treat him with respect and do not denigrate him. Take him to one side and converse with him in a low voice and with a grave face: this will give the appearance of thinking deeply about the case. If the doctor coming into this situation finds that a mistake has been made then Zerbi advises that the correction should be made in private and never publicly. If you are obliged to disagree with your colleague, says Zerbi directly, tell only the friends of the patient and do not argue in front of others.

But there was an exception to Zerbi's expectation that given tact and a few rules of etiquette two learned doctors would act to preserve their common reputation. There is a danger, he says, of rich and proud doctors coming late to a case and while paying scant attention to the patient, imposing their own will and opinions. These were the practitioners, says Zerbi, whose practice it was to surround themselves with sycophantic empirics and plebians, who would shout down the learned and modest doctor. Who was Zerbi referring to? What group of practitioners were distinct enough from the university-trained, learned and rational group that Zerbi represented, to have a different system of internal rules, or ethics? Zerbi further describes such a practitioner as 'some professor of medicine to whom, by law and by merit, collaboration cannot be denied'.[18] So such a person professed medicine (Zerbi does not necessarily mean he taught it) and was clearly an able physician – to merit Zerbi's grudging admission, such a doctor must have met Zerbi's criteria of being learned and rational. Clearly, too, he had a legal standing at least equal to that of Zerbi's group. For Zerbi to mention the fact – and the resentment is clear – this was clearly some status, or even legal protection over and above that which Zerbi and his kind claimed as learned teachers and practitioners.

Zerbi's term for such one-sided collaboration is *collegium*. The activity itself is expressed by a verb, and Zerbi says those who *collegiant* publicly are damnable. What Zerbi is condemning is the tendency of the 'collegiating' physicians to aggrandize themselves at the expense of their own kind, and in front of third parties. This, says Zerbi, 'causes murmurs among the vulgar' and generates disrespect for doctors as a whole.

Zerbi's ethics here reflect a professional rivalry between politically different groupings of similarly educated physicians. Let us try to reconstruct his situation. Zerbi identified with the student *universitas* of Padua and its medical teachers. But the professional body in Padua was the College of Philosophers and Physicians, which gave degrees and licensed practice. It was not necessary to belong to the College in order to practise or even to teach. If Zerbi was not a member of the College, or, if a member, was not part of the powerful inner ring of older *numerarii,* he may well have resented the powers of granting degrees and of licensing practice – and for which they doubtless gave themselves airs – that the College had.

There is also another possibility. Padua was in the Veneto, under the control of rich and powerful Venice. Venice, too, had had a College of Physicians, from the early fourteenth century, which was concerned with the regulation of the professional practice of medicine. This, then, was an institution of a kind different to the Paduan *studium,* and was not at first concerned with education or the granting of degrees (there being no *studium* in Venice). But it claimed the right to give degrees at some time in the middle of the fifteenth century, and nearer Zerbi's time, at the visit of the emperor Frederick III in 1469 the Venetian College of Physicians was given the right to give eight degrees annually in arts and medicine. The ambition of the Venetian College was to extend its power and become a *studium,* examining students and granting degrees.

The *studium* of Padua clearly felt threatened. Almost certainly their statutes of 1468 (with which this chapter began) were designed to reinforce its privileges in the face of the ambitions of the Venetian College. By 1470 some Paduan students were indeed going to Venice for their degrees. (In the same way the professional College of Milan attracted students who had been educated in Pavia.) The student *universitas* in fact claimed the autonomy to co-operate with a professional College other than the Paduan for the granting of degrees to its students. There was intense rivalry between the Colleges of Padua and Venice on this account, and considerable strain between the Paduan College and the *studium.*[19] By 1489 the Paduan College was losing income and prestige to that of Venice. In other words Zerbi's 'collegiants' would have been especially 'damnable' if they came from the College of the politically dominant Venice, were the agents of the decline of the Paduan College and the seducers of the students of the *studium,* and were politically powerful within the profession in terms of practice and degrees. Zerbi's *ethical* dissatisfaction with their behaviour reflects perfectly the fact that the College was to an extent a *rival* grouping with its own set of values and behaviour. Indeed, the College in Venice had an explicit ethical code, with detailed advice on cases of which Zerbi complained, where two doctors were called.

In considering the doctor's behaviour to his patients, Zerbi seems to rely primarily on the Hippocratic sources. The 'ethical' doctor obeys the *Oath* when entering a house and avoids all injury to those therein.[20] Just as the Hippocratic ethical works seem to be sets of 'our' rules in opposition to those of 'them', so Zerbi has here a great deal of rhetoric against the flattering doctors, whose aim is to please by personal attention and agreeable treatments, and who succeed (says Zerbi) mainly with women and the vulgar, generating 'a hollow reputation'.[21] Perhaps Zerbi is drawing on Hippocratic sources with which he can, because of their authority, identify. It is not clear that he and his group were in fact facing a threat from such practitioners from outside the group. The same is true when he speaks of those doctors whose aims are simply evil. That is, there was much in the post-classical literature that was set out in the strongest terms against opponents who were necessarily 'evil', or in our terms 'unethical', and Zerbi can add to his rhetoric (for 'our' group) by quoting these sources. They are (in addition to the Old Testament) Averroes, Damascenus and Pietro d'Abano.

Women patients were a special sub-group. Not only were there the technical and ethical problems of women-related diseases (see above) but also the problems of the male doctor attending the female patient. Again, the source of Zerbi's ethics is the *Oath*. Do not even begin to think about libidinous approaches, says Zerbi.

Ethics and Learning

So far we have looked at Zerbi's advice to the doctor in situations into which the doctor's practice leads him, but which are not in themselves concerned with the technical content of that medicine. But the doctor's ethics did concern themselves with the technical content of medicine, in two ways. First, the doctor naturally believed that the kind of medicine he practised was the best. It would clearly be unethical to depart from the best medicine; and other kinds of medicine were also unethical. Second, Zerbi's kind of medicine was rationalist (in following Galen's natural-philosophical explanations) and learned. These two characteristics of medicine had been used in the high middle ages to justify the study of medicine in the *studia* as a true *scientia,* and Zerbi devotes much of his ethics to a defence of learning and to the training of the rational, learned doctor.

So Zerbi is defending *his* kind of medicine, taught in the university and battling to preserve its claims to monopoly in practice. Zerbi is at pains to demonstrate not only that this is the best kind of medicine, but that it is the only possible kind. It was consistent with, and linked to, other aspects of Zerbi's world, to his religion, his view of the social order and to his knowledge of other disciplines. To practise the best medicine, ethical medicine, meant to share these views.

To Zerbi, learned medicine was progressive. This was partly from necessity, for the physical decay of mankind, since the ancients, had allowed the appearance of new diseases unknown to the ancients (Zerbi was writing a few months after the first appearance of the *morbus gallicus*) [22] Old remedies were no longer always appropriate. Moreover, medical knowledge had been added to by a string of authors since Hippocrates and Galen had written, and Zerbi makes generous use of the Arabic authors and some of the commentators. Zerbi felt himself to be in a tradition of learned medicine, a tradition that had to be defended. He makes his defence by binding together all those aspects of his view of the world that would be shared by people of his group and class, who if not medical men, may well have been in a position to fight for the privileges which the learned doctor claimed. This binding-together is most evident in Zerbi's ethics, which show that the Good Doctor is ethical precisely because he behaves in accordance with a view of the world that a learned physician might be expected to have.

Let us look in more detail at the world-view of Zerbi's Good Doctor. He knows that it is of the utmost importance that the young should be introduced to good doctrine at an early age.[23] (Zerbi's elaborate analogy of a seed growing in good soil is founded on the Hippocratic *De Lege*.) The aim of education is to enable those who have completed it to lead a good life. This is a comprehensive goal, and includes medicine where the educated man wishes to become a doctor. The best way of living, says Zerbi, is by reason perfected by art. The sentiment is Aristotle's, and Zerbi has borrowed it from the *Metaphysics*. Good education, university education, was of course almost entirely Aristotelian. The reason that art perfected was the Aristotelian dialectic with which the arts course began. The student passed on to Aristotelian moral philosophy in the *Ethics* and *Politics*. Aristotelian natural philosophy, which normally came later in the arts course, contained the natural principles on which the theory of medicine rested.[24] Good medicine was an extension of natural philosophy, and good practice of medicine was informed partly by moral philosophy. For example, the doctor's ethical reluctance to discuss details of his patients' cases is overcome only by Aristotle's observation in the *Ethics* that discussion with someone capable of theoretical understanding should be completely frank.[25] Zerbi insists that the doctor's erudition begins with the grammar, rhetoric and dialectic of the schools and universities, with the four quadrivial arts of arithmetic, music, geometry and astrology, and above all, with natural philosophy. (Even his discussion of the medical *cautela* is informed by the four Aristotelian causes.)[26]

So the Good Doctor is *learned* in Aristotelian, and then medical knowledge, and he is *rational* in dealing in an Aristotelian way with the particulars of sense observation in his practice in relation to the universals that are in the mind. Do not, says Zerbi, give your attention only to universals, and despise particulars, for to do so is not the art of medicine.[27] Indeed, sensory observation will reveal to you things that cannot be put into words and cannot be written about in theoretical treatises.[28] The Good Doctor is he who has been well exercised as a young man in practice, having sought out hospitals and other places where there are many patients, diseases and skilful doctors. On the other hand, says Zerbi, do not give your attention wholly to particulars and despise universals, for that is empiricism.[29] In this way Aristotle furnishes the Good Doctor with both a theory of knowledge (what is first in the senses is not first in nature; there is nothing in the mind that was not first in the senses) and with a criterion for medical licensing (empirics have no knowledge of universals). Zerbi says, expressly from Aristotle's logical works, that nothing can be known without its first principles. But, he adds, while the foundation of medicine lies in its first principles, first principles are on their own useless unless brought down to particulars. (It is in acquiring new particulars that medicine was for Zerbi, as we have seen, progressive.)

The later part of this education of the Good Doctor, says Zerbi, takes place in 'celebrated universities'.[30] Zerbi has a great deal of rhetoric on the behaviour of students. He makes an elaborate simile illustrating that as the father is the cause in procreation, so the teaching master is the cause of the student learning a *scientia*. Zerbi's rhetoric, in its prefatorial and aphoristic style, enlarges upon how the students must learn from, respect and obey their teachers, paying due reverence to their authority and skill. Now, this is a natural thing to write for a man who has been a university teacher for most of his adult life; it is also something that would naturally appeal to those with power to help implement Zerbi's view of the doctor's duties and privileges. But it is more than this. In these words Zerbi is binding together other aspects of his view of the world. We can examine these by focusing on the central notion of trust, or faith. Ultimately the Good Doctor is the one who behaves 'faithfully' – he is *fidelis*. It is faith that the student shows to his teachers in accepting what they say, obeying them and revering them. It is this same faith that the modern, late fifteenth-century doctor gives to the old authors. Despite the change in the human body and the progress of knowledge, faith is to be given to the fathers of medicine – Hippocrates followed by Galen. When Zerbi was writing it was only a few years since Leoniceno had launched his attack on Pliny.[31] The result was a bitter dispute in which the defenders of Pliny argued that although he may have been wrong in places, it was improper to make such a violent and public attack on so great a name. Colenuccio,[32] the lawyer, pointed out that in a court a misdemeanor could be excused if the defendant was a great ornament to society. Leoniceno, in his opponents' eyes, lacked that faith and reverence that should be accorded to one of the fathers of the Latin tradition of learning, the *res latina*. Precisely the same thing was to happen when Vesalius attacked Galen when, after the bitter troubles of the early Reformation, Vesalius' opponents lent a distinct *odium theologicum* to their accusations that Vesalius 'lacked faith'.[33] Much of Zerbi's ethical advice centres on the 'faithful' doctor, who *erit non aliter quam fidelis*.[34] The doctor is the faithful companion of the body of his patient, suffers with him and rejoices in his health. To neglect him, to act improperly in his home, to do anything prohibited by common morality or special medical ethics, would be to break faith with the patient.

Another element that Zerbi is binding into his notion of 'faith' is the Hippocratic ethics of the *Oath* and *Law*. The *Oath* represents an initiation procedure. The entrant swears to obey it. He is enjoined to keep the secrets of the group he is joining. He swears to honour his teachers and to pass on freely the secret knowledge to their sons. Other Hippocratic ethical works suggest that this secret knowledge is believed to have had a divine origin: it characterizes the group that has it and is responsible for their success. Its origin and utility meant that it had to be protected from outsiders, the profane. Holy things are given only to holy men. The doctor who used the *Oath* in his own ethical system saw himself as being within a tradition of special knowledge that had to be protected and where the fathers of the discipline were the first teachers, to whom were due reverence and faith. It was in Zerbi's time that the medieval medical textbook, the *Articella,* came to include not only the *Oath,* but also the other Hippocratic ethical text that Zerbi used, the *Law.*[35] Both clearly – and *Law* expressly – relate to a time when there was no system of medical licensing, but because both deal with the initiation of doctors and the faith within the medical tradition, and because of the authority of the name of Hippocrates, Zerbi can use them to strengthen his arguments for learned medicine to be the way he wants it to be inside and outside the universities.

Another thread that runs through Zerbi's view of the world that goes to make up his ethics is religion. This too deals with 'faith' and the word never entirely loses its Christian meaning. We should not expect that it would, for in the fifteenth-century university there could be no division of kind between 'medicine', 'religion' or other similar categories. During the previous two centuries medical commentators (like Gentile) could rationally begin their expositions with an invocation of divine help on the grounds that God was the ultimate cause of everything, including the commentator and his text.[36] God (they said) followed Aristotelian causality in creating all things: we can see arts-course Aristotelianism as providing a deeper understanding of religious doctrine. Contemporary discussions of what constitutes knowledge often emphasize the singleness of 'philosophy' as all knowledge of the works of man and God. Its purpose was perfection of the soul of man in anticipation of temporal and eternal happiness.[37] This is consistent with and an extension of Aristotle's belief that the end of moral philosophy is happiness.

Zerbi, like his medieval predecessors, places invocation of divine help in first place when giving his opening account of how to achieve the good life (reason perfected by art).[38] The second instrument for this end is erudition: the physician must immerse himself in study, day and night (that is, ethical medicine is *learned* medicine). The third and last is to preserve one's reputation by observing the medical canons. These are broad ethical rules that are parallelled, says Zerbi, by the evangelic law. Again, the first of these is the invocation of divine help, the help of the legislator who created all things. The parallel is the text of Matthew: ask, and it shall be given; seek and you will find. Second is dedication to the task: the narrow gate that leads to righteousness. Third, avoid false doctrine. Here the text is the biblical injunction to avoid false prophets, that is, 'heretical doctrine'.[39] The parallel is a fine one: heresy and the teachings of false prophets are, of course, *other* people's systems of thought and belief and so, in the sense we are using the word here, deeply *unethical.* Medical heresy for Zerbi was empiricism, that is, unlearned and so unlicensed practice.[40] Here[41] Zerbi is tying tightly together 'correct', ethical, medical and religious belief by making a common enemy in medical and religious heresy.

Having discussed the natural attributes and acquired skills of the Good Doctor, Zerbi's second chapter is concerned with the most important *cautela* of practice, the doctor's behaviour to God. Again, medical and religious belief are not to be distinguished: the doctor, says Zerbi, is like a priest, and is divine in using the medicines that God has created on earth; and he is divine also in being he to whom divine things are revealed, in being, that is, a Hippocratic. Part of the ethical training of Zerbi's Good Doctor is to be made fit to receive such revelation. The revelation is the special knowledge of the doctor (Zerbi quotes the Hippocratic *De Lege* through the commentator Nicholas) but the training is late fifteenth-century Christianity.

The doctor was like a priest also in his practice. Urge the patient to confess, says Zerbi, arguing that a secret sin may be at the root of the patient's illness[42] (and so may be evil demons, the *alabin*). Zerbi says the Good Doctor invokes divine help in compounding his remedies and in writing *consilia*; before beginning treatment he says 'May God liberate you'; he remembers that it is God who cures, not the physician; in using antidotes he always completes his treatment by saying 'If God so wishes'; in making prognostications he is careful not to appear to usurp God's foreknowledge.

Prognosis

While taking care not to usurp God's foreknowledge, the rational physician nevertheless had good professional reasons for relying a good deal on prognosis. Prognosis was display. It was a display of technical knowledge and techniques that impressed the patient. It was a display that showed that the doctor knew about the kind of disease that the patient had, at the point where the patient's interest was at its greatest, that is, about what was going to happen. For Zerbi it was an essentially Galenic technique, for it was a display that demonstrated that the physician knew all about the patient's disease from its symptoms down to the fundamental facts of nature. Prognosis, that is, was part of the rational doctor's Good Story, by which his reason and learning impressed the patient. Rational medicine competed in the market-place partly on the basis of prognosis. It was an *ethical* practice in the sense we are using the term in this chapter: that it was controlled by an explicit set of rules (about when to do it and when not: see below); rules that characterized a group and contributed to its success.

Zerbi's ideal rational, learned and prognosticating physician made a careful entry to the sickroom. He did not hasten round to the patient's house, run up the stairs and make an unexpected entrance, hot and sweaty, but waited until both he and the patient were prepared for the encounter. Meanwhile he kept his eyes open for any signs of earlier treatment that might give him a hint about what the patient or a previous doctor thought the disease might be. The inspiration for Zerbi was Galen's account, in *De Locis Affectis*, of how he had immeasurably impressed the patient with his skill in prognostication on the basis of chance observations of things left in the sickrooom. Zerbi then advises the prognosticating doctor to take the patient's pulse, noting down the hundred and more differences he will feel. Contemporary medicine was well supplied with distinctions within the kinds of pulse and amply furnished with technical terminology. The doctor was making a display of his mastery of these technical matters, and Zerbi's advice is to spend a great deal of time doing it.[43] Then, says Zerbi, touch the patient's chest and abdomen, examine his tongue and teeth and if you like, smell his breath. Then with everyone present and the patient listening, describe the great medical usefulness of taking the pulse and say 'I will now examine the urine, for it is principally by these two things, the pulse and the urine, that the type of fever is understood, together with the origin of their cause, the *ratio* of life and the *professio* of death.' In other words, this is the patter of the rational physician selling his medicine by claims of rationality and a learned tradition: the audience is arranged, the name of Galen is invoked, the display of pulse-taking is rationalized by reference to causality, and finally it is claimed that this learning and reason lead to the solemn business of prognostication.

The benefits of making a correct prognosis were considerable. Zerbi calls them honour and glory. But the dangers were also great, and the doctor had to handle things carefully. Never discuss the significance of your findings about the pulse and urine in front of the patient, advises Zerbi. Leave the sickroom and let a little time pass. Consider everything you have been able to learn about the patient, from his symptoms, from his friends, by looking about the house, from any earlier medical attendant. Be very cautious about making a prognostication, says Zerbi, especially of death, for the patient's state of mind may make such a prophecy self-fulfilling. Indeed it is best not to make absolute predictions, he adds, and the wise medical man, like the astrologer, makes his prognostications conditional, saying something like 'Certainly it seems to me if things remain as they are and nothing supervenes ...'[44] The model for Zerbi is Galen's highly conditional judgement that a patient will escape the disease if he has a good doctor, is himself obedient, has diligent servants well prepared with all external necessities and if nothing unexpected happens.[45] If the doctor is uncertain about the outcome or if the disease is changing the doctor could take Zerbi's advice and answer questions obliquely: change the subject, reply indirectly or let drop a significant but uncommitted word or two. Zerbi concludes that on the whole it is best to make a rather gloomy forecast when uncertain. If the outcome is good, the doctor gathers up the glory.[46] If it is bad, the doctor avoids blame, either because he saw the danger early, or because the blame can be attributed to the failure of one of four conditions suggested by Galen – the failure of the patient to obey, the servants to be diligent, the external necessities to be correct, or the arrival of the unexpected.

Anatomy and Ethics

Six years after Zerbi produced his tract *De Cautelis Medicorum,* there appeared his textbook of anatomy.[47] Both publications are in many senses very novel. It is claimed that there were earlier works on ethics, but they are not so explicit or even so big as Zerbi's small tract. As for the anatomy, the contrast with what had gone before is more striking. The statutory text was Mondino's brief *Anathomia,* but this did not generate published commentary until Berengrio da Carpi in 1521. Most other anatomical work was limited to commentaries on the Canon by expositors like Matthaeus de Gradibus, Jacobus de Partibus and Gentile da Foligno.[48] Zerbi's *Liber Anathomie* is quite different. Nearly half of a million words long, designed for use in conjunction with public dissections, drawn from a wide range of sources, it is clearly intended to make some major statement about the nature of university anatomy.

What can Zerbi's anatomy tell us about his view of the world, which we have explored in locating and explaining his ethics? Let us return to Padua. The statutes of 1468 and their revised version of the early sixteenth century use unusually strong language on insisting on the suppression of unlicensed practice, and on the regular performance of the public anatomies. Some urgency was clearly felt about both matters, and mention is made of previous laxity. When Zerbi returned to Padua in 1494 after periods in Bologna and Rome, he was an *ordinarius* teacher, the teacher who gave the principal lectures. He was directly concerned with the teaching, the practice and the defence of university medicine. As we have seen, what made university medicine different from any other sort was primarily that it was learned. It claimed its authority from a tradition of learning that seemed to stretch back to Hippocrates and Galen. It was on a basis of this learning that the university doctor claimed also that his medicine was more effective than others and that this in turn gave him the right to claim a monopoly of practice. Galen, as a Rationalist, had constructed a medicine on the foundation of structure, from which a discussion about function, malfunction and treatment could link the patients' symptoms to the fundamentals of the natural-philosophical world picture.[49] Anatomy was the touchstone of learned and rational medicine. The spectacle of public dissections was much more than a way of teaching the Paduan physicans and surgeons about the inside of the human body. It was a statement about the kind of medicine that was taught and practised and about the identity of the people who taught and practised it. Nothing could be a more arresting spectacle than, in tightly controlled circumstances, placing a dead human body on a table and cutting it into small pieces, beginning with a sweeping incision along the length of the abdomen.

The place of anatomy within rational and learned medicine is reflected in Zerbi's book on the human body. It opens with a declaration of the nature and purposes of anatomy. These are largely philosophical. Anatomy of the human shows to the highest degree the skill and providence of nature, says Zerbi; knowledge of its parts is knowledge of a high order and is of benefit to the soul. Zerbi does not need to say that Nature is the mode by which the Creator worked and works in the world any more than he needed to say that academic study of Nature was a major component of the arts course and the main way in which rationalist medicine reached back to the fundamentals of the world picture. His readers would have been well aware of this consonance between Christianity and Greek philosophy.

In this way Zerbi saw that anatomy was fundamental to the kind of medicine (and of course it included surgery, for which anatomy was necessary) which he was trying to defend. It may be that the perceived threat was simply fom unlicensed practice. But he may also have been convinced of the importance of the *teaching* of proper medicine – his medicine – within the *studium*, where it would inform the practice of future doctors. The teaching of medicine was not part of the functions of the Colleges and perhaps Zerbi was trying to defend his kind of medicine against that of the

Collegiants. His defence was essentially practical. The anatomy text was practical, designed to accompany a dissection. The dissection itself was practical: not only would such an image, a characteristic of rational medicine, be much more memorable than mere arguments; but also Zerbi was taking effective action through his book and its associated dissections, to follow the urgings of the new statutes. His ethics too were practical – he says so in a formal discussion about their place in medicine.[50] And one of the ethical rules themselves is that the intending doctor should not waste his life in the theory of medicine. We can recall that another section of the new Paduan statutes reveal anxiety about the level of unlicensed practice, or in other words, the learned and rational physician was facing competition from other doctors. Zerbi's *De Cautelis Medicorum* can be seen as consistent with, even if not inspired by this corporate nervousness about external groups with their own systems of ethics. It explains to the university doctor above all how to promote and defend his own kind of medicine. It would make perfectly plain to anyone who had the power to promote Zerbi's ideal on what grounds rational, learned and university medicine claimed superiority. To summarize, anatomy, and public dissections of the human body, were very powerful displays of the fact that the medicine they represented was learned and based on a rationalist view that the structure, function and malfunction of the body was intelligible. Its practitioners also thought that this kind of medicine was also ethically the best, if only because it was clearly unethical to allow the practice of a different, and therefore worse, kind of medicine. For Zerbi and the men who gave emphasis to these parts of the statutes, learning and rationality were to be defended and promoted as much by anatomy as by ethics.

Conclusion: Ethics Old and New

We have seen that Zerbi's ethics were written down in all probability in response to a threat he saw to his kind of medicine in the 1490s. If these were historically 'local' causes, can we speak of an earlier history of ethics, perhaps even a genre or tradition? We probably cannot, certainly if we limit ourselves to written materials in which we might find explicit discussions of the physicians' professional behaviour. Even though Zerbi makes a virtue of naming his sources, his book is a compilation of fragments by other people on other topics.

One example must suffice. For Zerbi the Good Doctor was the *medicus canonicus*. It is this 'canonical physician' whose serious-mindedness was, as we have seen, sometimes punctured by the coarse wit of the vulgar. It was he, also, who suffered from the high-handedness of the 'collegiates', and in this case, Zerbi argues, there is a *modus canonicus,* a proper method of procedure to be followed by the canonical physician. The canons of medicine that he follows in the same way as he follows the evangelic law (see above) would thus seem to no less than ethical rules. But the *modus canonicus* is derived from the first book of Avicenna's *Canon.* At the point in the text indicated by Zerbi (fen 1, doctrine 1, chapter 1: de *subjectis medicine.*)[51] Avicenna discusses not ethics, or behaviour, or reputation, but how medicine can only be effective if based on the first principles of (an Aristotelian) natural philosophy, and that upon the 'first philosophy' or metaphysics. In emphasizing what the physician must know – and anatomy is very important – Avicenna tells us more about the history of what in this chapter we have called rational medicine, but is not writing about ethics. The 'ethical' use to which Zerbi puts his source is thus derived from its technical superiority, and is not inherited from an ethical component of Avicenna's medicine.

In the period after Zerbi and before that to which the later chapters of this book are devoted, we can look for a history of medical ethics primarily in the sense that it was naturally considered ethical to practise the proper kind of medicine – one's own – and unethical to do otherwise, or to allow other – unethical – groups to succeed. In the sixteenth century, especially, there were more groups, readily identifiable, to be considered than in the earlier period. Following Leoniceno's attacks on Avicenna, there were many who would not have considered Avicenna's medicine to be *canonicus.* These were the 'skilled Hellenists' as Zerbi and Berengario da Carpi[52] called them, who objected to all things medieval, to commentators and even to the Latin language. Perhaps even as early as Zerbi's book on anatomy, one of these Hellenists, Alessandro Benedetti, had written an entirely Hellenist anatomy (it was rather slim).[53] Undoubtedly the sponsors of the revived Greek medicine of the Hellenists and humanists rejected much of medieval medicine, and so their views of what it was 'ethical' to practise must have changed in part.

But in part, too, there were continuities that reflect the other aspects of the physician's life, the power of his religion, his defence of the learned tradition and his need to protect the reputation of physicians as a whole. These things are reflected in the structure of a set of medical ethics of an author a generation later than Zerbi,

Clementi Clementini, writing in 1535. His *Lucubrationes* are similar enough to Zerbi's *Cautela* for us to guess that by the sixteenth century there was in fact a recognized topic of 'medical ethics' in medical education. The inclusion of the Hippocratic ethical works in the essentially medieval *Articella* presupposes some form of commentary on them during teaching. And even though the new classicism of the Hellenists had led to the end of the publishing history of the *Articella* (almost at the same time that Clementini's book appeared) they would have had little reason to exclude from their teaching a discussion of Hippocratic ethics.

Almost everything that Clementini wrote can be related to Zerbi's work. There is space here to draw only a skeletal parallel. Clementini begins with the sacred nature of medicine. It is partly that the curative powers of medicines are God-given (the physician merely administers them); partly that the doctor should, at his first contact with the patient, use some of the formality of the priest to reconcile the patient with God, the author of disease as well as of medicines and health; and partly that the physician piously emulates Christ the Healer. Indeed, the physician should be to his patient as another God, benign, merciful, charitably treating the poor for no reward and even the well-to-do for Grace rather than fees. Be confident, urges Clementini, that such charitable treatments will be rewarded by God, who will provide the charitable doctor's necessities (and punish the uncharitable's sins) and, in fact, will act to the doctors as the doctor acts to his patients. But the professional demands of reputation and financial respectability are not to be ignored and Clementini slides easily and without irony into the practical results of charitable practice. *Constant* charitable practice will through experience produce a better doctor, and so a charitable spirit often leads to a better reputation and richer financial rewards; one grateful patient may well meet in his fee the lapses of others. As with Zerbi the basis of the doctor's relationship with the patient is 'faith' which the doctor keeps with his patient, involving charity, love and just treatment. Moreover, says Clementini, again without irony or conflict of ideals, such medicine cures more quickly; from duties and liberality the doctor gathers up praise and thanks.

Like Zerbi too Clementini places emphasis on the learning of the doctor. It is limited to advice to study hard and in particular to be certain of what the medical literature says about the variations in disease that occur in different places and at different times. However, in a striking contrast to Zerbi, Clementini argues that ultimately the Good Doctor is born, not made. It is by the influx of the stars that the best doctor is almost divine, with sound judgement and an ability to predict. To be sure, learning is a necessary part of the process, and Clementini says he has seen many a man born full of vice under a bad astrological sign and yet made good by a study of letters. Indeed, some such thing is hardly avoidable for, as he says, theoretical medicine is subject to Taurus and practical to Scorpio: both signs make medical men jealous and malevolent among themselves, and only a commitment to philosophical learning and to moral discipline can overcome these astrological disadvantages.

Although it was a commonplace of medical thought that the good doctor had certain natural attributes (such as a retentive memory and capable hands; Zerbi discusses such things) it was quite another thing to claim that a physician, as physician, was born rather than made. An extreme form of this view was held by Paracelsus: that medicine was God-given and traditional learning useless. No discussion of Reformist thinking is in order in this chapter, but again we are reminded that as the sixteenth century progressed a protestant way of thinking about the best, *ethical,* way of practising medicine was added to the other groups we have identified. Clementini hovers between the 'almost divine' nature of the attributes of such a physician and the very human similar ones that Zerbi had offered direct injunctions about acquiring. Such a physician does not become inebriated; does not mix with the ignorant or the rustic but, self-contained and solitary, avoids the contempt that is bred by familiarity; he uses knowledge of letters and especially of philosophy to avoid vices to so to stand out from the ignorant crowd and even to govern it; to such a man incurable cases do not happen, perhaps because of the near-divinity of his prescience.

But Clementini is as explicit as Zerbi and no doubt for the same reasons on what to do if the doctor does find himself with a hopeless case on his hands: do not tell the patient (it will only make him worse), but make clear the prognosis to the assistants. Having seen them now in Zerbi we can understand what is behind the rest of Clementini's related ethical injunctions. Do not, he charges his readers, make prognostications more than necessary, and certainly not before those who are merely curious. The outcome of diseases, like that of wars, is uncertain; and Clementini, like Galen and Zerbi, warns that the doctor cannot be certain of the obedience of the patient or the assistants. Clementini took the Hippocratic view that judgement is difficult and *experimentum* fallacious: although there is great fortune in prognosticating at times of great danger, and although he who can see what will happen on the basis of learning and experience, collects the greatest glory, it is best, concludes Clementini, to keep quiet rather than risk it. He, too, recognized the doctor's device (like all of these devices, expressed at more length by Zerbi) of representing a case as more serious than it actually was in order to avoid the blame of a death and to collect large fees and much glory if the outcome were favourable.[54]

So – finally – Zerbi's ethics seem to be one of the earliest expressions of a group's self-regulatory rules of the renaissance period. They incorporate, for obvious historical reasons, the rather more fragmentary internal rules of regulation of the various groups represented in the Hippocratic corpus. They give the historian more insight into the group-rules of physicians as a society than do the earlier 'pathway of physicians' of Gentile da Foligno or the equation between ethical and technical superiority made by the New Galenism, described by Luis Garcia-Ballester. After Zerbi the appearance of new groups of medical men suggests not only the below-the-surface formulation of new ethics for each of the groups, but also – as in the case of Clementini – the historical appearance (or continuity) of a self-conscious discussion about how medical men should behave.

Notes

1. Thus *Ancient Medicine* can be interpreted as a defence of experiential, dietetic and (its self-image) proper and originally divine medicine against fluent and personable opponents with a resembance to the sophists. The *Oath* can be seen as representing an admissions. procedure into a group very like that portrayed in *Ancient Medicine.*
2. See R. K. French, 'Gentile da Foligno and the via medicorum', in J. D. North and J. J. Roche, *The Light of Nature* (Dordrecht: Nijhoff, 1985) 21–34.
3. *Statuta Almae Universitatis D. Artistarum et Medicorum Patavini Gymnasii* (Venice, 1589). The reference to Zerbi is on f.61r. The statutes about unlicensed practice are at f.69r, where the civil authorities are urged to take new action. The new anatomy statutes are at 67v. It was directed that the new statutes should all be read out publicly in Italian to the sound of trumpets.
4. See J. R. Lind, *Studies in Pre-Vesalian Anatomy. Biography, Translations, Documents* (Philadelphia: The American Philosophical Society, 1975) 141–56.
5. Gabriel de Zerbi, *Opus perutile de Cautelis Medicorum, in Pillularium omnibus medicis Necessarium clarissimi doctoris magistri Panthaleonis* (Lyons: 1528). According to Lind (1975) 151, Zerbi's was the first systematic account of medical ethics, preceded only by more

fragmentary accounts by Arnald of Villanova, Alberto de' Zancari, Cristoforo Barzizza and Alessandro Benedetti.

6. f.lxiii r.
7. f.lxiii r.
8. f.lxxii v.
9. f.lxxii v.
10. f.lxx v.
11. f.lxxiii r; lxxii v.
12. f.lxviii v.
13. Jacopo Berengario da Carpi, *Commentaria cum amplissimis additionibus in Anatomia Mundini,* (Bologna: 1521), ff 307v, 310r.
14. f.lxviii v.
15. f.lxix v.
16. f.lxii v.
17. f.lxx v.
18. f.lxxi r.
19. See the useful account by R. Palmer, *The Studio of Venice and its graduates in the Sixteenth Century* (Padua: Lint, 1983).
20. f. lxi r.
21. ff.lxi r–v.
22. The widespread notion that mankind had degenerated was compatible with the respect shown for the classical authors by the humanists and hellenists. It was to be developed by the Parisian anatomists Sylvius and Riolan to explain how the modern body was different from that apparently described by Galen. See J. Sylvius, *In Hippocratis et Galeni Physiologiae partem Anatomicam Isagoge* (Venice: 1556), e.g. f.7v.
23. f.lvi r.
24. Natural philosophy in the universities began traditionally with the text and a commentary of the 'Eight books of the Physics', *Octo libri physicorum.* These general principles of natural change, were then explored through a range of Aristotle's *libri naturales* that dealt with subject matter of increasing complexity – generation and corruption, the heavens and earth, meteorology and finally the workings of the soul in animals.
25. f.lix r.
26. f.lv v.
27. f.lix v.
28. f.lvii v. There were two areas where it was generally agreed that theory was inadequate, and only empirical observation would suffice: the actions of certain drugs, and the complex shape of some parts of the body. See French, note 2 above, 21–34; also *idem,* 'Berengario da Carpi and the use of commentary in anatomical teaching' in A. Wear, R. French and I. Lonie, (eds) *The Medical Renaissance of the Sixteenth Century* (Cambridge: Cambridge University Press, 1985).
29. ff.lvii r; lix v.

30. f. lvii r.
31. N. Leoniceno, *De Plinii et plurium aliorum Medicorum in Medicina Erroribus* [Ferrara: nd.(*c.*late 1492)].
32. P. Collenuccio, *Pliniana Defensio* [Ferrara: nd.(*c.* early 1493)).
33. See Sylvius, *Isagoge*, note 5 above. See also B. Eustachio, *Opuscula Anatomica* (Venice: 1563). 165–73.
34. f.lxi v.
35 For example, *Articella nuperrime impressa cum quamplurimis tractatibus pristine impressione superadditis* (Lyons: 1525): *De Lege* is at f.x, the third work of the collection. The edition of Venice, 1523 contains *De Lege* towards the end.
36. See Gentile da Foligno, in beginning his commentary on Avicenna (note 48 below).
37. In this it was like the philosophy of many medieval accounts of 'the sciences'. Perhaps the best known and certainly one of the earliest is that of D. Gundissalinus (Gundisalvi), *De Divisione Philosophiae* (edited by C. Baeumker and G. von Hertling in *Beitrage der Philosophie des Mittelalters* (Munster: 1906) vol 4.
38. Prologue.
39. f.lv r.
40. f.lvii v.
41. f.lv r.
42. f. lxii v.
43. f. lxiii v.
44. f. lxv r.
45. f. lxv v.
46. f. lxvi r.
47. Gabriele de Zerbi, *Liber Anathomie Corporis Humani et singulorum Membrorum illius* (Venice: 1502).
48. *Tertius Canonis Avicenna cum dilucidissimis expositoribus Gentile fulginate nec non Jac. de partibis Parisiense,* 3 vols, (Venice: *c.*1499); *Tertius Canonis Avicennae cum amplissima Gentilis fulg. expositione. Demum commentaria nuper addita videlicet Jacobi de Partibus super fen vi et xiii. Item Jo. Matthei de gradi super fen xxii quia Gentilis in eis deficit,* in 2 vols, the first without date or place, the second being *Secunda pars Gentilis super tertio Avic. cum supplementis Jacobis de partibus parisiensis ac Joannis Matthei de Gradi mediolensis ubi Gentilis vel breviter vel tacite pertransivit,* (Venice: 1522).
49. See P. Brain, *Galen on Bloodletting* (Cambridge: Cambridge University Press, 1986).
50. f.lv v.
51. *Principis Avic. Libri Canonis necnon de Medicinis Cordialibus et Cantica* (Venice: 1527) 3.
52. Zerbi (*Anathomie* 7v) discusses the *Periti Elleni,* as does Berengario, *Commentaria,* 49r.
53. It seems likely that the first edition of Benedetti's anatomy was that

of Venice, 1502. Lind (1975) discusses the problem of identifying supposed ealier editions.

54. Clementius Clementinus, *Lucubrationes* (Basel: H. Petrus, 1535). All of these remarks on ethics are contained in Clementini's preface (unpaginated). Much of the text is concerned with the logical processes related to the gaining of medical knowledge. It may be part of a discussion involving scholars like Leoniceno on the opening words of Galen's *Tegni.*

4

Medical Ethics in Early Modern England

Andrew Wear

Early modern England had no codified medical ethics, there was no *Handbook of Medical Ethics* of the type that the British Medical Association publishes nowadays. Instead, there was available a body of Hippocratic writings, for instance the *Oath, Decorum,* the *Law,* which described how a doctor should behave both with the patient and with other doctors (the two bases of much of modern medical ethics) and which was often cited in the early modern period. Other more general ethical value systems also influenced medicine.

Christianity was a major influence, as was Aristotelian ethics which formed a general context for the Hippocratic texts familiar to early modern physicians. In a sense, what we have here is ethics in medicine, whilst medical ethics can be found in the Hippocratic and Galenic texts which refer to specific norms of conduct as they relate to the details of medical practice. The distinction is, however, one that would not have been recognized in the sixteenth or seventeenth centuries.

Ethics were used in early modern medicine by competing groups of practitioners to argue for the rightness of their practice and the wrongness of that of their opponents. Ethics formed part of the epistemological, economic, political and legal weapons that were employed by the competing factions in English medicine at this time. The context for medical ethics was, therefore, assertive rather than deliberative. The polemical writings of the learned, university-educated physicians and those of their competitors indicate how ethics were put to work in the struggles of a medical market-place largely unregulated by law, and this is the focus of the chapter. However, the fact that ethics were put to such use should not lead to the inference that they were not strongly believed in. It is too often the case that historians diminish the force of people's beliefs whilst placing such beliefs into larger economic and social frameworks, and I do not wish to do so. The two opposing sets of ethics, one based on the classical tradition, the other on Christianity, which I will be discussing in this chapter represent two strands of thought and of belief which were central to the culture of the sixteenth and seventeenth centuries. It is difficult to overestimate their force and reality.

Tradition and the Good and Learned Physician

The learned physicians, who had invested time and money being taught the medicine of Hippocrates, Galen and other classical writers in Latin, if not in Greek, naturally based their medical ethics on classical sources. There were not many of them in sixteenth century England and they often give the impression in their writings of feeling beleaguered and surrounded by competitors. The founding of the College of Physicians of London in 1518 gave them an institutional home and also some authority, for the college regulated the practice of physic (internal medicine) in London and seven miles round it by issuing licenses to practise, by prosecuting unlicensed practitioners and by punishing instances of dangerous practice. The College could also supervise the activities of apothecaries and surgeons. At a formal level, therefore, the learned physicians were at the top of the medical ladder in status and authority. However, in practical terms all this was precarious. The College was limited geographically (it was founded on the model of the college of physicians in Italian cities), its powers of supervising and prosecuting irregular practice in London were never very effective and over time these became more and more diluted till by the beginning of the eighteenth century they had become practically non-existent.[1] In reality, the learned physician was faced with effective competition from a wide variety of sources. Illness was often treated by other members of the family: mothers and wives undertook to cure and care for the most serious of illnesses. Informal medical care was available from neighbours, clergymen and their wives and the charitable ladies who treated the sick poor. Wise men and women, empirics, uroscopists, astrologers, herbalists and others provided cheaper medical treatments than did the learned physicians.[2] In such a context of a largely unregulated medical market-place and with different views of what constitutes medical knowledge it is not surprising to find ethics being used to justify one group or another.

The learned physicians were mostly concentrated in London,

their clientele was relatively prosperous, yet they still felt threatened by competition. Their attacks on their competitors were fuelled by the knowledge that the rich (and even royalty), as well as the poor, patronized empirics. They were united by a shared medical education based on Hippocratic and Galenic writings which defined the good physician and in which, especially in the latter, there was a constant criticism of empirics and empirical medicine. Not surprisingly, therefore, the classical traditions, until at least the later seventeenth century, were used by the learned physicians to define the ethical behaviour of a physician at the bedside and to characterize the bad practitioner. John Securis' *A Detection and Querisome of the Daily Enormities and Abuses Committed in Physic* (1566) provides a typical example. A close examination of its contents illustrates how, in a very rennaissance manner, ancient opinions and injunctions were made relevant to contemporary concerns and provided an ethical value system.

Securis was an orthodox physician concerned with upholding the position of learned medicine. He practised in Salisbury and had been a pupil in Paris of Sylvius, the ultra-conservative physician and anatomist. Securis began his book by describing the good ethical, physician, he repeated the *Oath,* and enumerated the evils of unlearned medicine. His aim was a reformation of medicine, and he appealed in support of this to the Hippocratic principle of doing no harm to the sick and to the related one of achieving monopoly in the profession (i.e. only the doctors who do no harm should be allowed to practise). Securis asked:

> What doth it prevaile for us that be lerned to procede (as I saide) in any degree of maister, of bacheler, or doctor, and so to be allowed and have authoritie to use our science? When every man, woman, and chyld that lyst, may practice and use phisicke *(idque impune)* as well as we? And so, many tymes not only hinder and defraud us of our lawfull stipende and gaynes: but (which is worst of all and to much to be lamented) shall put many in hasarde of their lyfe, yea and it be the destruction of many. Is this tolerable? Will the magistrates alwayes wynke at this? Shall there never be no reformation for suche abuses? God of his great mercy graunt that ones they may be reformed. For if they be not, verily it wyll greately discourage men of learnying hereafter to apply them selves to the studye of Physyke, whereby the healpe, succour and safegard of many of sick man, woman, and chylde shall be hyndered and secluded....[3]

A way of highlighting abuses in medicine was to present as a contrast a composite picture of the good physician and his good practice. Securis wrote 'before I speake of ye abuses and enormities of phisike, I wil shew and declare first, what is the part office and condition of a good Phisition.'[4] Securis gave in Latin and English the central part of the *Oath* which directed and confined the actions of the physician to a virtuous path. He then went on to cite the *Law,* which, in a fashion to be echoed by Aristotle and Galen, had emphasized that a long period of study in medicine constituted an ethical requirement for the proper practice of medicine.

> Who soever saith, he wyl truly get him the knowledge of phisicke, he must satisfie his mynd, and as it were be accompanied with these guides, with nature, science, a place mete and convenient for study and learning, an institution from childhood, a labor and peinful diligence with a long time.[5]

A look at the beginning of the text of the *Law* shows why it was still relevant. Securis, who saw all around him empirics, mountebanks and quacks making money, and who deplored the government's weak and limited laws against them, must have identified with the situation described in the *Law:*

> Although the art of healing is the most noble of all the arts, because of the ignorance both of its professors and of their rash critics, it has at this time fallen into the least repute of them all. The chief cause of this seems to me to be that it is the only science of which states have laid down no penalties for malpractice. Ill repute is the only punishment and this does little harm to the quacks who are compounded of nothing else. For a man to be truly suited to the practice of medicine, he must be possessed of a natural disposition for it, the necessary instruction, favourable circumstances, education, industry and time. The first requisite is a natural disposition, for a reluctant student renders every effort in vain. But instruction in the science is easy when the student follows a natural bent, so long as care is taken from childhood to keep him in circumstances favourable to learning and his early education has been suitable. Prolonged industry on the part of the student is necessary ...[6]

Securis cited other Hippocratic works which defined the body and the character of the doctor, from *The Physician* he learned that 'the physician must be of a good coloure and comely countenance and of a good disposition of the body: he muste also be had in estimation among the common people, by commonly apparell and by swete savours [smells] (so that he be not suspected of to much excesse) for by suche meanes the pacientes are wont to be delited.'[7]

This was no antiquarian copying of ancient texts. The charter of Charles I to the Barber-Surgeons stated that 'no such apprentice [wanting to enter into apprenticeship] be decrepid, deformed' as well as 'or have any corrupt or pestilential disease.'[8] Many of the classical qualities required of the physician had force in Securis' time, and perhaps they still do.

What Securis did was to bring together into one place many different passages from Hippocrates and Galen which originally dealt with different aspects of medical ethics. As well as purity in mind and acts (the *Oath*), study and learning (the *Law*) Securis adds the character of a doctor. He must have 'a modest and sobre mynde', be not only modest in his talk 'but also in other things concerning his behaviour, he must be wel disposed: for there is nothyng that getteth a man better estimation and authoritie than to bee endued with an honest lyfe and good manners.' The need for reputation, *doxa*, for getting trade, in the end joined both physicians and empirics, and medical ethics could be useful in achieving it. Securis added that the physician's 'countenance must be lyke one that is given to studye and sadde'[9] (cf. the Act of 1522: 'That no person ... be suffered to exercise and practise physic, but only these persons that be profound, sad and discreet, groundedly learned and deeply studied in physic'[10] – note the coupling of moral character with deep knowledge, which had Platonic and Aristotelian origins, and served to place classical learning in the renaissance in an ethical framework.) But the physician should not over-do this, for he could 'be taken to be stubborn and scornful', yet he should not always be laughing for then he 'is taken for a lewde person'.[11] Reputation was all. Securis repeated the advice of *On Decorum* on how the doctor should be gentle and courteous, brightly consoling yet firm with the patient at the bedside,[12] (advice to be repeated by John Gregory two centuries later, and indicating not only a long-lasting and common appreciation of how a scholar and a gentleman should behave, but also that the conjunction of manners with medical ethics was not present in the eighteenth century alone).[13]

Ethical injunctions also helped to convey some of the tricks of the trade. The physician should not 'minishe his gravitie, for unlesse the paciente have in reverence and estimation his phisicion as a god, he shall never follow and obey his councell'.[14] The monopolistic aspirations of orthodox learned medicine were put at risk by internal competition and advertising, and Securis advised fellow physicians not to do down fellow physicians:

> They be so covetous that they would have all, and do al them selfe, and they, have envy many tymes at other honest men having cures, when they have none. Thys doinge verelye they bringe them selves

> in greate contempte, and dothe as it were abate and blemishe the honorable science of phisicke, which requireth rather to be sought, earnestly with great sute, with humilitie, reverence and prayinge, then to be offered, and as it were objected undiscretely to every man, and in every place, lyke a blinde harpers songe or a Pedlars packe. The common proverbe saith, that offered service stynketh.[15]

Securis easily mixed traditional medical ethics with contemporary concerns, the classical past was still relevant to the present. The Northampton physician John Cotta also believed this. A conservative Galenist physician, perhaps a Puritan, Cotta relied largely on learning and study in the universities, as Harold Cook has pointed out, to distinguish a physician from an empiric,[16] though when describing 'The True Artist' [the good physician] Cotta also stressed the need for the physician to gain experience and to know nature for 'Without the knowledge of nature our life is death, our sight blind, our light darknese, and all our waies uncertaine'.[17] In his *A Short Discoverie of the Unobserved Dangers of Severall Sorts of Ignorant and Unconsiderate Practisers of Physicke in England* (1612), Cotta stated that he would not describe 'vertue' as it was 'beside my promised performance'.[18] Rather, he stressed the need for learning, industry and past authority ('precept'),[19] and from Galen he took his model of the best physician, the man who was rational, who combined reason with experience over a long period of study. In this, Cotta, in effect, does come near to 'vertue' for, as Aristotle wrote at the beginning of the second book of the *Nicomachean Ethics*, virtue is acquired by habit over time by a process of learning and is not innate – at this most general level there is a shared process for becoming virtuous and for becoming a good doctor hence Galen's equation of the two.[20] For my purposes Cotta's book is significant not only for its reiteration of the traditional values that identified the learned physicians and the empiric with regard to medical knowledge, but for its stress on the dangers in medical practice. It is this thread that I want to follow, and I shall consider what kind of ethical issues relating to practice troubled medical writers. Tradition provided a framework with which to categorize empirics, and given Galen's analysis of the poverty of experience in medical practice, it supplied the dialectical ammunition with which to shoot them down. It also provided a picture of the ideal physician that was suited to the world of the virtuous, scholarly, middling and respectable physician. But there was more to medical ethics than a restoration of tradition.

Danger, Choosing a Doctor and Reputation

At the end of the seventeenth century a call for medical reform, that echoed some of the earlier sentiments of the learned physicians, came from Hugh Chamberlen, the royal accoucher, the empiric fined by the College of Physicians, the member of the family famous for its use of the forceps and the projector of such schemes as a land bank – a typical larger than life entrepreneur of the long eighteenth century. In his *A Few Queries Relating to the Practice of Physick* (1694) before setting out his scheme for a rate-supported medical service, he asked:

> Whether the Practice of Physick doth not very much want a just and due Regulation, and is not capable of great improvements for the benefit of Mankind? And whether it doth not well deserve such Reformation, since it concerns Life and Health, the dearest earthly injoyments?

More specifically Chamberlen asked:

> Whether there can be contrived (if the Government please) any just and proper Test or Standard whereby to try the several Abilities of Physicians much more truly and certainly than any we have at present?

He replied:

> This were at least to be wisht, if there were no hopes to reduce it to practice, for not to know how to distinguish the skilful Physicians from the ignorant is next to having none.[21]

Here is one of the main reasons why ethics became involved in the very definition of good medical practice and runs so strongly, though sometimes hidden away, in the writings of opposing medical practitioners. Without a system of medical licensing that applied to the whole country or which had general public support and recognition, the qualities that made a good physician became a matter for debate and analysis. The definition might for some groups include elements which today we can easily recognize as ethical such as the charitable physician which I discuss later.

Other aspects of what made a good doctor are less easily fitted into our ideas of what constitutes ethics in medicine or medical ethics. For instance, the actual procedures used by doctors could indicate if one was a good doctor who cured, or a bad one that harmed the patient. This mix of the moral and the technical, of character and skill, was characteristic in early modern medicine and is one that, except for extreme cases, we find difficult today to recognize as subject matter for medical ethics. Obviously total ignorance or gross negligence come within malpractice and modern medical ethics. But in early modern England normal medical practice (which today is a defence in English malpractice suits) could be labelled bad, dangerous and hence unethical. The good doctor, therefore, was defined by the type as well as the extent of his technical knowledge together with his moral behaviour, as indeed Galen had written centuries before. This occured in a context in which there was no general consensus amongst the different groups in the medical market-place on what was normal medical knowledge and practice. The imputation of danger and harm could be placed on any medical practice, so that potentially all medical actions might be problematical and fall within the ambit of medical ethics. The issue was how to defend one's own practice, how to convince patients that it was safe and how to prove that the practices of one's opponents were dangerous. Rhetoric, advertising, and denigration became mixed with medical ethics.

The learned physician advertised his superior skill by stressing the lengthy and individualized treatment (and preventive care by means of regimen) he offered: how he judged the individual's constitution, how he recognized the cause of the illness, how he achieved a fine fit between the patient, the disease and the remedies and how he took into account the day-to-day progress of the patient. Eleazar Dunk in 1606 wrote of this personalised treatment:

> First the learned Physician is to search out the proper signes of this disease, and by them to distinguish it from others that hath some affinity with it: then he looketh into the cause of it ... he examineth the naturall constitution of the patient, his present state of body, his former course of life, his age, his strength, the time of the disease, the season of the yeere etc he considereth the qualities and quantity of the humors; from whence the matter of the disease floweth ... by what passages it moveth, whether swiftly, or slowly ... Out of an advised consideration of all these, first a diet is to be appointed: this cannot be the same in every one that laboureth of this sicknesse, but it requireth great variety and alteration agreeable to the foresaid circumstances. Then followeth the consultation of the meanes of the cure: what kinde of evacuation is fittest, whether opening a veine ...

Without the method and the judgement of the physician danger lurked:

> In the great variety of these doubts, difficulties and distinctions

> there is a necessary use of sound judgement, confirmed by long study and profound knowledge both in philosophy and Physicke. It is therefore cleere that the practise of Empiriks, being destitute of these helps, must needs be unfit and full of perill.[22]

The practitioners of this type of medicine, men like John Cotta, James Hart, James Primrose,[23] considered it, like Galen before them, the best and safest type of medicine (hence ethically the best). Yet the population did not always agree. As I have argued elsewhere there was a great deal of similarity between learned physicians and empirics, for instance, both in the end gave medicines and applied procedures.[24] The learned physicians realized that some members of the public believed that the empirics were more successful. One might be sure of the virtue of one's own particular form of medical knowledge and practice, but was the outside world so convinced? Reputation was all. In their analysis of why the world was not always convinced, the learned physicians used ethical arguements to attack the behaviour of patients, and the way they were influenced by the people around the bedside.

Cotta deplored how people chose their doctors:

> It is strange to observe how few in these dayes know, and how none almost labour to know with election and according to reason, or reasonable likelihood, to bestow in cases of their lives the trust and care of their crazed healths, but for the most part wanting a right notice of a iudicious choice, take counsel of common report which is a common lier or of private commendations which are ever partiall. The unmindfulnesse hereof, and the more minde of mindlesse things, do steale from men the minds of men.[25]

The arrogant, yet whining, complaint that the patients did not automatically realize that rational, learned, medicine was best permeates the writings of the rational physicians. If medicine needed to be reformed of its unethical practitioners, the empirics, there was also a need to reform the patient (the two were frequently seen as conspiring together). The ethical righteousness of the physician can only be real in a practical sense if recognized to be so by the patient. Yet the moral and intellectual superiority assumed by the learned physicians made a denigrating attitude to the public almost inevitable. Richard Whitlock in his *Zootomia. Or Observations on the Present Manners of the English* (1654) took the part of the learned physicians and wrote 'the people love to be cheated'. He listed their sins: being influenced by the novelties and boasts of their practitioners, trusting the judgement of incompetents when choosing a practitioner, being impressed by a pseudo-skill in diagnosis, not realizing that the accidental success of an empiric is no guarantee that it will happen again – it is 'no more a rule for curing the same againe ... then one Swallow bringeth a Summer', and the physician 'is the last or late sent for' and unjustly gets blamed for failure. Whitlock also blamed patients for refusing to take the physician's treatment and substituting their own, or that of their neighbours' 'kitchen Physick'[26]. Without the patient's obedience the physician's honourable success could not come about:

> Sicknesse posteth to us, but crawleth from us: happy it were for Patients, honourable for physitians successe of their labours, if men would but truly deserve the name of Patients, when sicknesse is on them, if they would take counsell timely, and obey it patiently.[27]

If patients did not choose rightly, if they did not obey, then much of the failure of learned medical practice was explained: 'To conclude, through the default of Physitians, the Theory of Physick is for the most part Conjecture, or Controversie, through the default of Patients, the practise is but Lottery.'[28]

The bedside was a place which could make or break a physician's reputation. Here women were especially blamed, for as well as having no authority to practise medicine themselves, they also threw doubt on the physician's practice. Cotta wrote:

> Here therefore are men warned of advising with women counsellors. We cannot but acknowledge and with honor mention the graces of womanhood, wherein by their destined property, they are right and true soveraignes of affection; but yet, seeing their authority in learned knowledge cannot be authenticall, neither hath God and nature made them commissioners in the sessions of learned reason and understanding (without which in cases of life and death, there ought to be no daring or attempt at all).... We may justly here taxe their dangerous whisperings about the sicke, wherein their prevalence oft being too great, they abuse the weake sense of the diseased, while they are not themselves; and make just and wise proceedings suspected, and with danger suspended. For it is not sufficient for the Physition to do his office, except both the sicke himselfe, and also all that are about him be prudently and advisedly carefull unto good reason: without which love it selfe may be dangerously officious, the error of friendship a deed unto death....[29]

Both patients and onlookers in early modern England acted at times as practitioners and were, in a sense, like the empirics, rivals of learned practitioners and could be accused like them, of doing harm. There is clearly an ethical dimension in Cotta's diatribe against women. He details acts made morally suspect: 'they abuse the weake sense of the diseased', the contrast with 'just and wise proceedings' and the result of 'danger', and 'death' (though the honour of the physician and of his office lies just below the surface in all this). The breaking of moral and technical norms leading to harm to the patient epitomizes medical ethics. Moreover, the sense of this being medical ethics is reinforced when we remember that what is going on here is an attempt at exclusivity in medical practice.

In defence of a doctor's reputation very general ethical norms or prejudices were also brought into play. The assumed superiority of men over women in matters of medicine was supplemented by references to the bad practices of the common people. Cotta warned in a tone reminiscent of that to be found in Elizabethan and Jacobean government references to the dangerous mass of the poor:

> Oft and much babbling inculcation in the weake braines of the sicke may easily prevaile with them, to forget both that which their owne good hath taught them, and also by a borrowed opinion from others indiscrete words, to corrupt their owne sense. It is the common custome of most common people thus ordinarily to molest and trouble the sicke. Their presense therefore is dangerous and carefully to be either prohibited or better governed. Common and vulgar mouthes easily incline scandalously to prejudice the things they know not.[30]

The mixture of superiority and underlying defensiveness lay at the heart of the defence of learned medicine. The art was not to be blamed, others were:

> Hence it is in thes daies a customary worke to disswade physicke, while men not making right choice of their Physition, or perverting good counsell by their owne peevish frowardnes, and thereby multiplying unto themselves continuall occasion of complaint, unjustly therefore accuse art, which they never duly sought, nor found, nor used, and therefore never know. The offences that men justly take, are the faults, the blots, the staines of unperfect workemen, not of art; whereof art is as guiltlesse as they are void of art.[31]

Wrong judgement, lack of reason and restraint, imperfect knowledge, all these accusations expressed in the emotive terms of social superiority of the early seventeenth century, bear some analogy with classical Aristotelian ethics that was part of the university education shared by the physicians. The choice of actions define the just man, so also in the case of medicine. The emphasis is on the individual rather than on the out-reaching relationship of the individual to society as in Christianity or on the parts of society as in utilitarianism. As Aristotle wrote in Book five of the *Nicomachean Ethics:* 'but how actions must be done and distributions effected in order to be just, to know this is a greater achievement than knowing what is good for the health; though even there, while it is easy to know that honey, wine, hellebore, cautery and the use of the knife are so, to know how, to whom, is no less an achievement than that of being a physician.'[32] In constrast to the more social values of Christianity as applied to medicine (discussed below), the learned physicians were, I feel, most at home with the Aristotelian ethical position that focused on the right actions of the individual qua individual as judged against 'justice' or in the case of the learned physicians 'the art'.

At a time when patients could easily dismiss their physicians, and when they had a wide choice of different types of practioner, the learned physicians were not in a position to persuade patients to accept painful or uncomfortable treatments through the authority conferred by a monopoly or quasi monopoly of practice, backed up by legislation. The patient's personal preferences and dislike of unpleasant procedures could be translated into dismissal of the learned physicians. The right actions in relation to the art might be subverted by the promise of more pleasant treatments than those offered by the physicians. Cotta wrote of how 'many ignorants may speake faire and pleasing and commend things that look smooth and smiling upon the liking of the sicke' and how it is usual for 'many unskilfull busie-bodies under colour and pretext of gentle and safe dealing, to make familiar and ordinary the use of perileous medicines.'[33] Clearly medicine could appear harmful and painful, and this view was held throughout the seventeenth century. Chamberlen referred to it when he asked whether "tis better for a Physician to be a knave and increase his Practice by humouring the Fools and letting them die their own way; or to be honest and lessen his practice in saving them with methods displeasing, because really there are no other can help them.'[34]

Again he asked:

> Whether 'tis not safer for a Doctor to let his Patients die their own way with a gentle wrong Method, than to endeavour to help them with a rough right one, and to miss?

He replied:

> 'tis very probable it is, for the gentle method displeaseth none, and

> the Doctor, though he never endeavoured to save the Patient, still continues his Interest and Credit in the Family, because the Patient and Friends believe he did, not being able to judge; but on the other hand the Doctor, that endeavours to save, and misses, shall be esteemed a murtherer, because of the seeming violent medicines used and be discarded and hated, though he used the best skill then known to save the Patient.[35]

Normal clinical practice today is largely out of the net of medical ethics. One reason is that clinical trials and statistical analysis decide in the end on whether and to what extent a remedy or technique is safe or effective (though there may be a wider ethical dimension, for instance, in the case of embryo implantation, or in the allocation of resources that goes beyond the mere question of safety). Moreover, there are legal procedures such as inquests or civil cases for malpractice which can decide how far a medical practitioner has gone beyond the normal and the accepted. In the early modern period such legal methods of discovery were largely ineffective or not used.[36] In his time as Cotta put it, the medical errors of the ignorant (and, one could add, of the learned) were 'for want of knowledge unespied, or by the privacy smothered. For if they kill, a dead man telleth no tales: or if by chance they save one life, that shall be a perpetuall flag to call more fooles to the same adventure.' Instead of being able to use the modern advertising power of science other means such as word of mouth recommendation had to be employed for gaining credit in one's practice. Living almost a century later Chamberlen was able to look forward in a Baconian fashion to 'a true History of Cures' which would register the outcome of cures.[37] Failing such a method (and even that is neither 'objective' *per se,* nor avoids all debate), a practitioner's reputation was at the mercy of the public, and ethical values were employed in attacking or defending it.

Christian Charity and Dangerous Remedies

Christianity provided medicine with a different set of ethical values. The ethics of the classical world had largely been individualistic rather than social and were often devoid of charity and of altruism in relation to the care of the sick (though as Vivian Nutton points out in this volume Galen did encourage the physician to be philanthropic). However, the care of the sick was one of the six works of charity of the early Church, and Christianity, which had ever before it the example of Christ healing the sick, the lame and the blind, emphasized the value of giving care both at an institutional level (in monasteries, and then in church-run hospitals) and at the personal level of providing for the poor and needy sick. Although the Protestant Reformation cast doubt on the efficacy of good works for getting to Heaven, charity and the duty of neighbours to look after each other was still emphasized by radical Protestants. The opponents of the learned physicians used such Christian values to attack the ethical basis of their practice.

Their attacks had added point, because Christian ethics were largely absent from the writings of the learned physicians and, at least until 1660, this was a time when Christian belief was extremely important for society at large. The sources for the ethics of the learned physicians were largely classical and founded on the need for both learning and exclusive practice and on the rectitude of a person's actions in relation to the art. If God was mentioned it was often in terms of natural theology and the study of God's workmanship rather than the social ethic of charity.[38]

Christian ethics were also used to support new medical doctrines and practices, and to attack those of the learned physicians. In 1585 Richard Bostocke published one of the earliest English Paracelsian works. In the title of his book he emphasized the heathen and unchristian origins of classical learned medicine: *The Difference Between the Auncient Phisicke, First Taught by the Godly Forefathers, Consisting in Unitie, Peace and Concord; and the Latter Phisicke Proceeding from Idolaters, Ethnickes and Heathens; As Galen, and Such Other Consisting in Dualitie, Discorde and Contrarite. And Wherein the Naturall Philosophie of Aristotle Doth Differ from the Trueth of Gods Worde, and is Iniurious to Christianitie and Sound Doctrine.* Bostocke pointed out that not only was Greek medicine and philosophy unchristian in doctrine, it was also unchristian ethically in that it lacked charity. He wrote that if the Galenists would no longer be under the 'Wings and protection of Princes, Privilidges and Charters', then 'the Chymicall doctrine agreeing with Gods worde, experience, and nature may come into the Scholes and Cities in stede of Aristotle, Gallen, and other heathen' and people could decide if 'Galen and other heathen or the Chimests were most to be followed and allowed. And whose writings and travailes were more available for mans health, either conserving or restoring, and who seeketh more paynefully, faythfully, sincerely, charitably and Christianlike for the certein helpe of his neighbour, and not for lucre or veine glory and pompe, the auncient Chemical Phisition or Gallen and his followers.'[39]

The Christian ethical values of helping one's neighbour and

giving charitable care were powerful. Despite the Reformation and the consequent breakdown in England of church-organized charitable care for the poor and sick poor, the feeling that one ought to help one's neighbour in adversity remained. Alan Macfarlane has shown that many witchcraft accusations were made because the accused felt guilty that he or she had not provided charitable help to the person subsequently accused of witchcraft (their reasoning was that the person who had asked for charity then bewitched them out of a sense of revenge or spite). Bequests to the poor, and donations to the parish poor box continued despite the creation of the secular poor law system based on the parish rates.[40] At the time of the Civil War, the importance of Christian charity as a major social value was emphasized even more. As Charles Webster has pointed out, various reformers of medicine of the 1640s and 1650s wished to have a medical care service that would encompass all the country or at least would provide medical treatment for the poor[41] (though parishes were already paying for the medical treatment of the sick poor).[42] A sense of charity underlay such proposals and this is reflected in the choice by Gabriel Plattes, in his utopian *Macaria* (1641), of ministers as providers of such care – for they would be embued with charity rather than profit.

At various levels, then, Christianity, the most potent belief system of the early modern period, whose influence extended from politics down to the details of the household economy, was used to attack orthodox medicine for being based on pagan learning and values (though, of course, for many Christians the medieval assimilation of classical knowledge into Christianity had got rid of the contradictions that were being pointed out). Greed was seen as especially unchristian and, as Luis García-Ballester has shown in an earlier chapter, it was a quality associated from the Middle Ages with the learned physician. The learned surgeon, William Clowes, advised in 1579 the young surgeon not to be greedy: 'not too covetous for mony, but a reasonable demaunder/Being good unto the poore, let the rich pay therefore.'

Nicholas Culpeper, in the mid-seventeenth century complained that physicians would not come 'to a poor mans house who is not able to give them their fee ... and the poor Creature for whom Christ died must forfeit his life for want of money'.[43] Culpeper, who was one of the most prolific writers of popular medical books, had fought on Parliament's side in the Civil War and he integrated his religion into his medicine. It supplied the ethics for his medicine. Culpeper also contrasted the cheapness of his native God-given remedies, appropriate to the means of the poor, with the expensive and often exotic remedies of the Galenic physicians.[44] Charity, alternative medicines and care for the poor were opposed to expensive, fleecing, physicians. Securis had revealingly quoted the saying 'that phisicke unles it be earnestly sought and well payde for, it will never prosper nor worke well with the pacientes.' He quickly added that he did not mean that physicians should not 'be alwayes liberall and mercifull to the poore, on whom his living dependeth not but on the rich'.[45] The many books on remedies for the poor, with their references to charitable physicians and their self-help approach carried the implied accusation against orthodox physicians of avarice and of a lack of charity. 'J.E.' wrote in support of Robert Pemel's ΠΤΩΧΟΦΑΡΜΑΚΟΝ or *Help for the Poor* (1653):

> What Herbs, Flowers, Min'rals,
> Trees the earth doth bear
> For men his use and help, prepared are:
> Intended them unto poor peoples good;
> As well as of rich Lords, and Ladies, Gent.
> Poor people in pain meet help and ease do want;
> But oh the love of gold and sordid gain,
> That doth the Lords rich bounty much restrain!
> Let a rich man lie sick, or pained be,
> Upon his least request, to him doth flee
> The Physick Doctor, or the Surgeon
> Their Soveraigne Medicines them to try upon;
> And him to cure, the love of rich reward,
> Which there he hopes, makes him the rich regard:
> But let the poor, sick or diseased lie,
> Let him send for them, let him call and cry,
> They are as deaf as Baal to his Priests;
> He hath no gold to grease them in their fists
> Loe here a pitiful Samaritan,
> That taking care for the poor needy man,
> Doth him provide of easie medicines
> Which nor are costly, nor are hard to finde;
> So his own Doctor in need he may be,
> Without the care of any Doctors fee....[46]

The learned physicians did not directly reply to the age-old accusation of greed and of a lack of charity but Cotta and others like him did realize that religion threatened their attempts at monopoly: God had given the gift of healing to the apostles, and this posed the possibility that it could be acquired without learning and application, especially by clergymen (as descendents of the apostles) or by wise-women and others as a 'natural' talent (on the latter see below). The learned physicians reiterated Calvin's claim that the age of miracles was past and that God's ministers could not heal miraculously any more. Cotta also cited Calvin's doctrine on keeping to one's calling as forbidding 'pastor physicians' and he pointed to the dangers to patients of ministers being called away from caring for them by the duties of their other calling.[47] The Calvinist concern with public order was congenial to the physicians. Cotta opposed charity with the imperative of one's calling, and contrasted private acts of charity with the public policy of the commonwealth (a very conservative and typically Calvinist position).

> It is indeed a deed of mercie to save and helpe the sicke, and a worke of charitie to advise them for their health and ease: but the common good and public weale and the law for both inhibit the doing of every good by every man, and both doth limit and refraine it unto some speciall and select sort of men, for necessary causes, and respects unto good government and policie, and for avoiding confusion which is the ruine of publicke weales. Shal then Divinitie teach and allow for private deeds, ends and respects of charitie and mercie, to break publicke edicts, to trangress lawes, to condemme magistracie, to confound and disturbe good order?[48]

Richard Whitlock also wrote in support of learned medicine and opposed the Christian ideal of charity and of helping the poor that motivated 'Shee-Doctors' with the effectiveness of orthodox medicine:

> The Physick of Almes I allow them, but am out of charity with their Almes of Physick (by their owne hands:) with the former they may feed Christians, but with the latter they too often with Christians feed the Wormes; Or if they would be charitable in this way, let them pay for the Physick of the poor, the noblest way of giving Physick, and will have its Fee from Heaven.[49]

However, in the later seventeenth century the feeling that the regular physicians lacked Christian charity did touch a nerve and the College of Physicians set up charitable dispensaries. When the apothecaries in the Rose case (1704) accused the physicians of wanting to create a monopoly so that poor people who could not afford a physician's fees would be unable to go to the cheaper apothecary, the physicians replied by pointing to their dispensaries for the poor.

The Christian picture of the 'compassionate physition' not only included charity but also humane, kind medical practice that did not involve dangerous, cruel and painful treatments The radical Noah Biggs asked Parliament to reform medicine and wrote in his *Mataeotechnia Medicinae Praxeus. The Vanity of the Craft of Physick* (1651):

> ... till the body of Physick [i.e. orthodox Galenic medicine] be changed and reformed there's little hopes that a better sanation of Diseases or a Melioration of the languid condition of men and women will follow then what has been hitherto, and what that has been let the clamours of the Sick, and standers by, the cries of Widows and Orphans and the ocular unsuccessfulness of Physicians in their own practice, decide whether the things that I now move for ... do not groan for a Reformation.[50]

Perhaps the 'unsuccessfulness of Physicians' does not fall within medical ethics, after all we all die. Yet as one reads Biggs' convoluted work it is clear that he was condemning orthodox medicine for malpractice. The nature of medicine, its theories, beliefs and remedies produced illness, diseases could be iatrogenic.

> Oftentimes a man is chain'd to his bed by small disease ... and [the Galenists] only make them rage more by their remedies, when they undertake to expell them.[51]

As well as being disease-making, medicine created death, it experimented recklessly and was tainted with cruelty:

> Speculation, the alone Patron of idleness, and lazinesse, which weakly understood, and violently put in practise, hath made a shambles, rather than a Sanctuary, to butcher men violently and devoure and destroy them insensibly, then give ease or succour. For there is nothing more hard, more inhumane and full of Cruelty, among all humane Arts, through so many ages undertaken and usurp'd, then that art, which by a concentrick subscription doth make new experiments by the deaths of men, where the Earth covers the vices, the errors and fraud of its professors.[52]

Biggs used religion as part of his condemnation of the cruelty of learned medicine. He stressed that the erroneous opinions were those of 'Pagans and Infidels' and wrote of the 'ruines, the dangers and dreadful effects, the ignorence, errors, abueses, impieties and cruelties of Physitians.'[53]

The ethical rhetoric of dangerous and tormenting remedies was common currency in the medical market-place and amongst learned physicians. Cotta had also written of:

> Quacsalvers, banckrupt-apothecaries, and fugitive Surgeons every where over-travelling the face of this kingdome ... do sell ... these

> generose and noble secrets carrying on the outside the titles of famous medicines, and being within infamous poysons. And by this means quicke and desperate experiments, with such as thus like to gaine them grow vulgar medicaments.[54]

Cotta also mentioned how medicines in the wrong hands could cause disease. Yet the force of the argument was not equal. Unorthodox practitioners, often using Christian values, developed further the view that their remedies were milder and less dangerous than those of the faculty. William Walwyn, the Leveller, advertised in his *Physick for Families* (1669) his medicines and their cures. He presented them as 'Kindly and Powerful' rather than being 'hazardous, painful and dangerous'[55] (he went into detail to show the danger and pain involved in Galenic practice).[56] Significantly, he justified his whole enterprise by the Biblical injunction 'to love our Neighbour as ourselves'[57] and more specifically he argued:

> The Scripture saith, a merry heart doth good like a medicine: And if so, in true consequence, ought not the Operations and Effects of kindly and real Medicines to resemble those of a merry heart; certainly it can be no absurdity to expect it.[58]

Walwyn also stressed that Christianity was above philosophy, it provided both a moral pattern for the physican and knowledge hidden from philosophy.

> So I conceive my charitable intentions, sufficiently justified by the Text: The truly Christian Vertu of Compassion, being as essentially needful in a physitian, as in the most tender hearted Samaritan....
>
> Nor did I decline the common Road of Physick, for any other cause Imaginable, but for its manifest uncertainty in Principles, Roughness, Harshness, and Cruelty in Methods, Impropriety, Impotency, and danger in Medicines. Nor found out any way to relieve my understanding, when at first at so great a loss, but by withdrawing my thoughts from out the wilderness of all the uncertain Notions and Guesses of Philosophy and giving them free liberty in the walks of Scripture; where the true Original of men the sole subject of Physick (hid from Phylosophy) being apparent....[59]

Christianity was a way for the unorthodox to reject philosophy, the classical tradition, and it could supply not only the ethical values of compassion and neighbourliness but also give insight into medicine. Morality and knowledge were very close together, something which is also clearly apparent in classical medical ethics. Christianity, moreover, provided the characteristics for the 'Conscionable

Compassionate Physitians'[60] who Walwyn had in mind as the model of what was best in medicine, and Christianity was used to make orthodox medicine appear unfeeling, that is cruel and barbarous in its remedies, avaricious and uncharitable in its human relations.

Thomas O'Dowde, one of the instigators of a society of chemical physicians which it was hoped would be set up in opposition to the College of Physicians, though in politics O'Dowde was not a political radical having followed the royalist cause, presented himself as a charitable physician in his *The Poor Man's Physitian or the True Art of Medicine* (1665). He used the Christian model of the good physician: '... and rather than not do good for Gods sake, I will traverse all the Streets, Lanes and Alleys of this great and glorious city, to find out the Poor and Necessitious, wanting help and Medicine; and leave the Rich to them'[61] [the Galenists]. The title of his book shows, again, how morality, 'poor man's physician', was related to a particular position on medical knowledge: in this case 'the true art of medicine' lay in O'Dowde's belief in chemical remedies. The morality helps to give credence to the knowledge, in turn the knowledge has ethical value (is not dangerous etc.). It is worth taking a closer look at O'Dowde's work for it exemplifies the way in which morality and medical knowledge and skill came within an ethical framework, though some might feel that his use of Christian ethics arose more from motives of gain than from conviction, and that he used them in order to attract patients.

The title page of his book cited the passage from Mark 5:26 which criticizes medicine for its pain, rapacity and lack of success, rather than the more usual one from Ecclesiasticus 38:1, 'Honour a physician with the honour due unto him, ... for the Lord hath created him'. The passage from Mark reads: 'And had suffered many things of many Physicians, and had spent all that she had, and was nothing bettered, but rather grew worse.'

The Biblical context, the assertion that physicians could make the patient worse, plus the allusion to their rapacity encapsulates the ethical framework that O'Dowde used to justify his own practice. The same combination had occurred when the law at one time opened the door for empirics. The statute of 1542/3, which allowed unlearned practitioners to practise in a limited way, has not been seen as containing ethical statements, but it did:

> the company and fellowship of surgeons of London, minding only their lucres, and nothing the profit or ease of the diseased patient, have sued, troubled, and vexed divers honest persons, well men as women, whom God hath embued with the knowledge of the

> nature, kind and operation of certain herbs, roots and waters, and the using and ministering of them to such as been pained with customable disease ... the said persons have not taken anything for their pains or cunning [skill] but have ministered the same to poor people only for neighbourhood and God's sake, and of pity and charity. For although the most part of the persons of the said craft of surgeons have small cunning, yet they will take great sums of money, and do little therefore, and by reason thereof they do oftentimes impair and hurt their patients, rather than do them good; in consideration whereof, and for the ease, comfort, succour, help, relief, and health of the king's poor subjects inhabitants of this realm, now pained or diseased, or that hereafter shall be pained or diseased.
>
> Be it ordained....[62]

From the statute (often dismissed as the 'Quack's Charter') a picture was drawn of the ethical, good practitioner practising charitably with God's means and more effectively than the unethical, bad, money-grubbing, monopolistic and harmful surgeons who would not cure someone unless they were sure to get more than the cure was worth and 'many rot and perish to death for lack of help of surgery.'[63] By being labelled harmful the practice of the surgeons was put into the sphere of ethics, and this was made doubly so by its association with greed and lack of charity.

To return briefly to O'Dowde. What characterizes the description of his cases is that they are, like the language of the statute, assertions of fact and opinion. There is no argument for or against a position; we are dealing, as in the prescriptions of the *Oath* (and in advertisements), with absolute values and judgements, often expressed in graphic and violent language. The context was not appropriate for the deliberative debating of issues of a Warnock Report. The cases did not give rise to ethical problems but to ethical condemnations.

O'Dowde, like Biggs, referred to the cruelty and barbarism of the physicians, their experimenting with people's lives and leaving them for dead when they could be cured. Here are some examples:

> Mr Savage, at the Queens Head ... afflicted with violent Convulsive Fits, and extraordinary Dropsie and Scurvy and past all hopes of either life or recover, was perfectly cured by me in four days of Medicine, to his great admiration, after being long the Experiment of the Galenick Artists.
>
> Mr Garret ... under so prodigious a Dropsie and Scurvy, as after the Experiment of some able Artists, left as a dying man, not able to

> eat, drink, sleep, walk, lie, sit or stand; and thus weary of life and the most dejected of all men, was perfectly cured by me in four days of Medicine, when before assigned a peremptory day to dye in.[64]
>
> Mr Rowley, a Baker ... under a five years Dropsie Lask and Bloody Flux, a Patient, whose story is so remarkable, as to call Angels and men to witness against the barbarous inhumanity of those persons that stile themselves Doctors.

There follows the gruesome story of twin incisions into the scrotum and the division of the foreskin 'to the end', but though left in agony O'Dowde cured him.[65]

O'Dowde continued:

> A merchant of good account, (this last Patients Neighbour) and under the like Distemper, method and Doctor, was cured by being sent to his Grave, according to Art and Method [keywords identifying an orthodox Galenist], Cum Privilegis, good Mr Doctor.
>
> In all this, I appeal to all the fair Ladies and good Wives of this Nation, whether the Galenist or the Chymist, is the true Artist and Friend to Nature and Health, that thus restores languishing Nature, and makes it erect, and servicable as ever, or those than thus inhumanely butcher a principal part.[66]

It is not enough to refer only to Christian values of charity (the language of the last quotation is perhaps nearer to advertising than to Christianity) to explain what lies behind these cases. O'Dowde was saying 'my treatments are better, safer, more efficacious than the treatments of my opponents which are deadly, cruel and unsuccessful.' The actual treatment used became an ethical issue. Both the Christian and the Hippocratic doctor agreed that the patient should not be harmed, the disagreement, however, lay in what was good for the patient, and what constituted harm. This was expressed through a mixture of technical medical language and ethical values, the boundaries between the two being, because of the nature of the disagreements, imprecise.

The Law

The involvement of the law in medicine often puts ethical norms onto a formal footing and signifies the presence of the State. Discussion of this and of the law in general provides a further context that helps us to understand the state of play in the relationship between ethics and medicine in early modern Europe.

In post-Reformation England outside legal authority or agencies did not exist that would decide whether one type of medical practice was ethical or not (they hardly exist today). In a society where the study of canon law had been abolished by Henry VIII, where explicit statute law covered few civil or criminal contingencies, and where the apprehension of criminals was left to the victims of the crime and to lay officials such as the amateur constables and justices of the peace,[67] it was not likely that the law would be involved in any major way with the enforcement of ethical medical practice.

Medical ethics were not codified in law, and the development of English law in the early modern period goes against such a development. Common law, with its piecemeal, precedent approach and its hostility to the codifying tendencies of the continental Roman law tradition, was not the instrument with which to forge a legal-ethical framework for medicine. The ways in which trials were conducted also argued against the creation of such a framework. There was a general lack of expert evidence, (and when it was presented it was not given special status), the jury was still 'of the country' with special knowledge of the local situation, if it was no longer, as in the Middle Ages, composed of neighbours who acted as evidential testators as to the accused, still it had not yet been transformed into the nineteenth-century jury having no prior knowledge of the victim and of the accused and concerned with assessing the objective truth of the evidence.[68] English law at this time was on the whole neither investigative, nor inquisitorial, nor concerned with a scientific approach where juries put aside local knowledge and decided solely in terms of the court room evidence, nor did the law attempt to set down in writing every possible contingency (the latter is still not yet with us in England, but no doubt the influence of European legal-systems as expressed through the Common Market will achieve this). Another way of putting the same point is that it was only in the nineteenth century that the State began to legislate in detail on the activities of its citizens. In the early modern period the English State kept to a hands off policy except on particular areas where its interests were involved as in religion, or where devastating crises such as plague or famine occurred or where it perceived danger to itself as with vagrancy and the poor. The implementation of the law was left to local lay officials or to assize judges travelling on the different circuits around the country. The legal system was simple and largely amateur, and it was usually the judges rather than Parliament who decided how the law was to be developed. It is only in the nineteenth century with, for example, the influence of utilitarianism in penal and welfare matters, that the role of the Parliamentary legislator becomes dominant. It is, of course, no accident that it was around this time that codified medical ethics were developed, though in England the *laissez-faire* approach was strong enough to keep such ethics on a voluntary basis.

Given this context it is not surprising that we do not find codified medical ethics let alone a code with legal force. What we do have are statutes, sometimes contradictory, which were limited to a local area, London, which gave power of enforcement and of judgement, not to judges and juries at large, but to corporations. Where the common law was involved its tendency was to limit the power of the corporations and also to leave the law on malpractice undeveloped.

In the statutes and charters setting up the College of Physicians, Company of Barber-Surgeons and Society of Apothecaries there was an acceptance of the superiority of the learned physician, a recognition of grades amongst medical practitioners, with the physicians having a supervisory role over the apothecaries, and being able to do surgery. Safeguarding the public was a constant theme. Guarding people from being deceived by empirics and from the dangers of their unskilful practices was often the expressed purpose of the law-makers. The language could have come straight from Securis and Cotta. Nevertheless, as we have seen there was an alternative in law. The Act of 1542/3 expressed a different set of values, emphasizing charity and alternative, non-elite knowledge. That such a body of ethics in medicine, separate from the official, College classical tradition, was recognized by sections of government is confirmed when one looks at the way patrons of empirics sought to prevent the College taking action against them. In 1581 Sir Francis Walsingham, Secretary of State to Elizabeth, interceded 'in favour of one Margaret Kennix an outlandish, ignorant, sorry woman', as Charles Goodall apologist for the College put it. Walsingham wrote:

> Whereas heretofore by her Majesties commandment upon the pityfull complaint of Margaret Kennix I wrote unto Dr Symmondes [the former President of the College] ... signifying how that it was her Highness pleasure that the poore wooman shoold be permitted by you quietly to practise and mynister to the curing of diseases and woundes, by the meanes of certain Simples, in the applieing whereof it seemeth God hath given her an especiall knowledge, to the benefit of the poorer sort, and cheefly for the better maintenance of her impotent husband, and charge of Family, who wholy depend of the exercise of her skill; forasmuch as now I am enformed, she is restrained either by you, or some other of your

> College, contrary to her Majesties pleasure, to practise any longer her said manner of ministring of Simples, as she hath done, wherby her undoing is like to ensue, unles she maie be permitted to continue the use of her knowlege in that behalfe. I shall therefore desire you forthwith to take order amongst your selves for the readmitting of her into the quiet exercise of her small Talent, least by the renewing of her complaint to her Majesty thorough your hard dealing towards her, you procure further inconvenience thereby to your selfe.[69]

Given such *ad hoc* pleading, it is clear that this was not a time for a legal framework of medical ethics. What we have here are two sets of ideals being used by two different centres of power. The ethical values used by Walsingham implicitly opposed those of the College, and appealed to God, to helping the poor and to natural knowledge or talent (royalty and its courts, despite Bostocke's comment above, often favoured empirics). The College in its reply referred to the danger to her Majesty's subjects, the weakness and insufficiency of Kennix, and it tried to incorporate Walsingham to its ranks and to its point of view 'most humbly beseeching your Honor, that as most excellent Virtues and Learning hath made you famous to the World and posterity, so it might please you to be a favourable patron to such as have been trained and brought up therein.'[70]

It is a trite but often true point that the law reflects the views of the public, and mostly of those in power. The College found opposition to its policing of medicine from powerful figures – the Queen on various occasions, Walsingham, Howard, Essex and others. The monopolistic values of the College were not held by everyone in power. The judgement of Coke in Bonham's case (1608/9) is indicative of this as, crucially for medical ethics, Coke broke the link between licensing and skill: 'but he who practises physic in London, in a good manner, although he doth it without a licence, yet it is not any prejudice to the body of man'.[71] The College could not, according to Coke, convict someone of malpractice merely because they were not licensed. (Coke felt that the learning of a university graduate was sufficient – so his ideal was still that of learning). The effect of the judgement was not long-lived,[72] what is significant about it is that it was one of the few cases in which the courts became involved in the area of medical ethics.

The law on malpractice was largely underdeveloped. The specific offence of malpractice was recognized by the public courts (the College believed its right to convict for malpractice was a private one). In Groenvelt's case (1697) the Court of King's Bench decided that:

> *mala praxis* is a great misdemeanor and offence at common law, whether it be for curiosity or experiment, or by neglect, because it breaks the trust which the party has placed in the physician, tending directly to his destruction.[73]

However, the criminal courts do not seem to have elaborated further on this. The detailed judgement of whether malpractice had occurred was left in the sixteenth and seventeenth centuries for the physicians to decide. As Chief Justice Holt held, in Groenvelt's action for false imprisonment against the College, there was no appeal from matters that fell to the College members to judge as experts:

> Though the pills and medicines were really 'salubres pillulae et bona medicamenta' no action lies against the censors, because it is a wrong judgement in a matter within the limits of their jurisdiction; and a judge is not answerable, either to the king or the party, for the mistakes or errors of his judgement in a matter of which he has jurisdiction.[74]

The College doctors did get some support from the law. And it is clear from the cases of malpractice tried by the College in the sixteenth and seventeenth centuries that its finding of malpractice depended on whether the practitioner had any education i.e. was he or she an outsider, whether wrong or poisonous sort of medicines had been used (in the sixteenth century these would often be chemical which Galenists opposed) and whether harm had occurred,[75] the threads of classical medical ethics came together when they were enforced by a body steeped in the classics.

The law on malpractice as developed by the common law was not all on the side of learned medicine. The balance of opinion by the beginning of the eighteenth century held that if a patient died and the practitioner was unlicensed this was not of itself sufficient to constitute a criminal offence. The supposed legal immunity of physicians could provoke bitterness. In Volpone there is:

> *MOSCA:* No, sir, nor [physician's] fees
> He cannot brook; he says they flay a man
> Before they kill him.
> *CORBACCIO:* Right, I do conceive you.
> *MOSCA:* And then, they do it by experiment,
> For which the law not only doth absolve 'em,
> But gives them great reward; and he is loath
> To hire his death so.
> *CORBACCIO:*It is true, they kill with as much licence
> as a judge.[76]

However, it is not enough to assess whether and how far the ethical standpoints of the College physicians were policed or received full support. What should be recognized as well is that although the law contributed little to ethics in medicine or in a more narrow sense to medical ethics, even here two ethical approaches can be discerned – that of learning and that of Christian charity. Allied to the latter, but not always, there was an anti-monopolistic sentiment (as seen in the Lords' judgement in the Rose case).[77]

Conclusion

Reference to continental Europe provides a confirmation and a contrast to England, and can serve as a conclusion. On the continent there were the same diatribes about the unethical nature of empirical practice, the same complaints about disobedient patients, about the undue influence of onlookers, and about the doctor being brought in too late to the harm of his reputation when the patient died. Laurent Joubert's *Erreurs Populaires au Fait de la Medecine* (1578) dealt with many of these issues in quite a systematic and focused fashion. As the previous chapter has shown, in Italy the same defences of learned medicine can be found, as indeed they can also in Germany, for instance, in the writings of Johannes Langius.

However, it often seems that more learning was employed than by English physicians, for instance, by writers such as Ioannes Siccus, *De Optimo Medico* (1551), Baptista Condrochius, *De Christiana, ac Tuta Medendi Ratione* (1591) and Rodericus a Castro, *Medicus Politicus* (1614). Perhaps the poverty of the classical tradition in medicine in England has something to do with the sense of a lack of developed argument. England, despite Linacre, Caius and Harvey was a relative backwater in terms of the European renaissance of classical medicine. The richness and elegance of Siccus' depiction of the best doctor contrasts with the crudity of Securis' paraphrases of classical texts, and Cotta's even balder use of the sources. Yet in terms of substance there was little difference between the Continental and English ethical defences of learned medicine. What was different was the Catholic and Canon Law context of much of the European writing. Paulus Zacchias, who was personal physician to Innocent X and Alexander VII and Protomedicus to the Papal State, in his *Quaestiones Medico-Legales* (1621–35) dealt with many issues that concerned Canon Law and lay on the border between medicine and Canon Law. Zacchias was concerned with topics such the viability of the foetus, the causes of foetal death, types of madness, poisoning, impotence, malingering, torture, witchcraft, miracles, virginity, types of wounds and so on. The medical-forensic nature of many of these subjects stemmed from the canon lawyers' need to produce answers to a wide variety of contingencies having both moral and physical components. This gave a sharper but also more dialectical character to Zacchias' work. He asked questions related to specific aspects of medical practice. For instance, could necessary and urgent amputation of limbs be carried out with a safe conscience when there was a risk of gangrene. Zacchias replied that it was better to leave the patient in the hands of God than attempt such a treatment, which promised no ultimate safety and whose horror and pain was obviously most troubling.[78]

Again, in England the lack of detailed codes of law such as the *Constitutio Criminalis Carolina* (1532) which Charles V wished to apply to all the territories of the Empire meant that there was missing the sense of legislative authority which was present in some Continental medical writing.[79] It was this sense of a relationship between the law and medicine that led Johannes Bohn to write his *De Officio Medici Duplici Clinici nimirum ac Forensis* (1704). For instance, he wrote that a patient's secrets should not be divulged to any busybody, but only to those with a legitimate interest such as magistrates and to those who would be less safe by coming into contact with the patient by reason of contagion, or when the unfit, the impotent, the mad, the epileptic etc. attempt to marry.[80] Medical ethics, clearly, sometimes develop in response to the presence (or the needs) of the law and the State. In England medicine was largely oblivious to both.

Notes

1. On the College of Physicians see G. Clark, *A History of the Royal College of Physicians*, 2 vols (Oxford: Oxford University Press 1964–6); on the College in the Seventeenth century see H. J. Cook, *The Decline of the Old Medical Regime in Stuart London* (Ithaca and London: Cornell University Press, 1986).
2. On the medical market-place and on recent social history of early modern England: Lucinda McCray Beier, *Sufferers and Healers. The Experience of Illness in Seventeenth Century England* (London: Routledge, 1987); Roy Porter (ed.) *Patients and Practitioners. Lay Perceptions of Medicine in Pre-industrial Society* (Cambridge: Cambridge University Press, 1985); Roy Porter and Dorothy Porter *In Sickness and in Health. The British Experience 1650–1850,* (London, 1988); Roy Porter, *Health for Sale, Quackery in England 1660–1850* (Manchester: Manchester University Press, 1989);

Doreen G. Nagy, *Popular Medicine in Seventeenth Century England* (Bowling Green, Ohio: Bowling Breen State University Popular Press, 1988).

3. John Securis, *A Detection and Querisome of the Daily Enormities and Abuses Committed in Physic* (London, 1566), sig B3 r–v.
4. *Ibid.*, sig A2r.
5. Gent., sig A3v.
6. G. E. R. Lloyd (ed.) *The Hippocratic Writings* (Harmondsworth: Penguin Books, 1978), 68. I have kept to the traditional title, *The Law,* rather than *The Canon* of Lloyd's edition.
7. Securis, *A Detection,* sig A3v – A4r.
8. In J. W. Willock, *The Laws Relating to the Medical Profession* (London, 1830), clxxxiii.
9. Securis, *A Detection,* sig A4r.
10. Willcock, *The Laws,* xi.
11. Securis, *A Detection,* sig A4r–v.
12. *Ibid.*, sig A4v–A5r.
13. John Gregory, 'Lectures on the Duties and Qualifications of a Physician' in *The Works of the Late John Gregory M.D.,* 4 vols (Edinburgh, 1788) vol 3, 21: the bad behaviour of patients can 'cloud his [a physician's] judgement and make him forget propriety and decency of behaviour' in this situation appears the advantage of a physician 'possessing presence of mind, composure, steadiness, and an appearence of resolution.' Gregory's lectures have been unjustly overshadowed by the emphasis placed on the work of Percival.
14. Securis, *A Detection,* sig., A5v.
15. *Ibid.*, sig., C6v.
16. Harold Cook, unpublished paper 'Intellectual Property and Propriety: Professional "Monopolies" and the Physicians of Early Modern London'.
17. John Cotta, *A Short Discoverie of the Unobserved Dangers of Several Sorts of Ignorant and Unconsiderate Practisers of Physike in England* (London, 1612), 116.
18. *Ibid.*, 132.
19. *Ibid.*, 125–8.
20. On Galen see Vivian Nutton's chapter in this volume and Galen, *Quod Optimus Medicus sit quoque Philosophus,* in C. G. Kuhn, *Claudii Galeni Opera Omnia* (Leipzig, 1821) vol I, 61.
21. Hugh Chamberlen, *A Few Queries relating to the Practice of Physick* (London, 1694), 68–70.
22. E. D. [Eleazar Dunk or Duncan], *The Copy of a Letter Written by E. D. Doctour of Physicke to a Gentleman* (London, 1606).
23. Like Cotta, Hart and Primrose wrote defences of Galenic medicine: James Hart *KAINIKH, or the Diet of the Diseased* (London, 1633); James Primrose *De Vulgi in Medicine Erroribus* (London 1638) translated by Robert Wittie into English as *Popular Errors* (London, 1651).

24. Andrew Wear 'Medical Practice in late Seventeenth and early Eighteenth-Century England: Continuity and Union' in Roger French and Andrew Wear (eds), *The Medical Revolution of the Seventeenth Century* (Cambridge: Cambridge University Press, 1989), 294–320.
25. Cotta, *A Short Discovevie*, 9.
26. Richard Whitlock, *Zootomia. Or Obsevations on the Present Manners of the English* (London, 1654), 86 and 110–22.
27. *Ibid.*, 124.
28. *Ibid.*, 133.
29. Cotta, *A Short Discoverie*, 25.
30. *Ibid.*, 28.
31. *Ibid.*, 28.
32. Aristotle, *Nicomachean Ethics*, Book v, ch 9 [1137a11–18] in the translation of J. L. Ackrill, *Aristotle's Ethics* (London: Faber and Faber, 1973), 110.
33. Cotta, *A Short Discoverie*, 31.
34. Chamberlen, *A Few Queries*, 67–8.
35. *Ibid.*, 93–4.
36. Catherine Crawford in a recent study has pointed out that there were very few malpractice suits in the early modern period.
37. Chamberlen, *A Few Queries*, 76–7.
38. It is significant that when Cotta does mention God in his description of the true artist or physician it is in the context of knowledge and not charity. The physician's calling to study God's workmanship, nature, is an added reason for gaining knowledge, and one can use God as a guide: 'Not to speake of his excellent subiect (which is the life and health of mankind), his divine direction in his calling (led by the unchanged order and wisdome of God himselfe, manifested and set forth unto him in the structure and frame of heaven and earth) doth exact and require in him all possible perfection to sound and fadome the depth and height thereof. For as it is manifoldly and unmeasurably infolded and wrapped up in the intricate wisdome of his universal workmanship, so must long dayes and time carefully spent, indefatigable studie, paines and meditation, restlesse vigilance, a cleare eye of understanding, and sincere affection worke and labour it out .... And this must the true Physition ever behold God as his guide, and be governed and directed by his hand. For God is nature above nature, and nature is his hand and subordinate power, he is the giver of health and life in nature....' *A Short Discoverie*, 120.
39. Richard Bostocke, *The Difference Between the Auncient Phisicke ... and the Latter Phisicke....* (London, 1585), sig., Fiiir–v.
40. Alan Macfarlane, *Witchcraft in Tudor and Stuart England* (London, 1970); Paul Slack, *Poverty and Policy in Tudor and Stuart England* (London, 1988).
41. Charles Webster, *The Great Instauration. Science, Medicine and*

Reform 1626–1660 (London: Duckworth, 1975) 246–64

42. On the parish care of the sick poor see Margaret Pelling, 'Healing the Sick Poor: Social Policy and Disability in Norwich 1550–1645', *Medical History*, 29 1985, 115–37 and Andrew Wear, 'Caring for the Sick Poor in St. Bartholomew Exchange' in W. F. Bynum and Roy Porter (eds), *Living and Dying in London, Medical History Supplement* II, (London, 1991).
43. William Clowes, *A Briefe and Necessarie Treatise touching the Cure of the Disease called Morbus Gallicus* (my ed, London, 1585), 42r. Nicholas Culpeper, *A Physical Directory or a Translation of the London Dispensary Made by the College of Physicians of London* (London, 1649) sig. A1V.
44. Nicholas Culpeper, *The School of Physick* (London 1659) 7–40; Culpeper was following, often verbatim, Timothie Bright's, *A Treatise wherein is Declared the Sufficiencie of English Medicine* (London, 1580).
45. Securis, *A Detection*, sig., C6v–C7r.
46. Robert Pemel, *Help for the Poor*, (London, 1653), sig., A1r–v.
47. Calvin, *Institutes of the Christian Religion*, Book iv, ch XIX, sections 18–21; also see Calvin's comments on the healing miracles in his commentaries on the Gospels. The denial of miraculous healing was related to the Protestant denial of the efficacy of the Catholic sacraments and the anointing of the sick 'the greasy sacrament of the Papists' as William Perkins, the outstanding Puritan divine, put it: William Perkins, *A Golden Chaine* (London, 1612), 501.
48. Cotta, *A Short Discoverie* 88.
49. Whitlock, *Zωotomia*, 55.
50. Noah Biggs, *Mataeotechnia Medicinae Praxews. The Vanity of the Art of Physick* (London, 1651) sig., b3v.
51. *Ibid.*, 8.
52. *Ibid.*, 14.
53. *Ibid.*, sig. b3v and 17.
54. Cotta, *A Short Discoverie*, 33.
55. William Walwyn, *Physick for Families* (London, 1669), 2.
56. Walwyn wrote that his medicines if taken by those in health should nourish and not harm them (*ibid.*, 21) whilst for instance: 'The next sore troubler of the sick are Vescicatories, or Raisers of small and great Blisters, by irksome fretting, if not venomous Pleisters, sometimes flaying off all the skin from the backs, otherwhiles the shoulders, leggs ... to extream torments, expecially when those new places are rubb'd and irritated for diversion of venomous inflammations, hidious Curses and Excrations having been noted the impatient Effects of such cruelties; of which Nature also are the use of cupping Glasses, drawing of Silk through the Neck-skin, Leeches, and Issues, all full of pain, hazard and dangers (*ibid.*, 18). Note the religious distaste of 'Curses' the result of cruel medical practices.

57. *Ibid.*, sig., A2r.
58. *Ibid.*, sig., A2v.
59. *Ibid.*, 3.
60. *Ibid.*, 6.
61. On O'Dowde see Harold J. Cook, *The Decline of the Old Medical Regime in Stuart London,* 148–50. Thomas O'Dowde, *The Poor Man's Physician, Or the True Art of Medicine* (London, 1665) 3rd edition, Preface, unpaginated.
62. Willcock, *The Laws,* clxxvii–clxxviii
63. *Ibid.*, clxxviii.
64. O'Dowde, *The Poor Man's Physician,* 15–6.
65. *Ibid.*, 20–1.
66. *Ibid.*, 21–2.
67. Ronald A. Marchant, *The Church under the Law,* (Cambridge: Cambridge University Press, 1969); R. H. Helmholz, *Roman Canon Law in Reformation England* (Cambridge: Cambridge University Press, 1990), Helmholz makes the point that although the faculties of canon law at Oxford and Cambridge were closed down manuscript sources indicate that some canon law was taught within a civilian context 152–4; good accounts of the investigative and judicial processes in England are in J. S. Cockburn, *A History of English Assizes 1558–1714* (Cambridge: Cambridge University Press, 1972); Cynthia B. Herrup, *The Common Peace. Participation and the Criminal Law in Seventeenth Century England* (Cambridge: Cambridge University Press, 1987); J. H. Gleason, *The Justices of the Peace in England 1558 to 1640* (Oxford: Oxford University Press, 1969); Norma Landau, *The Justices of the Peace 1679–1760* (Berkeley: University of California Press, 1984).
68. J. H. Baker, *An Introduction to English Legal History* (3rd ed. London: Butterworths, 1990); S. F. C. Milsom, *Historical Foundations of the Common Law* (2nd ed. London, 1981); T. A. Green, *Verdict According to Conscience* (Chicago: Chicago University Press, 1985). O. F. Robinson, T. D. Fergus, W. M. Gordon, *An Introduction to European Legal History,* (Abingdon: Professional Books, 1985).
69. Charles Goodall, *The Royal College of Physicians of London* (London, 1684), 316–7.
70. *Ibid.*, 317–9.
71. Willock, *The Laws,* lxxxvi (8. Coke's *Reports* 107–21).
72. Harold J. Cook has given an excellent account of Bonham's case 'Against Common Right and Reason: The College of Physicians versus Dr. Thomas Bonham' (American Journal of Legal History, 29, 1985, 301–22.
73. Willcock, *The Laws,* cxxxvi.
74. *Ibid.*, cxlix–xl.
75. Some of the cases appear very serious, for instance, that of the surgeon John Lamkin. He admitted practising medicine, but he was

also tried by the College for malpractice: 'He was afterwards charged for Mala praxis upon several Patients (as his dropping of Oil of Sulphur into a Patient's eyes, from whence an inflammation ensued .... which endangered a total blindness; His prescribing Stupefactive Pills to a Citizen troubled with an Iscury, by which he fell into a total suppression of Urine, and made not one drop of water for ten days, but died most miserably on the 11th) which being proved before the President and the Censors, he was forwith commited to prison propter malam praxin et immodestos mores, and fined 20l.' A year later Lamkin was again brought before the College and imprisoned for further illegal practice, the Archbishop of Canterbury interceded for him then withdrew, and then someone else interceded with the result that he was released on a bond of £40 that he would not practice in the future. Goodall, *The Royal College of Physicians,* 331–2. From this case and others it is clear (as in Bonham's case) that the College mixed together its attempts to have control or monopoly of medical practice with protecting the public from malpractice, self-interest with altruistic concern at patients being harmed. The lack of State involvement limited the College's effectiveness as a judicial body. This is clearly seen in the decision of the College in 1635 to remit John Hope, an apothecary's apprentice to the higher courts, when they found that he had given an infusion of Coloquintida from which the patient died. The Censors certified that 'it was evil practice [malpractice] in the highest degree, and transcending the Censure of our College; and therefore we remit it in all humility to the higher Courts of Justice.' Goodall, *The Royal College of Physicians,* 442.

76. Ben Jonson, *Volpone* 1.iv.26–33. I am grateful to Dr Gordon Campbell for this passage.
77. Willcock, *The Laws,* xciv–xcvi. See also Harold J. Cook, 'The Rose Case Reconsidered: Physicians, Apothecaries, and the Law in Augustan England' *J. of the History of Medicine,* 45, 1990, 527–55.
78. Pauli Zacchiae, *Quaestiones Medico-Legales* (3rd ed. Amsterdam, 1651), 635.
79. See Esther Fischer-Homberger, *Medizin vor Gericht. Gerichtsmedizin von der Renaisance bis zur Aufklärung* (Berne: Hans Huber Verlag, 1983).
80. D. Johannis Bohnii, *De Officio Medici Duplici Clinici nimirum ac Forensis* (Leipzig, 1704) 95.

5

Conflicting Duties: Plague and the Obligations of Early Modern Physicians Towards Patients and Commonwealth in England and The Netherlands

Ole Peter Grell

'Physicians can never discharge their Duty with greater Applause, than by contributing their aid to popular Diseases, which at this season is the prime movent of these Meditations.' This statement by the Dutch born and Leiden educated physician, Gideon Harvey, which strikes a modern reader as perfectly reasonable, would not have been unqualifiedly embraced by the majority of Harvey's colleagues within the medical profession in England in 1665. Neither, for that matter, would this passage in Harvey's preface to the pamphlet, 'A Discourse of the Plague', have been wholeheartedly accepted by most physicians in the Netherlands. But then Harvey, who had settled in London during the Interregnum and become a denizen in 1660, remained an outsider from the medical establishment throughout his life. Thus he never became a member of the College of Physicians in spite of becoming Royal physician to Charles II in 1675.[1]

Should they have been intellectually attracted to the ethical values expressed in Harvey's preface, most of the fellows and licentiates of the College of Physicians would still have found it difficult to adopt them in practice. The College had a bad record when it came to fighting epidemics, especially plague. Most members had continually demonstrated a preference for flight rather than exposing themselves to the dangers of what was perceived as a highly contagious disease. The Lord Mayor and Aldermen of London were unable to obtain any assistance from the College of Physicians until the outbreak of plague in 1625 when two doctors finally agreed to be employed by the City to look after plague victims.[2] In the last epidemic to occur in London in 1665, the College, however, was able to improve on its record. In June it responded positively to the request of the Lord Mayor that the College should nominate six or more physicians for the jobs of plague-doctors to the City. The College supplied a list of eight members from which two were eventually chosen – Nathaniel Hodges and Thomas Witherly. Another two from this list, Nicholas Davis and Edward Deantry, later volunteered their services 'upon principles of honour and conscience'. Most members of the College, however, stuck to the tradition of self-interest and self-preservation, taking to their heels in times of plague, even if no less than seventeen of the twenty-four physicians who remained in the City in 1665 were members of the College.[3] In other words, there was still a long way to go in 1665 before a majority of physicians would have fully accepted Gideon Harvey's statement or have adhered to the ideals of utopian writers such as Tomasso Campanella, Johann Valentin Andreae and Gabriel Plattes, who considered the proper role of physicians that of 'devout public servants'. At most they would have felt defensive about their behaviour during the crisis, like Dr Jonathan Goddard. According to Samuel Pepys, at the first meeting of the Royal Society after the epidemic, Dr Goddard 'did fill us with talk in defence of his and his fellow-physicians' going out of town in the plague-time; saying that their particular patients were most gone out of town, and they left at liberty – and a great deal more, etc.'[4]

That a majority of medical men, in England as well as The Netherlands, found it difficult to honour these basic moral demands should, however, not surprise us. Plague was, after all, the most terrifying disease which could hit a community in the early modern period. Major epidemics devastated urban communities in England and The Netherlands at irregular intervals between the 1560s and the 1660s. In Amsterdam and London major epidemics often killed between 10 and 20% of the population in less than six months.[5] To stay and attempt to tackle such dangerous diseases with minimal hope of success was a tough demand to meet for all but a nucleus of medical practitioners who possessed the strongest moral and religious fibre.

Furthermore, the lack of understanding of this disease, what caused it and how it was transmitted, must have added to the dread, and the feeling of impotence it generated. The Reformation had changed very little in the perception of plague. It was still considered a primarily supernatural disease, sent by God to punish man for his sins. Contemporary terminology continued to equate sin with disease. God, however, was perceived to work mainly through secondary causes, according to the Law of Nature, and natural explanations of epidemic disease, with their Galenic emphasis on contagion and miasma, formed part of a useful circular argument. Thus supernatural and natural explanations constituted 'two interlocking parts of a single interpretative chain' which helped to provide the rationale for plague.[6] Consequently, religious remedies such as prayer and repentance came first. Only in conjunction with these godly remedies could medicine be properly used, and more importantly, expected to have a chance of success. Medicine was considered part of God's Creation and accordingly could only work through the grace of God. Together, the natural and supernatural constituted a most covenient double-track rationale which encouraged the use of medicine while simultaneously providing convenient explanations for the shortcomings of such remedies.

Apart from a continuous debate about the relationship between first and secondary causes of plague – between God and Nature and the role of Providence – most Dutch and English tracts written before the mid-seventeenth century were concerned with the difficulties of reconciling private and public interest. How could self-interest be reconciled with social and ethical obligations towards society and Commonwealth? In this connection the overriding issue of concern to contemporaries was the question of flight. Who, if any, might justifiably flee the danger? This was a particularly complex question for physicians, as well as ministers, whose separate callings were so intimately intertwined in this period. Obviously, physicians of the soul and those who ministered to the body, had similar if not identical obligations towards those who caught this disease, which fell within the supernatural, as well as the natural domain. Consequently, most tracts on plague used a terminology where medical and theological expressions were deliberately mixed. Medicine and theology represented closely connected approaches to the same problem. Experience and the medical teachings of Hippocrates and Galen pointed unambiguously to flight as the best way of avoiding epidemics. The Bible, however, was more ambiguous and provided ammunition for supporters and antagonists of flight respectively.[7]

This general, ethical concern was reflected in the growing number of tracts on plague, which were published in England and The Netherlands in this period. The conventionality and derivativeness of this literature, which for the greater part was written by ministers, was considerable.

The fact that the London bookseller, Richard Smyth, translated Gabriel Biel's fifteenth century sermon, *De fugienda Peste* in 1665, underlines that in some respects little if anything had changed in the debate about plague since well before 1500.[8]

In what follows I shall focus on the ethical and moral obligations of physicians and, to a lesser degree, clergymen in times of plague, as they were perceived in the contemporary medico-religious tracts published in England and The Netherlands. Owing to the close intellectual and social links between doctors and clergymen in this period – many held degrees in theology, as well as in medicine, not to mention the many ministers who practised medicine and theology simultaneously – the two professions are inseparable. Likewise, both groups belonged to the same social stratum of society and their ethical obligations in times of epidemics were generally perceived to be identical.[9]

The overriding moral problem for the early modern physician was obviously how to reconcile the often quoted advice of Hippocrates and Galen to flee an epidemic as quickly as possible, to stay away as long as possible and return only slowly, with his Hippocratic deontology.[10] Was the physician expected to advise those of his patients who had not yet caught the disease to flee while he himself stayed behind to help those who had fallen ill? Did his obligation towards the Commonwealth – society at large – take precedence over his obligations towards the individual patient? Or, re-phrased in the language of medical ethics: was his beneficence constrained by his duty of justice?[11] This dilemma was further complicated by related issues such as whether or not the physician could morally justify making social distinctions and give preference to those of his patients who belonged to the upper social strata, and whether or not he was allowed to benefit financially from an epidemic. Did not Christian charity and Hippocratic ethics oblige the physician to offer his services to rich and poor alike in times of crisis, as stated in *Precepts?*

'I urge you not to be unkind, but to consider your patient's wealth and resources. Sometimes you will give your services for nothing, calling to mind a previous benefaction or your present reputation. If there should be the opportunity to serve a foreigner or a poor man, give full assistance to him; for where there is love of man there is also love of the art.'[12]

Finally, of course, there was the problem of whether or not to tell the truth. Might the physician be morally entitled to keep the truth from those of his patients who had caught the plague when the outbreak of the disease had yet to become common knowledge, if he perceived it to be in the interest of the Commonwealth? Or might he withhold his suspicions about an oncoming epidemic from the general public for the sake of peace and stability? These were among the most important ethical problems which confronted Dutch and English physicians in the late sixteenth and early seventeenth centuries.

In 1527 Martin Luther wrote his highly influential tract *Ob man vor dem Sterben fliehen möge,* which not only went through numerous translations and editions, but which continued to be quoted by subsequent writers on plague well into the seventeenth century.[13] Luther had recent first-hand experience of a serious epidemic by the time he published this work. Plague had broken out in Wittenberg in the summer of 1527 and Luther had decided to disregard the Elector's orders to leave the town for the safety of Jena. Instead, he remained in Wittenberg together with Bugenhagen and ministered to the sick and frightened population. In accordance with his own and Bugenhagen's example, Luther expressed admiration for the Godly who refused to run away: 'They uphold a good cause, namely, a strong faith in God, and deserve commendation because they desire every Christian to hold to a strong, firm faith.' He added, however, that such devotion could only be exhibited by a few and emphasized that the weak could not be expected to carry the same burden as the strong. On the other hand, Luther had no doubt that pastors and those who held public office were under obligation to remain 'steadfast before the peril of death'. Only where enough ministers and members of the magistracy were available, or where adequate substitutes could be appointed, might some be permitted to leave. The same applied to all individuals who were bound by service or duty to people who had been infected with the plague. In this connection Luther specifically mentioned the duty of 'paid public servants such as city physicians' *not* to flee.[14]

For the individual physician Luther's message was simple. A doctor was ethically bound to stay and look after his patients, unless he could guarantee that a colleague would take over his responsibilities. Christian charity obliged him to fulfil such minimal demands. This was a natural consequence of Luther's theology with its emphasis on faith and grace. For Luther the individual came first and the Commonwealth second. This did not mean, however, that Luther rejected the use of medicine or normal precautions and health regulations. He was, in fact, a keen advocate of both, but considered them subject to Christian charity.

Physicians were, according to Luther, not obliged to offer their services free in times of plague. They were, as under normal conditions, to be remunerated and suitably rewarded, 'inasmuch as every labourer is worthy of his hire'. Those, who transgressed these basic rules because of greed, would be punished by God, while those, who did their duty, could rest assured that God would act as their 'attendant and physician'.[15]

Apart from giving priority to the individual over the Commonwealth, Luther also differed from most of the Dutch and English writers on plague of the late sixteenth and early seventeenth centuries, by pointing out 'that God's punishment has come upon us, not only to chastise us for our sins but also to test our faith and love'.[16] Most authors, writing within the framework of the Second Reformation, saw plague solely as God's punishing hand, applied for the sins of Man, which would only be removed through true repentance. The emphasis on sin and more importantly, on a sinful society, meant that Christian charity, which was geared towards the individual and the sick, had to be tempered by considerations for the healthy and society. This was to a large extent based on Aristotelian principles of justice which served to switch the balance towards the Commonwealth in general and the healthy in particular, rather than the individual and the sick.

Only a minority of later writers differed from this line, which was promoted primarily by Reformed theologians. One such was Johann von Ewich, physician to the city of Bremen, whose tract on plague was quickly translated into English in 1583 and the minister, Henoch Clapham, who in 1603 went as far as to argue that a Christian who died of plague showed lack of faith.[17] Another was 'the Dutch Hippocrates', the physician, Pieter van Foreest who had received his doctorate from the University in Bologna in 1543 before he commenced practising medicine in Alkmaar, his birthplace, in 1546. Twelve years later Pieter van Foreest accepted the position of town-physician in Delft, at a time when the town was suffering from a serious outbreak of plague. His experiences while serving the community in Delft, attending the poor and advising the magistracy, which he included in his *magnum opus, Observationes et curationes medicinales,* helped secure him the position as this period's most famous physician in The Netherlands. Van Foreest, however, did not have to wait until the publication of his work in 1588 for public recognition. In 1572 he was appointed physician to William of Orange and later, in 1575, he lectured briefly at the newly founded University of Leiden.[18]

In book 6, entitled 'Public fevers, epidemic diseases, malignant, contagious and pestilential fevers, and plague' of his *Observationes et curationes medicinales,* Pieter van Foreest adopts the Lutheran position on whether or not a Christian can flee the plague. He is adamant that physicians and ministers are obliged to stay and look after their patients and parishioners. It is the duty of the 'pious physician' to stay with the sick, if there are any; if not, the best remedy is a swift flight and a slow return. Van Foreest then adds a prayer to the effect that the outbreak of plague will not see an end to brotherly love and Christian charity; for him, not only the physician's duty, but also the individual citizen's obligation, is to the individual, whether patient or neighbour.[19]

By the late sixteenth century, however, Van Foreest's ethical view had become the exception in The Netherlands. Obligations towards the sick had by then been supplanted by concerns for the Commonwealth. This is evident from the changing role of town-physicians in the Northern Netherlands during the sixteenth century. Originally, in the first half of the sixteenth century, the duty to stay and treat the plague-stricken had either been implicitly understood or directly stated in the contracts between magistrates and town-physicians. Often the physicians were offered double their normal salaries to guarantee that they honoured these obligations and did not run away. This all changed in the United Provinces during the second half of the sixteenth century, when town-physicians to an increasing degree were specifically excused from attending plague-victims.[20]

Later, towards the middle of the seventeenth century, a reaction set in against this emphasis on the Commonwealth which had been generated by orthodox Calvinism. A movement within the Reformed Church in The Netherlands, underlining the value of individual piety and re-emphasizing the importance of faith, was inspired by the Utrecht professor, Gijsbertus Voetius and his pupil, Johannes Hoornbeek. Their theology, signified a return to neighbourly love and served to re-focus on the duty of ministers and physicians towards the individual citizen as a natural consequence of Christian charity.[21]

Among the first in England to write about plague after the Reformation was Bishop John Hooper, who in 1553 published *An Homelye to be read in the tyme of pestylence.* Hooper, who had spent years in exile in Zurich during the reign of Henry VIII, was on his return in 1549 heralded as the 'future Zwingli of England'.[22] His Zwinglian theology led him to focus on sin 'the chiefest cause of all plagues and syckenesse'. He pointed out that Galen's advice to flee the plague was only a viable way of escape if those who fled repented and changed their ways. Likewise, repentance was also needed by those who were prevented from flight by their calling and bonds of Christian charity. Apart from ministers of the church, they included those who 'haue places and offices of truste for the commune wealth'. Undoubtedly Hooper included physicians in this group whose regard for the Commonwealth could only be demonstrated by their Christian charity towards the poor and the suffering.[23] Hooper's insistence on the obligation of leading members of the Christian Commonwealth to stay and assist the afflicted population proves how strongly he was rooted in the ethics of the First Reformation. Only his strong emphasis on sin links him with later authors who wrote within a Calvinist tradition, most potently espoused by Theodore Beza. Likewise, it is noteworthy that Hooper does not envisage anyone being released from their calling by the appointment of substitutes or proxies, a possibility left open by Luther, as long as the office-holders retained a supervisory capacity.

Evidently the sense of community and Christian charity was strong among the early champions of the English Reformation, but time and self-interest, individual as well as institutional, served to dilute this emphasis. The Prayer Book of 1552 stated that ministers should visit the sick during epidemics. Limitations were, however, quickly applied to such open-ended Christian charity. By 1578 Bishop Aylmer instructed the clergy in London that they should select a few volunteers for this duty in order that the majority could avoid the dangers. Finally, in 1604 the new Canons specified that ministers were not obliged to visit if the sick suffered from or were suspected to suffer from an infectious disease.[24] Already in 1598 the later Archbishop of Canterbury, George Abbot, had attacked those who disregarded the dangers of plague and exposed themselves to infection. This was, according to him, worse than fatalism. It amounted to suicide and was therefore a temptation of the devil. Abbot acknowledged the Christian duty of ministers and physicians to stay within their communities, but he saw their roles as supervisory rather than directly involved with the sick. Instead, middlemen, i.e. plague officers, were to be appointed in order not to endanger valuable members of the community.[25]

The Dutch Reformed churches demonstrated similar characteristics. In 1574, only three years after the first National Synod had met in Emden, the Provincial Synod of Dort found it necessary to instruct its ministers to stop making distinctions between plague and other diseases. They were instructed to visit all sick members, but at the same time told not to run any unnecessary risks. It was obviously an agonizing problem for the Synod, for which only an ambiguous statement offered an escape.[26] The Alkmaar minister, Adolph Venator, was evidently not an isolated case when, in 1599, he refused to visit plague victims, excusing himself by referring to the three ministers in Nijmegen, among them his brother, who had died visiting the plague-stricken.[27]

The growing reluctance among the Reformed clergy to perform this duty went hand in hand with a decline in religious commitment and the institutionalism of Calvinism in The Netherlands. Among its consequences was the creation, and growing importance, of the position of visitor of the sick. This position, which initially had been created to help and assist ministers in times of crisis, eventually became a buffer between pastors and infected. During the early seventeenth century visitors of the sick appear to have taken over most of the pastors' obligations in this respect, eventually, as in the case of the exiled Dutch Reformed church in London, leading to further institutional proliferation in the form of the post of extraordinary visitor for the plague-stricken. A similar differentiation materialized within the Dutch medical profession during the same period. Town-physicians, as we have already seen, were by the second half of the sixteenth century often contractually exempted from attending plague victims, while magistracies, as was the case of Utrecht in 1597, by then felt obliged to employ medical men for plague purposes exclusively.[28]

Theodore Beza's highly influential tract on plague, which was translated into English by the Heidelberg educated schoolmaster and divine, John Stockwood, in 1580, stressed the value of flight and self-preservation as long as it was regulated by 'the common bond of humaine societie or by any other kinde of friendship'.[29] For Beza, precautionary measures such as flight were not only ethically sound but also the best remedies, especially when performed with 'earnest repentence' since 'our sinnes are the chiefe and the true cause of the plague'.[30] To illustrate this point Beza referred to his personal experience of plague:

> When as I my self about 28 yeeres past was sicke of the Plague at Lausanne, and that both others of my fellowe ministers, and amongst the rest, that singular man of blessed memory Peter Viret was prepared too come vnto mee: and that Iohn Calvin himselfe also sending a messenger with letters offered to me all kynd of curtesie, I suffered none of them to come vnto me, least I might

> haue beene thought too haue prouided for my selfe with the losse of the Christian common wealth, which was manyfest would haue been very great by the death of so worthie men: neyther doth it repent me to haue doone so, althugh peraduenture in the like case of theyrs they should not haue obteined the same at my hand.[31]

Where Luther, centring his theology around faith and grace, had focused on Christian charity and neighbourly love, Beza with his emphasis on predestination, providence, sin and repentance gave prominence to the Commonwealth. Self-preservation via flight was no longer a possibility left open solely to the weak, it became an obligation for the average citizen who held neither public nor ecclesiastical office. Some English Calvinists took his message even further. The minister, James Balmford, who, in 1603, dedicated his tract on plague to his parishioners in St Olave's Southwark, held that physicians who were not 'public persons' ought to flee the plague. The same applied to ministers and other 'profitable members of Church and Commonwealth' who were only obliged to find substitutes in times of epidemic disease.[32] Balmford's tract may have taken Beza's view to extremes, but orthodox Calvinists, such as Willem Teellinck and Andreas Rivet in The Netherlands and Arthur Hildersam and William Gouge in England, would have found very little with which to disagree.[33]

Three years after his translation of Beza, John Stockwood published an English edition of the Bremen physician, Johann von Ewich's pamphlet on the duties of the Christian magistracy in times of plague. Ewich, who had been appointed 'Stadtphysicus' in Bremen in 1562, drew on his personal experiences as a hard working doctor in Bremen in the mid-1560s when the city had suffered a serious outbreak of plague.[34] Johann von Ewich, who was heavily influenced by Luther's tract of 1527, had no doubt what the Christian citizen's moral obligation was when plague broke out. 'He greatlie offendeth against the rule of charitie, whosoeuer according to his abilitie doeth not seek and bring some ayde, as it were a preseruative' during an epidemic.[35] This was a moral axiom which obliged the Christian physician to stay and look after his patients. Practical experience, however, made Ewich realize that reality fell desperately short of such expectations. While he encouraged magistracies to employ physicians and surgeons in times of crisis, 'such as for yeares, fame, experience, honestie of manners, virtue, and feare of God, they shall iudge to bee best lyked and fitte', he acknowledged that 'it is an harde thing to finde such, and so perfect, especially in so dangerous times'. A decent salary was, according to

Ewich, the only way to guarantee the loyalty of town-physicians during severe epidemics – 'such is man his weaknesse'. Likewise, it fell to the magistracy to supervise the activities of the physicians they employed: 'If they do anye thing through errour or deceite, that it shal not be unpunished'.[36] It is significant that Johann von Ewich, who was himself a physician, saw the need for an external, as well as independent, body to police the medical profession in order to guarantee that physicians adhered to the necessary standards. He might well have envisaged a body on a par with the Health Boards of Northern Italian cities such as Milan, Florence and Venice. These Boards, which exercised considerable power over physicians and which battled to enforce minimum standards and control over the medical profession in times of plague, would have been ideally suited to ensure that ethical standards were met.[37]

Furthermore, Ewich warned physicians against greed. They were entitled to charge their patients for their labour, but not, as opposed to 'Experimenters, Jewes, Paracelcists' and 'Alchimists' who were not bound by their Hippocratic Oath, to 'hunte after gaine'.[38] For Ewich Christian charity and Hippocratic deontology gave precedence to the individual patient over considerations for the Commonwealth. Ethically his views were similar to Luther's whose work on plague from 1527 he cited at great length. A similar strong commitment to assist suffering fellow-believers and citizens, which characterized early Protestantism, can also be found in the immigrant, Amsterdam doctor, Jacob Viverius's work on plague from 1601.[39] Physicians, who belonged to immigrant Protestant communities, such as the Dutch and Walloon Reformed churches in London, often displayed a stronger and more lasting commitment to such ideals than did their native English and Dutch colleagues. Raphael Thorius, Johannes Brovaert and the two Baldwin Hameys, father and son, all stayed in London and served the 'stranger' communities during epidemics in the early seventeenth century.[40]

A few physicians, such as Van Gerwen in The Netherlands and two members of the College of Physicians in London, Francis Herring and Stephen Bradwell, also advocated against flight. Like Herring, they acknowledged that plague was 'the stroke of Gods wrath for the sinnes of mankinde' and considered flight futile or destructive, as opposed to proper medical precautions. Likewise, they argued that those who had the means to flee were obliged to stay due to their responsibilities towards their poor fellow-citizen. 'Stay then, you that are Rich, to helpe the Poore, and you that haue skill in Physicke to helpe the sick' was Bradwell's exhortation to his readers.[41] Most physicians, however, towed the line of mainstream Reformed theologians, as laid down by Theodore Beza, and later promoted by Willem Teellinck and Andreas Rivet in The Netherlands and William Gouge in England. To put the interest of the Commonwealth and the healthy before that of the infected, who more often than not were indeed the poor, was, after all, in the interest of the establishment which included physicians, as well as clergymen. The fact that the non-Calvinist theologian, Lancelot Andrews, and the crypto-Catholic physician and poet, Thomas Lodge, held similar views would indicate that the social effects of a gradual institutionalism of Protestantism were of greater importance in promoting such attitudes than were Reformed theology.[42]

Thomas Lodge, who belonged to an influential City family – his grandfather, Sir Thomas Lodge, had been Lord Mayor in 1563/4 when London had suffered a serious outbreak of plague – had received his medical training at the University of Avignon, graduating in 1598, before being incorporated MD at the University of Oxford in 1602. Lodge had already been practising in London for some years when another plague-epidemic hit the City in 1603. Paraphrasing and translating a continental source, Lodge quickly produced *A Treatise of the Plague,* which he published with a dedication to the Lord Mayor and Sheriffs of London at the height of the infection. Lodge claimed to have been moved by his sense of 'Dutie and loue which I owe this Citie' and 'charitable remorse' for paupers who suffered most from the plague. He had written his pamphlet for the benefit of the poor and requested the magistracy 'that this charitable intent of mine may be furthered by your discreet orders, in such manner that these bookes may be dispersed among those families that are visited, to the end they may find comfort and cure by their owne hands and diligence'.[43]

Lodge, however, was in total agreement with most Reformed theologians and doctors in emphasizing the doctor's duty towards the Commonwealth rather than the infected patient:

> When as (by the will of God) the contagion of the Plague is gotten into any place, Citie, or Countrey, we ought to haue an especiall regard of the generall good, and by all meanes to study for their preseruation who are in health, least they fall into such inconueniencie.[44]

Consequently, Lodge recommended flight as the best preservative against plague, quoting Galen's *De Differentius Febrium* and Hippocrates's *De Natura Humana.*

Like most of his colleagues in the medical profession. Lodge unequivocally condemned the activities and crass commercialism of mountebanks. Thus he reported, that a number of people had sought his assistance, mistaking him for a neighbouring quack who had been advertising his merits in the City. This experience had aggrieved Lodge 'because of that loathsome imposition which was laide vppon me, to make my selfe vendible, which is unworthy a liberall & gentle minde, much more ill beseeming a Phisitian and Philosopher, who ought not to prostitute so sacred a profession so abiectly, but be a contemner of base and seruile desire of money'.[45] Lodge's contempt of commercialism and advertising would undoubtedly find strong support among modern medical practitioners. Whether or not such high standards were generally met is, to say the least, questionable. That English Renaissance literature is packed with references to greedy physicians can hardly have been a result of the writers' imaginations. It must have been based on reality. Otherwise, Ben Jonson's satirical statement in The Poetaster: 'You make more haste now, than a beggar upon pattens; or a physician to a patient that has no money' would neither have been comprehensible nor funny.[46]

According to Lodge health regulations should be strictly enforced in the interest of the Commonwealth, but primarily against men 'of seruile and base condition' whereas 'men of note' were considered to 'haue the meanes, and obserue the methode to preserue themselues'. One is left in no doubt that the author is voicing the opinion of the establishment. Likewise, concern for the Commonwealth made Lodge argue in favour of deception:

> And if by chance, or by the will of God the Citty becommeth infected, it ought not incontinently to be made knowne: but those that haue the care and charge of such as are attainted, ought in the beginning to keepe it close, and wisely conceale the same from the common sorte, imparting it onely to such, who by their good aduise and counsaile may assist them in the time of danger, which counsaile and aduise diuine Hipocrates setteth downe in his oath and attestation to Phisitians, and consequently to all those that haue the charge of the sicke, forbidding them to reueale that which ought to be hidden for the common profit: which being considered by the diuine Philosopher Plato, in the third booke of his common weale, he auoweth that it is lawfull for Magistrates & Phisitians to lie for the safety and conseruation of their Citty. For oftentimes to conceale a truth to this intent, is no error in such men, whenas by such means the common weale is conserued and profite.[47]

Lodge's case for deception in the interest of the Commonwealth can undoubtedly be supported by Book III of Plato's *Republic*, whereas any Hippocratic corroboration of his position is dubious. The Hippocratic Oath committed physicians to benefit and not harm their patients, an obligation which overrode any requirements of not deceiving them. It is, however, difficult to see how, according to Hippocrates, beneficence to the Commonwealth might justify deception of individual patients.

Similar justification of the use of flight, and precedence of the interest of the Commonwealth over those of individual plague-casualties, can be found in the writings of orthodox Reformed clergymen, such as Willem Teellinck and William Gouge. In accordance with the publicist, Henry Holland, they maintained that flight was a sensible precaution against plague:

> Depart speedily, farre off, and returne slowly. As this is Physically prescribed, so it is diligently practised, as daily experience teacheth, of all sorts of men, yea of the Physicians themselves.[48]

Flight without proper repentance, however, was recognized to be useless or even dangerous, since one could not flee the wrath of God. For the Godly it was 'foolish presumption, rather than a prudent resolution, either to accompany those that are as it were in the fire of Gods judgement, or not to go from them when a faire and warrantable opportunity is offered'. People such as magistrates, ministers, soldiers, doctors and nurses, however, were obliged to adhere to their callings. They could only leave if and when they had appointed willing and able substitutes. For Gouge the Commonwealth took precedence over the individual. Accordingly, neither physicians nor ministers were obliged 'to hazzard their life in particular mens cases. They are set over a Society, not over one or two particular persons. Indeed every particular member of the Society belongeth to their charge: and they ought to do what they can to the good of every particular person under their charge, so farre as may stand with the good of the whole body, and prove no prejudice thereto.'[49]

Willem Teellinck agreed with his English colleague, but he took matters further when he pointed out that not only were valuable members of society obliged to preserve themselves for the sake of the Commonwealth, but the plague-stricken must show restraint. They 'should not allow any such valuable citizens to attend them, whose services are so necessary to the community, in order that these individuals should not become infected and society denied their invaluable service'.[50]

The Leiden professor of Theology, Andreas Rivet, struck a similar note in his pamphlet, *Epistola ad Amicum*, which published together with Beza's plague tract saw several editions in The Netherlands. Rivet emphasized that the most learned and important ministers ought not to visit plague victims because their value to their congregations was too great to risk. He shared the opinions of the Heidelberg theologians, Hieronimus Zanchius and Zacharias Ursinus, 'that the general welfare took precedence of the particular and the majority over the minority, and that you do not place the commander in the first battle order and expose him to the greatest danger'.[51] Rivet warmly recommended the Genevan model where in times of plague a couple of doctors were elected to look after the infected only. Likewise, ministers were chosen by drawing lots to care for the sick in order to limit the risk to the whole Company of Pastors.[52] That the Genevan model also appealed to Dutch physicians can be seen from the writings of Anton Deusing of Groningen, a leading Dutch doctor, who was in the unusual position of being appointed professor of Medicine at the University of Leiden two days after his death.[53]

These were ethical positions which, while serving the interests of the establishment, helped to legitimize the prevailing habit of self-preservation and flight among physicians and ministers. That the physician's beneficence towards plague-stricken individuals should be tempered by his duty towards the Commonwealth was undoubtedly connected with the social bias which plague began to display to an increasing degree in the early seventeenth century. The astrologer, John Gadbury, only emphasized a well-known fact when in 1665 he claimed: 'how small a number of worthy generous persons this Pest prays upon, in comparison of the vast multitudes of the vulgar that are swept away by it'.[54]

Other factors also helped to promote the Commonwealth-view. The unwillingness of 'profitable members' of society, such as ministers and physicians, to attend plague victims, began to occur, not only at a time when plague had started to display a social bias towards the poorer members of society, but also at a time of social ascendancy of the medical and clerical professions. Towards the end of the sixteenth century, the medical profession, like the Church and the legal profession, was perceived to be a métier for gentlemen. This improved social position of the physician underlined his role as a highly valued member of society whose life should not be risked in times of crisis. Furthermore, the physician's value to society was seen to manifest itself through his knowledge and experience, acquired through long and expensive studies at university. He was, in other words, an exclusive commodity, who needed a fair amount of protection. The result of such considerations could often take on farcical aspects, as it did in Bologna during the plague of 1630. There the local physicians suggested to the magistracy that they should try to cure patients in the plague-hospital at a distance, since recent experience had shown that doctors who served within the lazarettos were highly likely to die. Instead, the physicians suggested that they should be consulted at a safe distance, standing outside the hospital while the barber-surgeon shouted out of the window 'the quality, sex, condition of the patient and the stage of the illness'.[55] That this peculiar approach was not only restricted to Italy can be seen from the writings of the above-mentioned Groningen physician, Anton Deusing. He pointed out that physicians should avoid visiting the infected while informing themselves about their condition from a safe distance, preferably by offering medical advice to the plague-stricken and their helpers from outside the infected houses.[56]

Thus by the late sixteenth century, Aristotelean principles of justice were used in England and The Netherlands to emphasize the medical practitioner's duty towards the Commonwealth rather than the patient. The importance of charity and neighbourly love which had characterized the First Reformation was rapidly disappearing, as can be seen from Beza's tract, written in 1579. To what degree this shift, away from beneficence to the individual and towards duty to society at large, was inspired by the theology of the Second Reformation, rather than a gradual secularization and fall in religious commitment brought about by the growing institutionalism of Protestantism, is difficult to determine. Luther, while pointing to the godly physician's and clergyman's moral obligation to stay and provide care and consolation for suffering brethren, had acknowledged that such staunch demands often faced practical difficulties and were reserved for the strong, who, by definition constituted a minority. In other words, he recognized that such ethical demands were extremely difficult to meet.

The prominence given by Beza and his Dutch and English successors to the Commonwealth at the expense of the individual also served to rationalize the moral shortcomings of doctors and ministers who fled and left their parishioners and patients to fend for themselves. No wonder it proved popular with those whose calling might so easily expose them to the dangers of plague.

Notes

1. Gideon Harvey, *A Discourse of the Plague*, (London: 1665), 1; for Harvey, see *Dictionary of National Biography* (Oxford: Oxford University Press, 1917 onwards).
2. Paul Slack, *The Impact of Plague in Tudor and Stuart England*, (London: Routledge & Kegan Paul, 1985), 276.
3. J. J. Keevil, *The Stranger's Son*, (London: Geoffrey Bles, 1953), 142–54 and W. Birkin, 'Dr. John King (1614–1681) and Dr. Assuerus Regemorter (1615–1650)', in *Medical History*, 20 (1976), 292.
4. Charles Webster, *The Great Instauration, Science, Medicine and Reform 1626–1660* (London: Duckworth, 1975), 288; for Samuel Pepys' comments, see R. Latham and W. Matthews (eds), *The Diary of Samuel Pepys, A new and complete transcription*, vols I–XI (London: Bell Hyman, 1970–83), vol VII, 211.
5. Paul Slack, *op. cit.*, 144–72 and Leo Noordegraaf and Gerrit Valk, *De Gave Gods. De Pest in Holland vanaf de late middeleeuwen*, (Octavo Bergen 1988), 233–6.
6. Paul Slack, *op. cit.*, 29.
7. For flight and prudential action, see Gen. 27. 42–3, Proverbs 22. 3, and Ephesians 5. 29. Against flight and stressing the role of Providence, see Ezekiel 9, II Kings 20, Chron. 16. 12 and Psalm 91.
8. Paul Slack, *op. cit.*, provides an excellent survey of the plague-literature in England during the first half of the seventeenth century compiled from the STC; during the epidemic of 1603/4 28 tracts were published out of which 15 were devotional; in 1625/7 36 pamphlets were printed out of which 21 were devotional; 1636/7 22 tracts were published out of which 12 were devotional; 1665/6 46 pamphlets were printed of which a third were of a devotional nature. It is considerably more difficult to get a precise picture of the number of Dutch tracts on plague in this period, W. P. C. Knuttel, *Catalogus van de pamfletten verzameling berustende in de Koninklijke Bibliotheek*, vols 1–2, (The Hague: Algemeene Landsdrukkerij 1889), offers some assistance, as does *De slaende Hant Gods over de voornaemste Steden van't Christenrijck, in't besoecken met de pestilentiale sieckten, sedert het jaer 1600 tot aen't jaer 1664* (Amsterdam, 1664); see also the considerable collection of plague-tracts in the University Library in Leiden. For Smyth's translation of Biel, see Paul Slack, *op. cit.*, 41.
9. Andrew Wear, 'Puritan perceptions of illness in seventeenth century England', in R. Porter (ed.), *Patients and Practitioners, Lay Perceptions of Medicine in Pre-Industrial Society* (Cambridge: Cambridge University Press, 1985), 69 and G. Groenhuis, *De Predikanten; de sociale positie van de gereformeerde predikanten in de Republiek der Verenigde Nederlanden voor ca. 1700* (Groningen: Wolters-Noordhoff, 1977), Historiche Studies uitgegeven vanwege het Instituut voor Geschiedenis der Rijksuniversiteit te Utrecht, 33, 179.

10. Compare the classic statement: *Cito, longe, tarde* with Hippocrates, *Epidemics*, I, II, and the Hippocratic Oath.
11. For a discussion of this aspect of medical ethics, see R. Gillon, *Philosophical Medical Ethics*, (Chichester: Wiley, 1985), 74–9, 86–91.
12. Hippocrates, *Precepts*, Chapter 6.
13. See *Luther's Works*, Jaroslav Pelikan and Helmut T. Lehmann (eds), vol 43 (Philadelphia: Fortress Press, 1968), 115–38; for an English author citing Luther, see Henry Holland, *Salomons Pest-Hovse*, (London: 1630), 51–2; see also the English editions of the Lutheran, Andreas Osiander, *How and whither a christen man ought to flye the horrible plague of the pestilence* (London: 1537, 1538, 1563/4).
14. *Luther's Works*, vol 43, 120–2. That Luther, attending the Marburg Colloquy in 1529, decided to flee the city with the other theologians when an epidemic of the 'English sweat' occurred, does not undermine the reformer's position, as claimed by P. A. Russell. Luther, after all, had no pastoral duties in Marburg and was therefore free to leave, see P. A. Russell, 'Syphilis, God's Scourge or Nature's Vengeance?', in *Archiv für Reformationsgeschichte*, 80 (1989), 289 note 12. Philippe Melanchton did not divert from the Lutheran position, see E. Wickersheimer, 'Les Recettes de Philippe Melanchton contre la Pest', in *Janus*, 27 (1923), 1–7.
15. *Ibid.*, 129; for Luther's theology, see G. Ebeling, *Luther Einfürung in sein Denken (*Tübingen: 1964).
16. *Luther's Works*, vol 43, 127.
17. John Ewich, *Of the dutie of a faithful and wise Magistrate, in preserving and delivering of the common wealth from infection in the time of the Plague or Pestilence* (London: 1583), and Henoch Clapham, *An Epistle discoursing upon the present Pestilence, teaching what it is, and how the people of God should carrie themselves towards God and their Neighbour therein* (London: 1603).
18. See H. L. Houtzager (ed.), *Pieter van Foreest. Een Hollands medicus in de zestiende eeuw* (Amsterdam: Rodopi, 1989).
19. Pieter van Foreest, *Observationum et curationum medicinales* (Leiden: 1591), Book 6, 99–100. I should like to acknowledge the assistance of Dr Vivian Nutton in locating this reference.
20. See M. J. van Lieburg, 'Pieter van Foreest en de rol van de stadsmedicus in de Noord-Nederlandse steden van de 16e eeuw', in H. L. Houtzager (ed.), *Pieter van Foreest*, 46–9.
21. For Hoornbeek, see *Nieuw Nederlandsch Biografisch Woordenboek*, 10 vols, Leiden: 1911–37: A. W. Sijthoff's Uitgevers-Maatschappij N.V. for Voetius, see *Biografisch Lexicon voor de Geschiedenis van het Nederlandse Protestantisme*, vol 2 (Kampen: J. H. Kok, 1983), 443–9 and J. Dort, De Onbekende Voetius (Kampen: 1989).
22. John Hooper, *An Homelye to be read in the tyme of pestulence, and a moste piesente remedye for the same* (London, 1553). See also Paul Slack, *op. cit.*, 43 and Andrew Pettegree, *Foreign Protestant*

Communities in Sixteenth-Century London (Oxford: Oxford University Press, 1986), 30).

23. John Hooper, *An Homelye,* A IIIr, B IIr & C IIr–v.
24. Paul Slack, *op. cit.*, 228.
25. George Abbot, *Questiones sex, totidem praelectionibus* ... discussae (Oxford: 1598), see the fifth question. This part of Abbot's pamphlet was translated into Dutch in 1637 by Adrian P. Ravesteyn, see *Van de Peste,* (Delft: 1637).
26. See O. P. Grell, 'Plague in Elizabethan and Stuart London: The Dutch Response', *Medical History,* 1990, 34, 424–39 especially note 32.
27. Leo Noordegraaf & Gerrit Valk, *op. cit.*, 124.
28. See O. P. Grell, 'Plague in Elizabethan and Stuart London: the Dutch Response', in *Medical History,* 1990, 34, 424–39 and M. J. van Lieburg, 'Pieter van Foreest en de rol van stadtmedicus in de Noord-Nederlandse steden van de 16e eeuw', in H. L. Houtzager, *Pieter van Foreest,* 49.
29. Theodore Beza, *A shorte learned and pithie Treatize of the Plague, wherein are handled these two questions: The one, whether the Plague bee infectious, or no: The other, whether and howe farre it may of Christians bee shunned by going outside, trs. by John Stockwood,* (London: 1580), DIr.
30. *Ibid.*, D IVv.
31. *Ibid.*, D IVr.
32. James Balmford, *A Short Dialogue concerning the Plagues Infection,* London: 1603), 26 and 72; see also Paul Slack, *op. cit.*, 43.
33. For Willem Teellinck & Andreas Rivet, see *Biografisch Lexicon voor de Geschiedenis van het Nederlandse Protestantisme,* vols 1–2, (Kampen: J. H. Kok, 1978 & 1983), I, 373–5, II, 375–8; for Hildersam and Gouge, see DNB.
34. John Ewich, *op. cit.*, It was first published in Latin in Neustadt in 1582; that year Johann von Ewich also published a devotional tract on plague: *Die Pestilenz, ob sie eine anfällige Seuche sei, und inwiefern ein Christenmensch ihr weichen möge* (Basel: 1582); for Ewich, see *Biographisches Lexikon der hervorragenden Aerzte,* vol 2, (Wien: Urban and Schwarzenberg, 1885), 318–19.
35. John Ewich, *op. cit.*, 4r.
36. *Ibid.*, 13v & 14r. In Protestant Switzerland town-physicians in general appear to have honoured their obligations to their local communities and stayed during severe epidemics in the sixteenth and seventeenth centuries, see H. Koelbing, 'The town and state physicians in Switzerland from the 16th to the 18th centuries', in A. W. Russell (ed.), *The Town and State Physician in Europe from the Middle Ages to the Enlightenment* (Wolfenbüttel: Herzog August Bibliothek, 1981), 151–2.
37. C. M. Cipolla, *Public Health & The Medical Profession in the Renaissance,* (Cambridge: Cambridge University Press, 1976), 8–9 and 35.

38. John Ewich, *op. cit.*, 16v. & 56r.
39. No copy of the first edition from 1601 appears to have survived; for a reference to that edition, see Jacob Cool, *Den Staet van London in hare groote Peste* (ed.) J. A. van Dorsten & K. Schapp (Lieden: E. J. Brill, 1962), 31 and 61; Jacob Viverius, *De Handt Godes of een Christelick verhael vande peste of Gaeve Godes* (Delft: 1624), especially 13; for Jacob Viverius, an immigrant from the Southern Netherlands born in Ghent, see Nieuw Nederlandsch Biografiswch Woordenboek.
40. See O. P. Grell, 'Plague in Elizabethan and Stuart London: The Dutch Response' *Medical History*, 1990, 37, 424–39.
41. I. van Gerwen, *Moedt-gevinghe ofte ernstighe overdenckinghe voor de vluchtende ende alle die meer voor de peste als de sonde vreesen*, (Leiden: 1636); Stephen Bradwell, *Physick for the sicknesse commonly called the Plague. With all the Particular Signes and Symtoms, whereof the most are too ignorant* (London: 1636), especially A 3r. See also Francis Herring, *Certaine Rvles, Directions,* or *Advertisements for this time of pestilentiall contagion,* (London 1603, reprinted 1625), especially A3r–v. Herring's instructions for how to behave while visiting the plague-stricken would have made it near impossible for a physician to examine patients:
    'If any man be bound by Religion, consanguinitie, office, or any such respect to visit the sicke parties; let him first provide, that the chamber be well perfumed with odoriferous trochiskes or such like, the windowes layd with herbes aforenamed, the floore cleane swept, and sprinkled with rose-water and vineger: that there be a fire of sweet wood burning in the chimney, the windowes being shut for an houre, then open the casements to the North. Then let him wash his face and hands with rose-water and rose-vinegar, and enter into the chamber with a waxe candle in the one hand, and a sponge with rose-vinegar and wormwood, or some other Pomander, to smell vnto. Let him hold in his mouth a peece of Mastic, Cinamon, Zedoarie, or Citron pill, or a Clove. Let him desire his sick friend to speake with his face turned from him.
    When he goes forth, let him wash his hands and face with rose-vinegar and water as before, especially if he haue taken his friend by the hand as the manner is: and going presently to his owne house, let him change his garments, and lay those where in he visited his friend, apart for a good time before hee resume them againe.' (B 2r–v).
    The lack of proper examinations of patients would also help to explain why Dr John Symcotts was unable to diagnose plague in a patient in 1637, see F.N.L. Poynter and W. J. Bishop (eds), *A Seventeenth Century Doctoor and his Patients: John Symcotts, 1592? –1662,* Publications of the Bedfordshire Historical Record Society, vol 31, 1951, 62–3.
42. For Lancelot Andrewes' attitude to plague and flight, see Lancelot Andrewes, *A Sermon of the Pestilence. Preached at Chiswick 21 August*

1603, (London: 1636); see also Paul Slack, *op. cit.*, 234–5. For Thomas Lodge, see below. During the early seventeenth century the commitment among Catholic priests and physicians in London towards plague-stricken co-religionists demonstrates similar characteristics to those of minority Protestant groups such as the stranger churches in the City, compare Philip Caraman, *Henry Morse. Priest of the Plague* (London: Longmans, Green and Co, 1957), 77–114 with O. P. Grell, *Dutch Calvinists in early Stuart London* (Leiden: E. J. Brill, 1989), 93–105.

43. See Thomas Lodge, *A Treatise of the Plague*, (London: 1603), A 2r–v. For Thomas Lodge, see E. A. Tenney, *Thomas Lodge* (London: 1935), 1–15 & 155–91; for Lodge's dependence on a continental source, see Paul Slack, 'Mirrors of health and treasures of poor men: the uses of vernacular medical literature of Tudor England', in Charles Webster (ed.), *Health, Medicine and Mortality in the sixteenth Century* (Cambridge: Cambridge University Press, 1979), 242.
44. Thomas Lodge, *op. cit.*, C 3v.
45. *Ibid.*, A 3r.
46. Cited in P. G. Brewster, 'Physician and Surgeon as Depicted in 16th and 17th Century English Literature', *Osiris*, XIV, (1962), 28. See also William Bullein, *A Dialogue against the feuer Pestilence*, M. W. Bullen & A. H. Bullen (eds), (London: Early English Text Society, Extra Series No. 52, W. Trübner & Co., 1888), 55, where Medicus provides the following statement: 'He loued me as I loued hym, He me for health, and I hym for money.'
47. Thomas Lodge, *op. cit.*, F 1v.
48. Henry Holland, *Solomons Pest-Hovse or Tower-Royall*, (London 1630), 2; for Henry Holland, see DNB.
49. William Gouge, *Gods Three Arrows. A Plaister for the Plague*, (London: 1631), 23 & 101–04. Gouge's tract was translated into Dutch in 1666, see C. W. Schoneveld, *Intertraffic of the Mind* (Leiden: E. J. Brill, 1983), 202.
50. Willem Teellinck, *Wraeck-sweert. Bepleytende Het recht van Gods Verbondt door Bloedithe Oorloghe. Diere tijdt Bleecke Pestilentie*, (Amsterdam: 1624), 64.
51. Andreas Rivet, *Epistola ad Amicum, in Variorum Theologici de Peste* (Leiden: 1655) and in A. P. Ravesteyn's collection, *Van de Peste* (Delft: 1637), especially 36, 38 & 39.
52. See A. P. Ravesteyn, *op. cit.*, fol. 20 and W. C. Innes, *Social Concern in Calvin's Geneva* (Allison Park, Pennsylvania: Pickwick Publications, 1983), 134.
53. For Deusing, see G. A. Lindeboom, *Dutch Medical Biography* (Amsterdam: Rodopi, 1984), 432–4. See A. Deusing, *Twee diepzinnige en heilzame onderzoekingen nopende de Pest* (Amsterdam: 1964), 52.
54. John Gadbury, *Londons Deliverance Predicted*, London 1665, 30.

55. See C. M. Cipolla, *Public Health & the Medical Profession in the Renaissance* (Cambridge: Cambridge University Press, 1976), 72–5 and C. M. Cipolla, *Cristofano and the Plague* (London: Collins, 1973), 26.
56. A. Deusing, *Twee diepzinnige en heilzam onderzoekingen nopende de Pest* (Amsterdam, 1664), 55.

6

Ethics in the Eighteenth Century: Hoffmann in Halle

Roger French

Introduction

In an earlier chapter in this book it was argued that medical ethics can be seen, like the ethics of any group, as an activity that not only characterizes the group but that is also a code of behaviour that, if successful, tends towards the survival of the group. The group we are concerned with in these two chapters is that of the learned and rational physician, and in this chapter we shall see that although separated by two centuries, the strategies adopted by the two subgroups that we are examining were very similar. We shall also see that where they differ, it was owing to the different circumstances in which they found themselves.

Hoffmann in Halle

Friedrich Hoffmann was a well-known name in the medical literature of the eighteenth century. He was the first professor – or one of the first two professors – of medicine of the new university of Halle, founded in 1694.[1] By 1730 there were 529 medical students in Halle, a large number by European standards.[2]

A new university provided an opportunity for a teacher to teach a new curriculum, and Hoffmann took it, presenting in his writings a reasoned account of the relationship of medicine to religion and philosophy. The wider aspects of this are dealt with in his *On the Best Way of Philosophizing* and his medical ethics are presented in a tract that compares the duties of the physician and the theologian, and in his *Medicus Politicus.*[3]

Hoffmann was one of the few medical writers of the seventeenth and eighteenth centuries to set down a system of ethics. (His publisher stressing the novelty of the *Medicus Politicus* after

Hoffmann's death, seemed to think it unique.) Although it was clearly his own synthesis, for use in a new university, yet much of it is equally clearly common to other medical men of his kind and represents the ethics of the learned physicians as a group.

There are also special sources of Hoffmann's medical ethics, historically more local. First, his own 'group' was not coterminous with learned physicians as a whole. He was, for instance, a Protestant, and a particular kind of Protestant, a Pietist. The moral apparatus of the Catholic Church, from Canon Law to the church's interpretative role and learned tradition, was not available to him. Yet in the late seventeenth century the church, of whatever sort, lent a good deal to any ethical system, and we shall see how Hoffmann's church was a resource for him.

The second local source of Hoffmann's ethics lay in Halle's political circumstances. Hoffmann's career at Halle covered the period when Brandenburg-Prussia was becoming increasingly an absolutist and military state. Control of the medical profession by court edicts, the founding of medical boards and in general the rules issued by the State for medical credentials[4] made the boundaries of the practice of internal medicine important. These rules had the effect of separating the physicians from other healers and emphasizing their university training. Clearly, in a new university and teaching the State's doctors, Hoffmann found ethics an important topic. What the State wanted was the new Rational, enlightened, 'scientific' medicine, based on anatomy, precisely what Hoffmann taught.[5]

The Prudent Physician

Hoffmann's ideal ethical doctor had, or had to adopt, certain fundamental character traits. Each of them was ethically good in a direct and simple sense but each of them, too, combined to improve the reputation of doctors as a whole. Hoffmann's ideal doctor, like that of Zerbi, is not arrogant, but can talk equally with nobles and plebians. His talk is, moreover, guarded and he does not disclose secrets he may have learned from patients (particularly women) nor does he discuss their diseases, especially when they are disgusting ones. He is attentive to his patients and visits them as often as necessary. In short, he leaves behind him an image of a doctor that will encourage the patient and the family at the bedside to call the doctor or his successor again when illness strikes.

Hoffmann's *Medicus Politicus* is, of course, an idealized set of ethics. It was designed for and taught to the medical students at Halle (and it was published from notes taken down from his lectures). As we might expect of a rational physician Enlightened in the eighteenth-century way, Hoffmann finds reasons for what must so often in professional life have been the simple moral rules that resulted in the benefit of the group. One way of making rationalized rules attractive was to make them intelligible to the reason of, and apparently in the self interest of, the member of the group. (In contrast, the similar rules of Zerbi were presented in an aphoristic, injunctional style, with an unselfconscious moral loading.) Hoffmann is addressing the young medical man with a set of 'rules of prudence', where 'prudence' is an Enlightened intellectual exercise by which the young man is advised to organize his studies and life 'if he wishes to quickly acquire and keep a reputation and a satisfactory practice'.[6] The moral aspect of these ethical rules does, however, (as in Zerbi's case) appear in the odium incurred on breaking them. We shall see in a number of places that the explicit appeal to rational self-interest in place of direct moral admonition does not entirely hide the implicit benefit that accrues to the group, sometimes at the individual's expense. Even the individual's interest in acquiring a reputation, so often pointed to by Hoffmann, is of benefit to the group.

The 'political' doctor is he who can live and work in proximity and harmony with other groups, an 'urbane' man in an *urbs or polis.* The *Medicus Politicus* lays down rules for how the physician should behave when he comes into contact with other groups of people. These other groups are the other kinds of practitioners, chiefly the apothecaries and surgeons; lawyers, in cases where medical evidence is required; and patients in different categories.[7]

Medical 'prudence' was more than enlightened self-interest. The 'prudent' or 'political' man was a creature of the Enlightenment, rational and philosophically detached even in the face of pain and illness, worldly-wise and not without cynicism. The *politicus* belonged to 'polite' society, important in which was the image of the Prussian nobleman as a military officer, cool and detached even in leading his men into action.[8] The cynicism could become 'political' in a fairly direct sense in what Geyer-Kordesch calls '... the double dealing world of court and bureaucracy where dissimulation was a stage requisite'. It was also a medical requisite: in Hoffmann's aphorism 'He who cannot dissimulate cannot cure.' We shall see why below. Prudence was taught in universities, and Alberti, Hoffmann's colleague, writing on medical jurisprudence, lists prudent books in medicine, theology, law and philosophy.[9] There was even a book teaching how to be a politic patient.

The Physician and Surgery

The division between the roles of the physician and surgeon, emphasized by decrees of the State, is clearly marked for Hoffmann by ethical considerations (so notably absent from Zerbi's ethics). It is, he says, below the dignity of the physician to cut, burn and plaster: these are the concerns of the barbers, bath-house keepers and lithotomists. (Chapter 2, section 2.) Nor should the physician, he says, undertake the ordinary, *vulgares,* operations of the regular surgeon, which include venesection, lithotomy and amputation of parts affected by sphacele. Hoffmann is claiming for his kind that the superior dignity of the physicians is based on their rationality and erudition, and the effect of these rules is to make the division between the two branches of medicine obvious in practical terms. Other ethical questions about this boundary are likewise involved with obvious behaviour: Hoffmann insists that surgeons must not give internal remedies, the reserved practice of the learned physicians. To be sure, in the absence of a physician and in an emergency, says Hoffmann, the surgeon may give some that relate to surgery, like decoctions of wound-plants, wound-powder and crab stones, and even light purges like senna or rhubarb. In Halle as elsewhere (mostly outside Italy) the physicians claimed (here with State backing) the right to control surgical practice, and Hoffmann advises the physician not to be too stern with surgeons, but to advise them gently. He assumes that a physician can effectively prevent a surgeon from giving internal medicines in his presence, and from ever giving any kind of heroic remedies such as opiates and strong purges. These are like a sword in the hands of the unskilled, says Hoffmann. He explains that only the erudite physician, by virtue of his knowledge of how the body works, can tell if a patient is strong enough to stand surgery. It was similar knowledge that enabled the physician to understand and so regulate the effect of internal medicines upon the body; and Hoffmann further claims that lack of this knowledge made it improper for a surgeon to conduct post mortems and judge on the lethality of wounds in cases that relate to jurisprudence. A surgeon may be allowed to open the body, says Hoffmann, but it is only the physician's systematic knowledge and exploration of the other organs that could provide a judgement in these important cases. So extensive was the erudition of the physician, in Hoffman's view, that it actually included surgery, and the physician might want to practise this after all noble art in difficult cases. Hoffmann accordingly gives hints on performing a trepannation. One of them was to give the patient analeptic drugs: these were heroic pain-killing opiates that only physicians could administer.

In Halle, whether or not the physician had as much power over the surgeon as Hoffmann found ideal, in practice they cooperated in providing the two sides of medical practice. Hoffmann advises the physician always to work with the best surgeon in order to be accepted in town and to secure a sound reputation. Erudition on its own is, he says, insufficient for the purpose. Yet close collaboration had its dangers for Hoffmann, and part of his ethics at this boundary of his profession is to urge the young doctor not to become too friendly with surgeons. Familiarity breeds contempt, he says, and it would not do to have surgeons looking down their noses at physicians.

One of the duties of the physician in Hoffmann's picture of the ideal is to examine the knowledge of surgeons, particularly new ones. This is not 'ethical' in the usual sense, but it is very much part of the behaviour of a group, behaviour that characterizes the group and by which it asserts its relationship to others, here in competition with it. In Hoffmann's picture, the examinee is examined in the College of Surgeons by physicians and surgeons. He is asked about the names, positions and connections of the principal muscles, about the route taken by the arteries and nerves, so that he may avoid cutting them in letting blood. He is expected to know something of the structure of joints, for the reduction of dislocations, and about the signs and cure of inflammation of wounds. He is asked whether wounds to the major organs are invariably fatal. He is not asked, that is, about anything that lay outside a severely practical knowledge and inside the learned physician's store of erudition. According to Hoffmann it is even the physician's duty to inspect the surgeon's instruments, and if he suspects that they have been used indifferently on infected as on uninfected patients, to ensure that they are washed.

The Physician and Pharmacy

The other important boundary that Hoffmann's ethics help to define was at the point where the physician met the pharmacist. (Here the similarity to Zerbi's ethics are marked.) Hoffmann's physician claimed superiority and even more than in the case of the surgeon, the physician's ethical rules serve to define the boundary between the two trades. Again it is the case that familiarity breeds contempt and it is for that reason that Hoffmann's ethical doctor does not fraternize or play games with the pharmacist. The ethical doctor must preserve his reputation, which among pharmacists relies on superiority. No doubt partly social, it is clearly for Hoffmann also financial – it is proper that the learned physician is better off than the pharmacist. It is for these reasons that in Hoffmann's eyes one of the most unethical things a doctor can do is to enter into an agreement with a pharmacist in which the doctor overprescribes for his patient in return for a share of the pharmacist's excessive profit. In doing so – and Hoffmann says this odious and damnable practice is not uncommon – the doctor was not only fraternizing with the pharmacist, but losing much of his freedom of action, losing his reputation, especially among the pharmacists, and risking his proper financial superiority.

In other words the doctor with such an arrangement with a pharmacist was crossing the boundary and, given the reason for the existence of ethical systems, was necessarily being unethical. To share the ethics of another group, in however small a way, was to do disservice (to be 'disloyal') to one's own group. To maintain a reputation was important, but nowhere more important than among members of the rival group. As Hoffmann says, it is very unethical, *turpe,* to ask a pharmacist about the reasons behind (or the course of) a disease or treatment, precisely because it reveals ignorance on the part of the doctor and would reduce the physicians' reputation among the pharmacists. Again, when Hoffmann urges the young doctor to write his prescriptions elegantly, it is to guard against the pharmacist thinking them unlearned. Here as elsewhere the physician relied above all on his erudition for his reputation. As in the case of surgery this amounted to the physician subsuming the theoretical part at least of another part of medicine within his own knowledge. Manual operations of the other trades may have been below his dignity, but the rational and learned physician had to know – ideally – as much of the theoretical part of pharmacy as the pharmacist. Indeed, he had to know more. As Hoffmann had declared that the physician, with his knowledge of the workings of the body, was in a better position than the surgeon to make a judgement about the lethality of wounds, so he argued that the physician's knowledge of diseases and their causes was necessary to judge the effects of drugs and to estimate their doses. In no other way, asserted Hoffmann, was *rational medicine* possible. The pharmacists did not have this knowledge, he said, and must not practise internal medicine; although the vulgar imagine that the pharmacists know all about simples, such knowledge (says Hoffmann) is mere empiricism.

Hoffmann had another and rather personal reason for deriding the pharamacists' knowledge of simples. It was that in his view they pay no attention to chemical remedies, which he thought important. Hoffmann presents himself here as the up-to-date and knowledgeable physician whose enlightened views were frustrated in practice by the obstinacy and ignorance of the pharmacists. The latter stuck by the traditional remedies of the ancients, with a deep attachment to polypharmacy. Hoffmann argued in vain (he says) that the ancients had been ignorant of chemistry; and that modern discoveries had added greatly to the range and effectiveness of modern medicine. But the pharmacists were content with their plants, either because it was an area where their own erudition successfully maintained their reputation among the lower classes, as Hoffmann suggested, or because there was civil control over what they sold. Hoffmann complains of the fact that modern chemical preparations, cheap and effective, were not approved by the magistrates for sale in the pharmacies. Without action by the magistrates or of a prince, says Hoffmann, the physicians can do nothing to improve the pharmacopoeia. And (he argued) it badly needed reform. Fully half of the multitude of things stocked in the pharmacy could, in his opinion, be thrown away. Traditional theriac was an example: although compounded of fifty ingredients, Hoffmann reckoned twenty would suffice; indeed (he said) much of its action could be ascribed simply to the opium it contained. Here Hoffmann is doing what he urged others to do – displaying his learning by the wise selection of a few simple drugs rather than by a display of polypharmacy. It is expressly a reputation-building exercise: Hoffmann says so, and to what he says we can add that in using a few chemical remedies he is seeking to make the physicians' erudition of a different kind, and better, than that of the pharmacists.

The physicians had the right of visitation over the pharmacies (derived from the *Collegium Medicum* in Berlin by way of the local medical board). Their power did not extend, as we have seen, to introducing new items into the pharmacopoeia, but was limited to determining that the medicines had been properly prepared and that the ingredients and simples were fresh and effective. The young doctor addressed by Hoffmann was urged to determine if the oils were rancid, the spirits phlegmatic, the distilled waters acetic. Has the rhubarb been too long exposed to the weakening effect of the sun and air? The doctor's interest was in the purity of the ingredients, so that he could work out appropriate doses for his patients. Again, in this boundary between two parts of medical trading, we are not concerned with 'ethics' in the usual sense, particularly when and if such inspections were unproblematic. But these actions of the physicians were certainly internal rules that the group had succeeded in having recognized by external authority. The same thing may be said of the physician's apparent right to examine the new pharmacist's qualifications to sell drugs. The questions asked were on the same level in pharmacy as those asked in surgery by the physicians: he was examined on his knowledge of poisons and medicines that were poisonous in excess, like strong vomits and purges, of abortifacients, of the means of preparation, and of the principles of chemistry.

We come closer to ethical problems in the more usual sense with Hoffmann's insistence that the pharmacist should know enough about doses to be able to make up medicine of the right strength in the absence of a doctor. The danger of overdosing with heroic remedies was matched by the danger of confusing two remedies. It was for the latter reason that Hoffmann urged his young doctors to write down his prescriptions rather than deliver them orally. It was also essential, he said, never to allow the pharmacist to substitute one item for another. Failure to observe these rules led to situations that were ethically disastrous. Hoffmann relates the case of the daughter of Pastor Merckius of Halle, who went down with a petechial malign fever. The physician prescribed *nitrum antimoniatum* to reduce the fever and the girl began to recover rapidly. But the standard of care slipped. The following day the physician did not personally deliver a prescription to the pharmacy, and the pharmacist was not there. In his place his servant sent *vitrum antimonii* in error, and the patient was poisoned, dying horribly.

As in other parts of Hoffmann's ethical system the rules are rational and their moral loading apparent only when they are broken. Hoffmann also deals in midwives in a similar way. They are to have certain qualities, are to be taught and examined in a certain way. They should have special knowledge on topics like infanticide and pregnancy. The ethical importance of these rules is underlined by Hoffmann's prefatory remarks on the sadness occasioned by the current high infant mortality.

The Physician and His Fees

The handling of money is an area that we readily see as ethically sensitive. It was less so in the eighteenth century, but was still as central to our Enlightened doctors' rules of behaviour as it had been to Zerbi's. The physicians as a group had indeed a set of rules that had succeeded in putting them into a dominant position in the medical market, in being able to command a higher level of monetary return. Indeed, as we have seen, financial superiority was itself ethically desirable for the physician as part of the circumstances that enabled him to maintain his reputation – and so his very earning ability.

The ethical problem for the doctor was how to secure his fee. As a gentleman, the physician preferred to see his fee not as a wage, the product of a money-for-work contract as practised by people lower in the social scale. This was how surgeons and empirics worked, agreeing a fee before beginning work. But Hoffmann saw this as a vice, a sordid wrangling over money; instead, the physician's fee was an honorarium. This is the term used by Hoffmann, who wanted to make sure that the patient knew the difference. An honorarium was a gift from a grateful or an anxious patient, and its size depended on how the *patient* felt about his treatment. It was certainly in the physicians' interest to put no limit on its size, for it could often be very large. The difficulty was that if the patient forgot to pay it – in effect reducing the honorarium to nothing – the doctor as a gentleman found it unethical to pursue it. As Hoffmann says, the doctor receives but does not demand; an importuning physician generates contempt and (we add) reduces the reputation of the group. (It was of course, as Hoffmann points out, perfectly possible in the event of non-payment to secure the help of a third party: in this and in other aspects of the financial rewards of the physician, there is a strong parallel in Zerbi's case.)

The physician emphasized his gentlemanly status by treating servants free of charge. Hoffmann adds that often the physician would also treat the poor without charge, but that it was proper to accept payment from them. The ethical physician in Hoffmann's view should accept his honorarium without shame or sadness, irrespective of its size. To emphasize the difference he felt between the rational physicians and the surgeons and empirics, Hoffmann stresses that it is highly unethical to take a pre-arranged sum and then fail to perform a cure. The somewhat uncertain method by which the physician secured his fees, and the fact that they were sometimes not forthcoming, enabled him also to insist that, after all, the primary duty of the physician is health, not money. There is no reason at all to doubt that Hoffmann and others (including Zerbi) sincerely believed this, and acted accordingly. But it would also have had the effect of adding to the reputation of physicians as a whole.

The physician who was uncertain of his fee had a number of strategems he could employ. Not only was the attention of the physician unpriced, but so were the medicines he administered. As Hoffmann explains, what the patient paid on this account might be double or more their normal price, for the sick (he says) never demand medical help free of charge and are more liberal than strictly necessary when settling bills. Another device was the exercise of discretion as to the appropriate time to 'receive rather than demand' the honorarium. Hoffmann explains again that a patient in pain is quick to offer and ready to pay a large sum. It is proper to 'use the pain' in this way and accept the money, says Hoffmann, because such readiness to pay does not endure. While the patient is ill and in great pain he believes that the pain is a sign of approaching death, and will offer huge sums. Sometimes the merest anxiety will produce a generous honorarium. But, continues Hoffmann, when the pain is assuaged, then the offer, if not previously accepted, becomes smaller as the fear of death diminishes. Some patients send off a fee as soon as they are free of their disease, to avoid paying more after the doctor's later visits. Hoffmann advises the doctor to make his visits nevertheless; it will demonstrate that his business is health, not money (and, we can add, it will do his reputation no harm at all. In all these respects, the similarities to Zerbi's ethics are striking). Hoffmann here has harsh words for men not of his own religion: it is the Jews, he says, who often call the best doctor in town when they are ill, but who more often forget to pay him. Another strategy is open to the doctor in this situation, should he be called a second time. He dallies a little, finding that he has pressing business elsehere; at once the forgotten fees are remembered and sent: the doctor calls, having not stepped outside the ethics of a Christian gentleman. From the vehemence with which he condemns it, we may guess that some doctors in such a situation were tempted to prolong the cure for the sake of a larger fee.

The Physician and the Patient

The doctor's source of income was his patient. In most cases then, the interests of the two were identical. A patient who was cured was a better source of income and reputation than one who died. Most of Hoffmann's advice is accordingly technical in the medical sense – how to deal best with different categories of patient. But there were problems, and Hoffmann's rules take account of them. Perhaps the biggest was the patient who, like patients since Zerbi's time, was not satisfied with a single doctor. As Hoffmann suggests, such a patient may have a chronic disease, or is simply hasty in his search for a cure. Hoffmann sees it as an improper practice and one, therefore, that the physician discouraged. Hoffmann took a strong line with some of his patients, as we shall see, and here seems almost to be trying to force his code upon them. The difficulty was that two different doctors, given no chance of consulting each other, might well give the patient quite different accounts of the nature and treatment of the patient's illness. Hoffmann adds that two doctors should never discuss a case in front of the patient, who would be sure to have suspicions about their knowledge. Now, rational and learned medicine depended almost entirely for its success upon the erudition of its practitioners. What counted above all was that they could convince the patient they they alone knew about his illness. It is abundantly clear from what Hoffmann says that the one thing that the physician must never allow to fall into question is his erudition. By means of it the rational physician told a better and more convincing story to his patients; by means of it he persuaded society as a whole and the authorities who framed its laws that it was precisely by lack of erudition that the empiric was a quack and not fit to practise; it was by claiming that his own erudition was superior to and anyway included that of the pharmacist and surgeon that the rational physician claimed his superiority over them, his right to examine them and the right to practise, if he so wished, their form of medicine.

It was then of the first importance that the physicians should agree upon the nature of their erudition. This was the purpose of education, and most university-trained physicians in Europe not only spoke a common medical language, but agreed about many of the major points of medical doctrine. We have seen how central to Zerbi was the common education and the joint defence of the learned tradition, the purpose of which is laid out in the strongest language by the two authors. Yet at the level of practice, it was very easy for two different physicians to differ in diagnosis, prognosis and treatment of the same case. In circumstances where he was obliged to write down his first judgement of a case and follow it through to the end, often even a single physician found it impossible to be certain of the nature of the case.[10]

So if two physicians gave different accounts of a single case to the patient, for him the common wisdom and erudition of physicians as a class was open to doubt. It is this that lies behind Hoffmann's urgent recommendation that physicians should not take as patients those who cannot bear delay while awaiting a cure. If they go to another doctor, some disagreement among physicians will be made manifest. If they go to a quack and die as a result of his ministrations, then some of the blame will fall upon the physician who first treated him (and so upon physicians in general). If they go to a quack and survive, then the quack claims all the glory, and all his previous failures are hidden by one apparent success. Hoffmann adds to this the ethical command not to decry one physician in front of a patient whose case you hope to take: it can only result in the patient becoming uncertain about the wisdom of physicians as a class. Above all, says Hoffmann earnestly, never ever put your judgement in writing: if the patient is not satisfied and seeks a second opinion, then nothing is more damaging to the reputation of both doctors (and of course to the group) than a comparison of two written and differing judgements.

Hoffmann is here discussing prognostication from urine, in which for centuries the physician had had to guard against the tricks of those who sent into the physician's office urine of a source different from that stated. Hoffmann is aware of the danger to the physician's reputation in this and in other modes of prognostication. Do not, he advises, declare that a patient's case is hopeless, and abandon him: such a rash judgement may well be wrong, and if the patient subsequently goes to a quack, is cheered by his promise of a cure, and perhaps by his cheerfulness alone recovers, then what an appalling thing it would be for the physicians' reputation that a quack had cured a patient deemed by them incurable.

Also in defence of the erudition of the doctor are Hoffmann's rules governing the single doctor in charge of a case. It is essential, he insists, that the patient does not form a poor idea of the doctor's erudition. It is for this reason that the doctor, although grave and serious, is not to be taciturn or morose in the sickroom. He must explain the nature of the disease, its causes and remedies. (But on the other hand the doctor must not chatter, especially about other patients.) Hoffmann says that many physicians overplay their hand, and make too much of their erudition in front of the patient, boasting and promising things they cannot in the end perform. This too, warns Hoffmann, will ultimately damage the physician's reputation, making him like a boasting but unsuccessful quack. But worse than this in Hoffmann's view is the physician who does not use his erudition enough. Often enough he will be called to treat a literate man knowledgeable in natural philosophy who has read up his own disease in the medical books and who quizzes the doctor when he arrives. However difficult, the physician must be one step ahead of his patient and explain the nature of the disease and its causes, and explain why this or that medicine has been selected. Less elaborate answers are to be given to the semiliterate, and Hoffmann suggests that they are pitched at a level that is slightly too technical to be wholly intelligible. With the common people, says Hoffmann, use such phrases as 'the liver is blocked', 'the blood is corrupt' or 'the spleen is swollen'. We may compare Zerbi's little set-speech on prognostication from urine and the pulse. In both cases this is Rational Medicine working in the medical market-place. The erudite physician has in the end a better story to tell his patients about their condition than his rivals. He pitches it at a level appropriate to his audience and it is always impressive, if rather complicated.

In defence of the doctor's reputation, Hoffmann was firm with his patients. Not only did patients have the habit of seeking a second opinion, but they would often promise to obey the doctor's instructions about taking medicines, only to disobey once he had gone. Hoffmann's code allowed him to bully plebian patients into doing what he wanted, and to deceive them all, plebeians or not. For sometimes a patient would from fear or disgust refuse to take his medicines, such as mercury pills and heroic purges and vomits. Pretend they are something else, advises Hoffmann, and while soothing them with a 'I would not give you such things' mix them up under the appearance of something mild, which they will drink happily as a mere comforting medicine.

Hoffmann's ethical rules enjoin different behaviour to different kinds of patients. With the noble and powerful the physician must be especially careful, for the greater the patient, the greater the reputation of the successful doctor. But the difficulties are correspondingly greater, for the nobility cannot be bullied into taking their medicines and princes will not take being contradicted. Again, the doctor must deceive: 'he who cannot dissimulate cannot cure' is an aphorism to Hoffmann. For example, many of the vilest and commonest medicaments are the most powerful, for God, says Hoffmann, has arranged it so that they are readily available to the poor; but princes expect to be treated with rare and expensive medicines, and when the powers of the viler medicines are needed, they must be mixed with the expensive. (Compare Zerbi's aphorism that expensive medicines are effective by reason of their cost.)

Of all the multitude of pharmaceutical items available to the eighteenth-century doctor – about which Hoffmann grumbled – we may be sure that the opiates and the heroic vomits and purges were indeed powerful drugs. They were also just the kind of internal medicines, as we have seen, that Hoffmann's ethics reserve for the sole use of the learned physician. The physician's monopoly of their use was another strategem for preserving the physicians' common reputation: Hoffmann says so. Prognosis, he says, is even more dangerous with the famous and great than with ordinary patients, but there is one thing of which the physician can be certain. Like everyone else, the noble patient in great pain thinks he is near death; and by the use of opiates the physician is certain to reduce pain. The result is that the patient believes he has been snatched from death and, Hoffmann says, 'the physician unites fame and physician'.[11]

The prudent and political physician was matched by the prudent and political patient, at least in Longolius' *Der Galante Patiente* (1727).[12] The ethos we have met above in relation to physicians supplied the patient also with a set of ethics that directed him on the topics we have seen from the doctor's viewpoint. Longolius had been a medical student at Halle, and must surely have heard Hoffmann's lectures on the Political doctor. His own Political patient acted in a complementary way: he 'dissimulated' in facing pain without change in his bearing or conversation, but told the doctor the truth about his symptoms. He faithfully took his pills (and did not, like others, reserve his ethical behaviour for when the doctor was present). He used tact in changing from one doctor to another (which seems to have happened frequently). The honorarium he gave the doctor was more than was needed to buy a new pair of heels for an old pair of boots, and approximated to those suggested in published figures.[13]

The Physician and the Law

Hoffmann's ideal medical man knew what to do when called on to give evidence in a law court. The rational and erudite physician was an expert in matters of legal importance, such as poisoning, pregnancy, abortion, impotence, infertility, insanity and feigned insanity, contagion and epidemics. Hoffmann gave most of his attention to the lethality of wounds. There was a contemporary controversy over the question of whether the death penalty was justified in cases where the accused had inflicted on the victim a wound that would not have killed a healthy man. But if the victim was in poor health and died as a result of the wound, the wound was thus 'lethal' *per accidens* and not *per se*. The university lawyers of Halle and Erfurt decided that the death penalty was justified on the grounds that there was a cause and effect relationship between the wound and death. Likewise, was a wound (for example a blow to the head) lethal when the victim could have been saved had a surgeon been there (to perform a trepan for example)? In this case the physician, says Hoffmann, is best not to declare on the lethality of the wound, which was ostensibly a medical matter, but to describe the wound and give the secondary causes of death. We can recall that it was in such cases that Hoffmann insisted that it was only the learning of the physician, and not the skill of the surgeon, that could pronounce on the lethality of wounds. But on the boundary between the professions of medicine and law, Hoffmann is more cautious and advises the physician not to step into the territory of the juriconsults. But again, the reward of the doctor who is sagacious in his judgement of the lethality of wounds is an increased reputation, as Hoffmann makes clear.

Hoffmann's physician was doing more than offering technical advice in a process of law. He was sharing in a growing belief that law and medicine had a common concern with *nature*. Natural justice demanded a knowledge of the natural constitution of man, physical as well as moral. These, too, were the concerns of the physician. The 'law of nature and nations' was an Enlightenment synthesis that replaced topics that had been distinct in the seventeenth century. In fact, Hoffmann's *Medicus Politicus,* in explaining how the good, ethical, doctor acts towards different groups of people, is a specialized Natural Law text, for such things are very commonly set out in sections that deal with man's duties to himself and to different groups of other people, such as parents and teachers. We can take as an example the book of M. H. Otto, a colleague of Hoffmann at Halle.[14] The 'law of nature and nations' it describes is, as in Hoffmann's philosophy, an aspect of divine law. It specifies how a man should behave to his fellows, to parents, teachers, his spouse and to his rulers, just as Hoffmann directs his special duties as a physician to various groups of other people. It is wholly drawn from reason, and is Natural in being deduced from the nature of man and of things, again like Hoffmann's Natural Law. And, like Hoffmann's again, the Necessity of natural things arises from their *mechanismus.*[15]

The remainder of this chapter will examine how such a synthesis of 'Natural' topics is represented in Hoffmann's view of the world, and how this in turn shaped the ethics of his *Medicus Politicus.*

Physicians, Philosophies and Religions

The first chapter of the first part of Hoffmann's *Medicus Politicus* is about religion and the medical man. The first rule, the opening words of the work, is 'The doctor should be Christian'. Of course,

Hoffmann meant his kind of Christian. Not only should the doctor have the common Christian virtues of caring for and healing the poor and ill, and of living as well as believing in a Christian life, he should have virtues of the kind of Christian Hoffmann thought was the right kind. Hoffmann was an 'enlightened Pietist'[16] believing that merely to believe the teachings of Christianity and not to lead a matching life was 'practical atheism'. Hoffmann naturally saw himself, as a moderate Pietist, at the centre of Christianity, and those who disagreed with him at one or other extreme. There were firstly 'theoretical atheists', perverse followers of Descartes, and there was Spinoza, who all believed that the world ran like a clock without the continuing providence of God. At another extreme – secondly – were those who practised *enthusiasmus* by which Hoffmann meant those Pietists who claimed inner, personal revelation of God. Related were the Quakers and the neoplatonists who believed that the spirit within them was part of God Himself. All these people (and perhaps he meant Catholics as well) were 'superstitious'. Hoffmann thought that extreme Enthusiasm was the result of an organic disease of the brain.

Hoffmann's intellectual makeup was not shared by everone in Halle. Indeed, those influential in the founding of the university were more markedly Pietist than Hoffmann and sought to staff it with men of their own persuasion. Hoffmann's medical colleague was Georg Ernst Stahl, who as a Pietist made the soul the centre of his medical system in defiance of a wider move – in which Hoffmann shared – towards corpuscular and mechanical interpretations of the body. And from 1715 Stahl was first physician at court and the president of the State *Collegium Medicum* in Berlin. Even Hoffmann's colleagues Alberti and Thomasius, although far from being enthusiastic Pietists, thought that a medical system based on mechanism was untenable.[17]

Hoffmann's account of how his medical system differed from (and was better than) that of Stahl, his tracts on the best means of philosophizing, his notion of the lawfulness of nature and of man, can be seen as a defence of his whole philosophy. The ethical component of this, expressed in the *Medicus Politicus,* was founded in part directly upon his Pietism and partly upon his rationalizing position. In contrast to the enthusiam of the Pietists and the animism of Stahl, Hoffmann thought that he was at the centre of a *rational* Christianity. His ethical doctor stood aloof from disputes about religion and faith (rule two) and instead immersed himself in philosophy and erudition (rules five and six). Religion, philosophy and erudition were not separate issues for Hoffmann but aspects of a Christian view of existence (as they had been, in a different way, for Zerbi). Hoffmann rationally begins his exposition with God, the creator alike of man, medicine, philosophy and the physical world. Philosophy is a gift of God designed for man's perfection, and by it man may – partly from a sensory examination of the physical world – come to an inner conviction of the existence and attributes of the Creator. Many such expositions could have been described in just these words from the middle of the thirteenth century to the late seventeenth. What had changed by the time Hoffmann came to write down his was that the explanation of the nature of the physical world had *changed completely*. And, like that of the medievals, Hoffmann's 'philosophy' was wide and the things within it tightly connected, so much so that they too changed. In more direct terms, the university curriculum, still in the second half of the seventeenth century based on scholastic commentaries on Aristotle, suddenly switched to a wholly new world picture.

Looking at Hoffmann's philosophy can help us to understand how this change came about. Hoffmann's physician, who must also be a philosopher, knows that philosophy is double, physical and moral. The moral part of it, important for ethics, is also double, concerned both with the intellect and the will. That concerned with the will inculcates good actions leading to temporal and eternal tranquillity. Intellectual moral philosophy leads to the recognition of the Law of Nature, the *jus naturae*. Understanding this intellectual part was to understand why actions should be ethically good in relation to the natures of things and people. That is to say, a 'law of nature', conceived in a moral or almost legal sense and based on the *natures* of things, especially man, had been discussed since the Middle Ages, but now things were changing. Natural Law as accepted by the civil lawyers was defined in the *Digest* as the law of nature that made, for example, birds fly, fish swim, and large animals eat smaller. The Catholic reaction to this in the eighteenth century was that as a definition this was too wide and that Natural Law was the collection of precepts, such as the distinction between right and wrong, and a knowledge of Himself, that God had put into every man: it was in his nature.[18] But it was open to Protestants to enlarge upon the Roman Law definition and argue from the natures of animals as parts of Creation to the existence and attributes of God as Creator.

These were in part what Hoffmann was referring to when he says there were, when he was writing, several and contradictory principles of Natural Law. However, Hoffmann has a formula to solve the problem. His first premiss is that the *desiderandum* is human happiness (he means eternal as well as temporal.) This principle contains three laws. The first is 'revere God'. The philosopher rationally fears God (He who made us can as easily destroy us); honours God (as the Creator of the universe); and loves God (who preserves us). All this is clear, continues Hoffmann, from the light of nature, *ex lumine naturae.* Although the context is the moral part of philosophy, because philosophy is a whole, Hoffmann can use its physical aspect: the light of nature illuminates the Law of Nature.

Hoffmann's second law is 'preserve society'. This is the legal rather than the natural aspect of Natural Law and shows clearly how the Enlightened principle crossed earlier boundaries, as we saw in the case of medical jurisprudence. Historians of ideas readily recognize that successful intellectual systems support the existing social order and the two are mutually confirmed. Hoffmann's third law is 'preserve the order of nature'. He means first that man should lead a temperate, natural life and so reach a good age. But the order of nature also concerns all created things: the heat of fire, the qualities of foods and other things that effect us and in which a balance is needed. Here, too, Hoffmann uses physical philosophy to throw the light of nature on the moral aspect of Natural Law. When discussing the laws of motion of Huyghens, Hoffmann regularly uses the term *leges.* In a similar way, Newton's law of gravity is a *lex naturae* which never fails. Indeed, Hoffmann says, every finite entity acts according to certain *leges* imposed by an external cause: God.[19] In his theological tract Hoffmann says that it is in *lege naturae* (and in the Bible and the acts of Christ) that we see the will of God.[20] It may be that Hoffmann wanted to distinguish *lex* in the sense of 'a specific enactment' (the laws of motion and gravity) from *jus,* which is the term he regularly uses for the moral aspect of Natural Law and which might be construed as 'the body of law'. But within his single philosophy, both are attributes of nature and both derive directly from God. Perhaps for Hoffmann *lex* is a particular *jus;* it is clear at all events that Natural Law for Hoffman covered the physical as well as the moral world.

Since for Hoffmann the Law of Nature operates in both the physical and the moral (and so ethical) side of philosophy, we must ask how he saw nature. Hoffmann says the laws of nature are the object of the study, *scientia physica.* The good doctor must also, then, be a *physicus,* who knows the causes and phenomena of nature. The schoolmen would have agreed. But now – and it is tolerably clear that Hoffman had formed his views well before the end of the seventeenth century – the causes are different. What the *physicus* looks at, says Hoffmann, is 'all the machines occurring in the world, or what is the same, universal mechanism'. This *mechanismus* was formed by Hoffmann from what seemed illuminating in the experimental natural philosophy of the second half of the seventeenth century. It seemed to him that Descartes' account of particles in motion was the fundamental revelation of the way things worked; but as a practising Enlightened Pietist he could not follow the Cartesians into their providence-less world of clockwork that no longer needed the attentions of the clockmaker. As a doctor he believed in active powers of matter – drugs were by their nature active – and so could not agree either with his colleague Stahl's animism,[21] or with the particle-to-particle transmission of matter of Descartes. Moreover chemistry, which also seemed to demonstrate the active powers of matter, and which had never been a subject of absorbing concern of the Cartesians, interested Hoffmann deeply. It was 'the soul' of medicine. Indeed, chemistry and laws of motion drawn from mechanics were for Hoffmann the two components of experimental *physica.*

It was just this experimental *physica* that Hoffmann saw as the chief tool of natural knowledge, *scientia physica* (which was the causal rather than descriptive side of the natural part of philosophy). It was only experimental knowledge, thought Hoffmann, that was making progress, and it was this progress that so impressed him. Astronomy, physico-mechanics, anatomy and chemistry seemed to him by about 1700[22] to have left the rest of philosophy behind. Telescopes, microscopes and other instruments, experiment, observation and 'right reason' constitute Hoffmann's royal road from particulars to universals. On 'motion taken from mechanics' Hoffmann cites Leibniz, Wallis, Borelli, Gassendi and others; on general physical principles, Descartes, Du Hamel, Le Grand, Rohault; on particulars, Boyle, Sturm and the periodical literature; and for the proper relationship of natural philosophy to God, he is particularly attracted to English physico-theological works by Derham, Stillingfleet, Matthew Hall, John Ray and Boyle.

Natural Law in the Universities

One obvious name is excluded from this list. Hoffmann only rarely mentions Newton. His ideal erudite doctor would indeed learn English for its learned books, and among them read those of Bacon, the medical writers and those just mentioned; but not

Newton. I want to use the name of Newton here to introduce what I think is a new way of looking at the intellectual background of people like Hoffmann. For Hoffmann it is part of the explanation of his use of Enlightenment reason, in the form of Natural Law, in his religion and ethics.

When Newton came up to Cambridge the textbooks he read in natural philosophy were commentaries on Aristotle's physical works by what are normally called late scholastic commentators, among them Spanish and Portuguese Jesuits. Also available were the standard teaching texts of Dutch authors, popular in mid-century.[23] What the Protestant Dutch and the Jesuits had in common was Aristotle, and those works of his that had formed the basis of teaching natural philosophy in the universities since the middle of the thirteenth century. Comparatively suddenly in Cambridge this natural philosophy vanished and was replaced by one which rested on a mechanical view of the world. Historians have perhaps too readily seen the hand of Newton himself in this change.

If we think of medicine as a university subject, then this change is greater than might first appear. To understand this, we must first explain what the old curriculum was, and how it worked. The intending medical graduate, like everyone else, began his university career with the university arts course. Here he was first taught Aristotle's universal arts of argument, logic, dialect and rhetoric. These were techniques of argument capable of being applied to any of the substantive doctrines that followed. Natural philosophy was, then, a dialectical treatment of the natural world, beginning with the abstract principles of motion in the *Physics* and moving on to disciplines in which these principles were applied to a range of phenomena of increasing complexity in Aristotle's works on generation and corruption, on meteorology, on the heavens and earth, ending with the complex 'biological' topics of the *Parva Naturalia,* perhaps the works on animals and certainly that *On the Soul.*

This course in natural philosophy was paralleled by another in moral philosophy, based on Aristotle's ethics, politics and economics. Aristotle's ethics, a study of the distribution of Good in society, was readily used in a Christian civilization, and must have formed part of the basis of ethics of every learned man (including Zerbi).

The medical course, as a higher faculty, followed on naturally from the topics at the end of the natural philosophy of the arts course. The theory of medicine was essentially Aristotle's physical principles extended, originally by Galen, into the human body. 'Where the philosopher ends, the physician begins' was a common saying.[24] In educational terms medical theory rested on the natural philosophy of the arts course and was unintelligible without it. The erudition by which the physician from before Zerbi's time to the mid-seventeenth century defended his reputation and attacked that of 'quacks' was Galen's Aristotelianized medicine.

We have seen that less than half a century later Hoffmann was also defending his reputation by his erudition, but erudition of a very different kind. What has happened is that the *whole* of the arts course and the *whole* of the medical course have changed together. Their connections were too tight for it to have been otherwise. But what do they still have in common, that makes eighteenth century medicine still dependent on natural philosophy and the arts course?

The answer, I would venture, is Natural Law. Let us first go back to Hoffmann's single, universal philosophy. Its most principal part, he says, is mathematics.[25] For Hoffmann it is mathematics that extends the faculties of the mind into all aspects of the disciplines and arts. In other words, it is a universal mode of arguing that can be applied to all of the substantive disciplines of increasing complexity. Mathematics, then, has precisely the same curricular function as Aristotle's dialectics. Hoffmann is clear on this: true erudition[26] is obtained by 'right reason' which we get from logic. But this is not 'vulgar logic' (by which he means Aristotelian) but from mathematics. The 'proposition' and 'demonstration' involved in this 'logic' are those of geometry (he particularly admires Descartes' 'logic'); and the other parts of mathematics for Hoffmann are doubtless those used in conjunction with the study of motion, from mechanics. When he says *mathesis* is the mother of all the *scientiae,* he is emphasizing its fundamental role as a replacement for Aristotle's dialectic at the beginning of the arts course.

In a similar way, Hoffmann's moral philosophy, to which we have now been introduced, replaces the group of ethical, political and economical works of Aristotle. We have seen that the 'intellectual' part of Hoffmann's moral philosophy rests on the Law of Nature that gives all created things their 'nature', which is also the basis of their natural behaviour, the subject of natural or experimental knowledge.

Chemistry and mechanics are now the substantive *scientiae* to which the universal art of mathematical 'logic' is applied, exactly as the old arts course applied dialectic to physics. And just as the general principles of the old *Physics* were applied in turn to a series of actual physical situations, so Hoffmann's chemistry and mechanics supply the principles of natural phenomena, up to and including life. Medicine, based on these same principles, again follows naturally. The physician starts where the philosopher stops, remarks Hoffmann himself.

So in Hoffmann's case the whole of the Aristotelian apparatus has been removed. Its categorical logic has been replaced by mathematical; the teleology of its final causes has been removed from nature and put into the hands of God; local causes (formal, efficient, material, and form, matter and privation) has been replaced by Natural Law, the law written by God into the 'natures' of things, largely expressible in terms of particles and mathematics. In the history of natural philosophy this is generally called 'mechanism', as indeed Hoffmann himself calls it. (But to his colleagues in Halle, like Otto, mechanism was Natural Necessity, the Natural Law of material action.)

The story of the sources of Hoffmann's medical ethics has become tortuous. To clarify it let us return to the notion of ethics with which my two chapters have been concerned. It is argued that ethics are the rules that give coherence to and characterize a group. They may also contribute to the relative success of the group. For the rules to be effective they must be accepted by the members of the group as indicating proper behaviour, and where the rules include technical knowledge, as in medicine, that knowledge will be taken as true. The question of the actual truth of the knowledge is another and a lesser question. The question, too, of the historical sources of that knowledge is one that should in the first instance be kept separate both from that of truth value and from that of ethical value. Zerbi could take material from the Hippocratic ethical works, from Christianity and from the Aristotelian moral philosophy of the university arts course, believe it, and use it all in a medical ethics which largely functioned in the interests of his group of learned physicians. So with Hoffmann the sources were often very different – a Reformed religion, physical mechanism and Natural Law, but his belief in them was as great as Zerbi's in his sources, and they functioned in the same way in defending Hoffmann's learned medicine.

Natural Law and Religion

This adoption of a new curriculum in a new university is explained in a slightly different way in Thomasius' introduction to Alberti's medical jurisprudence.[27] How is it, he asks rhetorically, that two traditionally separate subjects, law and medicine, have come together in medical jurisprudence? The answer, like Hoffmann's, is that all the disciplines are part of a single body of knowledge and mode of life. The philosophy of the arts course was the basis of this. Not only was it a case of 'where the *physicus* stops the physician begins', but also 'where the ethical and political philosopher stops, the lawyer begins'. In just the same way, says Thomasius, the theologian (and of course he meant his kind of theologian) begins his work with the revealed knowledge of the scriptures where the metaphysician stops. Not your scholastic metaphysician, Thomasius is careful to add, but he who is concerned with natural theology. Thus the natural theology of the metaphysics of the arts course was matched by the natural law of the ethics and natural philosophy. Thomasius' point is that knowledge of all disciplines, including medical jurisprudence, produces a citizen who is watchful over the *salus* – meaning both physical health and religious salvation – of himself and of the body politic. The point for us is that this is another illustration of the total replacement of the late seventeenth century curriculum by one based on a new view of nature.

The novelty of the arrangement is expressed by Thomasius when he observes that in previous centuries the students were given 'insufficient or frankly wrong' doctrines. Thus in physical knowledge excessive respect for authority (says Thomasius) maintained an Aristotelian doctrine or produced a Cartesian, Stoic or Gassendist physics; in ethics and politics, Aristotle has scarcely been replaced. The new knowledge operative in the Halle curriculum was, of course, consistent with the civil and religious life of the community. It was aggressively Protestant. The insufficient or frankly wrong disciplines of medicine and law are attributed by Thomasius to the action of popes who had tried to suppress reason by the use of human authority within the universities. It was for this reason, he said, that medical men stuck to Galen and Hippocrates and the lawyers to Justinian and Canon Law. What made them do so was the seduction of 'good faith'. To have good faith to the old authorities of one's discipline was precisely the plea of the defenders of traditional medicine like Sylvius, Eustachio and Riolan against dangerous neoterics like Vesalius, and by Zerbi in defence of his view of the learned medical tradition. It was (for the opponents of Vesalius) a counter-reformation strategy, conflating medical and religious belief and referring both to a learned and interpretative tradition. As it was the Protestant Paracelsus who was called the *Luther medicorum,* so in anatomy more Protestants than Catholics can be counted among the defenders of Vesalius.

Thomasius took an equally Protestant view of the earlier

literature in medical jurisprudence. The work of Fortunius Fidelis (1603) contained not only ancient doctrine, owing to the 'indolence of the times' as Thomasius called it, but also wrong doctrine because Fidelis was 'an addict of the Pontifical religion and had to repeat the erroneous and false assertions of pontifical law' such as that relating to birth after copulation with demons. Not only were earlier texts vitiated by such 'superstitions', in Thomasius' view, but also by their medical doctrines being traditional (and so by implication Catholic). This was the case with the volumes (1621–52) of the great Zacchias; however, says Thomasius, because Zacchias 'cut much ice', *glaciem hic fregerit,* he should still be read.

For Thomasius, the unsatisfactory state of earlier medical jurisprudence was not only due to a great deal of it being Catholic but to the sects that had sprung up in the disciplines involved. The lawyers were divided into 'glossators' and 'humanists', and the medical men into chemists, dogmatists and empirics (to say nothing of the surgeons, bath-house keepers and midwives whom Thomasius says by their popularity threaten to swamp the learned physician, and against whom, no doubt for the same reason, Hoffmann's ethical code was directed). Now, the tool whereby all this was going to be put right was at root Natural Law. The Cartesians, Gassendists, Stoics and Aristotelians about whom Thomasius grumbled in natural philosophy and the chemists, dogmatists and empirics of the medicine that depended on natural philosophy, were all to be made redundant by the new Rational and Enlightened medicine. Thomasius recommends first a text (of 1614) by that exponent of Natural Law, Rodericus a Castro. This is his *Medicus Politicus,* designed like Hoffmann's later text of the same title, to set out the duties of the physician in his relations with other people. A Castro, from Portugal, was seeking (like Grotius) a code of law that was viable in any religious climate. In seeking a code from what was common to all men rather than from the commands of one system of belief, a Castro found Natural Law useful. In this text a Castro employs a similar technique and dismisses the chemists and other modern sects in favour of a Rational Medicine that appeared to derive from the reason that was common to all men and which was the basis of Natural Law in its legal sense. Thomasius, perhaps not recognizing a Castro's strategy, was puzzled to know whether a Castro was still a Catholic and why he dedicated his book to Lutheran consuls of Hamburg.

Second and more important, Thomasius recommends the medicine of Alberti, for whose book he wrote this introduction.

Alberti joins Natural Law in its legal sense to Rational Philosophy (as the successor of the dialectical arts) and to Natural Philosophy as the foundation of the knowledge of the medical juriconsult (thesis 6).[28]

Conclusion

We have in these two-chapters been concerned with a particular view of ethics, seeing them as a set of rules internal to the group and directed to the behaviour of its members, with results that have an effect on the group as a whole. We have not been concerned, as a moral philosopher might, with the ethical validity of those rules. Indeed, it is consistent with this anthropological, or perhaps better, biological view, to imagine that these rules were not consciously formulated or maintained with ethical ends in mind. They survived because they had the effect, but not the purpose, of ensuring the survival of the group. We need not suppose that this was visible to those who obeyed and enforced the rules.

This way of looking at ethics seems to be justified by the comparison that has been made between Zerbi and Hoffmann. Where their ethics were concerned with the defence of learned and rational medicine – their group at its largest dimension – they were strikingly similar. (Some, but by no means all, of these similarities have been referred to in this chapter.) Where the two sets of ethics differed, it was due to the different circumstances of the two subgroups that contained the two men, pre-Reformation Padua and Pietist Halle. Hoffmann's ethical behaviour to surgeons differed from that of Zerbi because of these local differences. His use of chemistry, his engagement with forensic medicine and above all his use of a natural philosophy based on Natural Necessity and Natural Law, were due to his fighting for learned and rational medicine in new circumstances.

Notes

1. See J. Geyer-Kordesch, 'German medical education in the eighteenth century: the Prussian context and its influence', in W. F. Bynum and Roy Porter, (eds), *William Hunter and the eighteenth-century Medical World* (Cambridge: Cambridge University Press, 1985). I am grateful to Dr Geyer-Kordesch for many instructive sessions on the topic of this chapter. She argues that Georg Ernst Stahl was at Halle from its foundation.
2. This can be compared to the 300 and more in Leiden in 1709. See Geyer-Kordesch (1985) 183.
3. See note 5 below for Hoffmann's collected works. We are here concerned with the *Exercitatio de Optima Philosophandi Ratione* and the *Dissertatio Theologico-Medica de Officio Boni Theologi ex Idea*

Boni Medici, published in the first part of the *Supplementum*, and in particular with the *Medicus Politicus, sive Regulae Prudentiae*, published in the second.

4. The *Collegium Medicum* in Berlin (established in 1685) was the State's executive arm for the control of the medical profession. Frederick William I established much tighter control over the medical profession by setting up the *Collegium Medico-Chirurgicum* in Berlin in 1725. One of his purposes was to ensure a supply of well-trained surgeons for the army. The professional association of surgeons and physicians was of course directly counter to Hoffmann's ethics. See J. Geyer-Kordesch, 'German medical education in the eighteenth century: the Prussian context and its influence', in W. F. Bynum and Roy Porter, (eds), *William Hunter and the Eighteenth-Century Medical World* (Cambridge: Cambridge University Press) 1985, 177–205; 204, and 'Court physicians and state regulation in eighteenth century Prussia: the emergence of medical science and the demystification of the body', in Vivian Nutton, (ed.), *Medicine at the Courts of Europe 1500–1837* (London: Routledge, 1990) 155–81.
5. Hoffmann's pupil and biographer, Schulze (and Hoffmann himself) emphasizes the place of anatomy in Hoffmann's medicine. The bibliography of the collected works is complex. For our purposes we need to note that the life of Hoffmann by J. H. Schulze, *'Commentarius de vitae Friderici Hoffmanni'* prefaces the first of the six volumes, which was published in Geneva in 1748: *Opera Omnia Physico-Medica.* The *Exercitatio de Optima Philosophandi Ratione*, the *Meditationes Theologicae quibus Summa Religionis Christianae breviter et perspicue traditur*, and the *Dissertatio Theologico-Medica de Officio boni Theologi ex idea Boni Medici* are in the *pars prior* of the *Operum Omnium Physici-Medicorum Supplementum in duas partes distribitum* (Geneva: Fratres de Tournes 1749). The tract on the difference between his medicine and Stahl's is in the *secunda pars* of this *Supplementum*, following the *Medicus Politicus*, both with separate pagination.
6. The full title of the work is *Medicus Politicus, sive Regulae Prudentiae secundum quas medicus juvenis studia sua et vitae rationem dirigere debet, si Famam sibi Felicemque Praxin et cito acquirere et conservare cupit.*
7. This section also contains technical medical hints that are ethical in the sense of belonging to one's own medicine.
8. See Geyer-Kordesch's interesting treatment of this question: 'Cultural habits of illness: the enlightened and the pious in eighteenth century Germany' in Roy Porter, (ed.), *Patients and Practitioners. Lay perceptions of Medicine in pre-industrial society* (Cambridge: Cambridge University Press, 1985), 177–204; 182ff.
9. M. Alberti, *Systema Jurisprudentiae Medicae* (vol 1, Halle: 1725) 17.
10. See R. K. French, 'Surgery and scrophula' in C. Lawrence, (ed.), *Medical Theory, Surgical Practice* (London: Routledge, 1992).

11. *et tali in casu Medicus Medico conciliat famam:* part 3, chapter 4, rule 2 (24).
12. Geyer-Kordesch, 'The enlightened and the pious', 184.
13. For Longolius, see Geyer-Kordesch, 'The enlightened and the pious', 184.
14. M. H. Otto, *Elementa Iuris Naturae et Gentium* (Halle: Officina Rengeriana, 1738). Man's duties towards his fellows are laid down at pp. 155ff. The definitions of natural law are on pp. 3ff.
15. Otto (1738) 10, 98. Otto's text is accompanied by postils in German. Thomasius also often taught in German, and Geyer-Kordesch argues that this marks the Enlightenment among the lawyers of Halle.
16. See R. K. French,'Sickness and the soul: Stahl, Hoffman and Sauvages on pathology' in A. Cunningham and R. K. French, *The Medical Enlightenment of the Eighteenth Century* (Cambridge: Cambridge University Press, 1990) 88–110.
17. See the prefaces by Thomsasius and Alberti in Alberti (1725) and note 28 below.
18. J. Hooke, *Religionis Naturalis et Revelatae Principia methodo scholastica digesta, in usum academicae juventutis* (Venice: J-B Pasquali, 1763). Hooke was a professor of theology at the Sorbonne; this is the Italian edition. Natural Law is dealt with on p 198. Hooke's mode of procedure is first to defeat atheism in a dialectical way. The God who thus stands revealed is the author of Natural Law and Hooke is mostly concerned with the argument *down* from God to nature. The Protestant argument in the other direction, from nature to God, is absent.
19. Chapter four of *De Optima Philosophandi Ratione,* 13.
20. *Meditationes Theologicae, quibus Summa Religionis Christianae breviter et perspicue traditur, in Supplementum ... Pars Prima,* first pagination, 61.
21. See note 5 above for Hoffmann's account of the differences between his medicine and that of Stahl.
22. This date is from the Leibniz letters, *Supplementum ...Pars Prima,* first pagination, 49.
23. According to R. H. Kargon, *Atomism in England from Hariot to Newton* (Oxford: Clarendon 1966) 1, Newton's textbook was J. Magirus, *Physiologiae Peripateticae libri sex* (Frankfurt: 1597, Wittenburg: 1609) etc. Magirus draws freely from the Jesuits, the medieval commentators and the neoterics. The only enemy is Ramus: see the 1609 ed., 12, 41. Even more reliant on the Portuguese Jesuits and the commentators is the *Axiomata Philosophica* of D. Sthal, the third edition of which was published in Cambridge in 1645. The Dutch authors, the sudden appearance of whose books probably signals some change in the teaching of natural philosophy in Cambridge in the 1640s, were principally Keckermann, Heereborde and Burgersdijk,

who wrote texts covering all aspects of the arts course.

24. See C. Schmitt, 'Aristotle among the physicians', in A. Wear, R. French and I. Lonie, (eds) *The Medical Renaissance of the Sixteenth Century* (Cambridge: Cambridge University Press, 1985), 1–15; 15.
25. Here Hoffmann is discussing the best way of philosophizing, and is not expressly thinking in medical terms. See note 5 above.
26. *Medicus Politicus:* see note 5 above.
27. Thomasius' preface in Alberti (1725).
28. Alberti (1725) p.10 says rational philosopohy does not include Paracelsus, Fludd, Scaliger, Cardan or van Helmont. Cartesianism, corpuscular philosophy and pre-established harmony bring more pain than light, *nihil lucis, plus crucis,* in medical jurisprudence. Sections 4 to 9 (pp 10–11) say an entirely mechanical or chemical medicine is also unacceptable; and that there are no spirits, auras or vital flames.

7

Infanticide and Medico-legal Ethics in Eighteenth Century Prussia

Johanna Geyer-Kordesch

Introduction

Although professional ethics have a long history, their modern form was a creation of the Enlightenment. Several developments were crucial for this step forward. One of them is the close association of legal thinking with the rise of empiricism in medicine. This important link was forged through a legal practice unique to the German states. The Carolingian code provided the overall framework of civil and criminal law, but its application depended on a referral system of the lower courts to law faculties, and, where required, to medical expertise. All documentation pertaining to a case was sent to trained jurists or medical faculties to seek an opinion. The practice was called *Aktenversendung* and the case review by experts was called a *Consilium.*

Medicine was firmly embedded in this system of supralegal advice since murder, assault, infanticide, paternity, consummation of marriage, poisoning, etc., were dependent on medical fact-finding. Moreover, as natural law theory changed the face of legal thinking, the cases became showpieces of Enlightenment ideology. In other words, case studies contain real indications of cultural change. Embracing the new thus means looking at both cases and their underpinnings in legal and medical theory.

Law and medicine established precedents that were wide-ranging indeed. Both innovations at law and the application of modern empirical methods in medicine are first discernible in cases but reverberate far beyond the case. This is particularly true in how the *Consilia* cases substantiate secular authority in judgements of facts and morals. Without this decisive step toward autonomous and secular professional authority, ethics would have remained within the domain of theology. Autonomous professional ethics were created through natural law theory, legal practice and medical expert witness testimony.

Ethics devolved from the duties and practices of the legal and medical profession do not, however, encompass the whole field of moral judgements. While professional ethics strove to assert their autonomy, they fed into ideological changes of a broader nature. Medico-legal authority was subject and indeed, challenged, by values evolved from the axiomatic use of reason particular to the Enlightenment. Natural law removed socially binding views of right and wrong from theological dictates. This typical and fundamental move toward secularization in the Enlightenment meant that eventually public opinion could exert a unique pressure on decisions made by professionals.

More than in any other period, Enlightenment ideology deregulated the sophistry of casuistic thinking. Casuistic judgements relied on principles of morality clearly defined in scholasticism. Common sense and reason, and indeed, the moral sentiments, were introduced as a better foundation for forming individual and communal judgements. Within this new framework new discussions evolved using the open forum of literary debate and the social mirror of case studies. Thus evaluations and rules applied within the self-defining obligations and duties of the secular professions became subject to larger cultural debate. Such discussions went well beyond the experts. In a tentative look at what may have happened when these extraordinary tensions took hold, this paper will examine infanticide cases, as a good example of an issue dependent on public opinion.

Professional Decorum and Medico-legal Authority

In 1691 Halle was on its way to becoming the central influence on Enlightenment thinking. Christian Thomasius was appointed to the Academy in 1691 before it became the University (in 1694).[1] Thomasius had already made his reputation in opposing orthodox university traditions and was to be of European significance in furthering the social and legal changes engendered through natural law theory.[2] As a member of the Law Faculty he was closely in touch with reform initiatives in medicine, with an anti-mechanist, anti-Cartesian position, influenced by the powerful pietist neo-platonism of his colleague, Georg Ernst Stahl, recently appointed professor of medicine.[3] By 1747 the medico-legal coalition was in place, though Stahl (d.1734) and Thomasius (d.1728) were dead, through the continuity of the publications and teaching of Stahl's successor, Michael Alberti, who had taught on Thomasian ideas, produced several volumes on medico-legal issues and was himself an ardent Stahlian.[4]

The University of Halle was founded in Brandenburg–Prussia's newly acquired province of Magdeburg. It swiftly attracted a juridical faculty toughened in intellectual battles against orthodox opinion. Departure from orthodoxy was an integral part of Prussian statesmanship, now on the verge of more than provincial political power under the Churfurst Frederick William (1620–88). The Prussian state councillors charged with establishing the university were told to spare no expense to acquire the eminent jurist Samuel Stryck (1640–1710), who came to Halle in 1692 with a 'princely salary' from orthodox Wittenberg.[5] His close colleague, in a relationship of creative tension, was Christian Thomasius (1655–1728), whose professorship predated Stryck's (1691) and who filled the post of Director of the University and Professor Primarius after Stryck's death. The other law professors, notably Justus Henning von Böhmer, Johann Peter von Ludewig and Hieronymus Nicolaus Gundling, were also jurists well-known for defending the new emphasis on natural law. The faculty was the largest, the most well-paid and with the highest student members for all faculties inside or outside of Halle.[6] It had close ties with the court in Berlin, but not to the extent of following its directives. This explains the independent weight and influence of its opinions. Here the tail wagged the dog.

In Halle the faculties of theology, law, medicine and philosophy (an innovation) were integrated to an astounding extent, considering the independent intellectualism of their respective members. This was due to Pietism, in its early and most powerful years concerned with innovation and social action rather than any dogmatic appeal.[7] Pietism was at first common to nearly all the teaching body. There was therefore something like a common cause in the university. This readiness for new thinking, coupled with phobia for authority, supported one of the most liberal of university statutes imaginable at Protestant universities.[8]

Liberalism allowed natural law theory, a literature developed previously in Holland, Scotland and England, to become a dominant concern in Halle. The key man responsible was Christian Thomasius who drafted the treatises and popular tracts arguing for secular morals. He defined the conceptual relation between *decorum* and control of the passions (*Affektenlehre*) essential to professional behaviour.[9] In 1705 he published his *Fundamenta juris naturae et gentium* based on the thinking of Hugo Grotius, Samuel Pufendorf and Thomas Hobbes, which he pitted against scholasticism, Aristotelianism and the school of Wittenberg. In challenging these central authorities and championing natural law, Thomasius pushed forward nothing less than a redefinition of the purpose and nature of civil society.

In the broadest terms, natural law theory redefined relations within the community. Thomasius unequivocally separated ethics (*philosophia practica*) from its base in theology.[10] He pushed forward an autonomous ethics of worldly behaviour. He did not deny religious faith, the relevance of the Old and New Testaments, nor the obligation to the Commandments. He did, however, argue that natural law did not reflect the truth of (*Offenbahrungswahrheit*) revelation. Natural law theory was based on the supposition that man's capacity to reason sufficiently equipped him to decide what was good. Goodness in practical terms meant happiness. The German term of the period is 'Glückseligkeit' or 'Eudämonie', a term one dictionary describes in English as 'well-being which consists in well-doing – an activity in accordance with the highest excellence (virtue) attainable by man'.[11] Any Greek residues of pleasure or hedonism are not included. Eudaimonia as a common good, or the common principle on which good is definable, looks toward self-evident truths which are recognizable through reason. The life of the community, including the contribution of the professions, is based on usefulness ('Nützlichkeit'),[12] not on the contemplative ideal of wisdom (*sapientia*). Usefulness and the well-being of a community are the practical aims of all learning and all university teaching.

This casts a new light upon the relation of learning to the professions. The guiding principle is not erudition but applied usefulness. In fact Thomasius goes a step further and calls the learned tradition pedantry.[13] Pedants hand down knowledge for its own sake, while Thomasius wishes to inject 'the critical potential of eclecticism'.[14] Eclecticism means choosing knowledge according to one's assessment of its usefulness, leaving no authority safe.

Dilthey has called the aim of the Protestant educational tradition 'civilizing through learning' ('Versittlichung durch *eruditio*'),[15] but in Thomasius' writings both these terms acquire a new meaning. 'To civilize' does not describe Protestant moral expectations in the tradition of Luther and Melanchthon, but the capacity to represent one's professional status in life in an urbane and worldly sense. This is the meaning of Thomasius' version of *decorum*, namely, the upgrading of the learned professional to a secure place in polite society. It was a new departure and set a new standard for polite conduct apart from (for example) court etiquette. It represented a social category of its own for the professional, competing on home ground with the aristocracy's self-assertion through elaborate social rituals. *Decorum* is thus not a set of moral rules or a strict code of professional conduct, but rather a newly invented way of behaving that anchors the dignity of the learned professional in his deployment of manners, while his professionalism is gauged according to the practical usefulness of what he knows.[16] 'Erudition', in this context, is then not scholarship but evidence of practical competence. The Thomasian emphasis on decorum vests authority in the professional himself, making him, rather than Aristotle, Aquinas, Melanchthon or anyone else, the arbiter of his action.

The great ethical guideline of *honeste vivere, neminem laedere, suum cuique tribuere* (to live honourably, to do harm to no one, to render to each his own)[17] in this view is thus neatly tied to professional competence, guided by the experience only a professional can have. Thomasius' definition of *decorum* as he derived it from natural law theory coincides with these traditional pillars of moral action. His subsuming honour (*honestum*), justice (to each his own = *justum*) and right conduct into the decorum of a separate development of secular professional conduct thus provided the Enlightenment framework for professional ethics.

The concept of *decorum* was complemented by Thomasius' influential writings on the *Affektenlehre*.[18] This 'teaching on the passions' maintained that although men were endowed with reason, the exercise of this capacity alone would not suffice to ensure well-being. Reason was not immune to the action of the will and the passions and therefore it was fundamental to community life to learn to guide and regulate the passions. Passions and feelings were to be finely balanced in accordance with the use of the other faculties (*'Gemüthsruhe'*) . In effect this restrictive cautionary tale on the passions accorded well with *decorum*. Thomasius' view of reason did not endorse its superman qualities, or its splendid isolation, as did Cartesian thinking. The passions were much more central to social conflict than the philosopher's metaphysical invocation of reason. The *Jurisconsultus* Thomasius had certainly not been spared reflection on human emotions: the flourishing passions so much in evidence in the *Consilia* bear him out.

This remarkable but unknown genre of sources bears witness to the social impact of natural law theory and its relation to the development of medical ethics. The genre is that of the *Consilia,* cases in law sent to a faculty for advice.[19] The advice given was based on case documents; legal fact-finding (legal inquisition) and citation of relevant textual authorities in law and medicine. The advice or *Consilium* sent back to the court in closely argued form represented a model for the assessment of the particular issues raised. The *Consilia* were thus judgements for the law courts at one remove. While courts of law in a particular region (for Halle the province of Magdeburg and the Earldom of Mansfeld) were bound to ask the advice of the law faculty, very many of the *Consilia* were sought without such strict necessity. In fact seeking law faculty or medical faculty advice was simply the usual thing to do. Because it was general practice, and the advice covered almost every aspect of civil and criminal litigation, the *Consilia* were interesting to everyone. In respect to Halle, approximately 4,000 of these *Consilia* of the law faculty were published in collections between 1693 and 1749.[20] They had great popular appeal and were written and published in the German vernacular rather than the usual language of the erudite, Latin.

The collections of *Consilia* reached a wide audience because they integrated legal or medical theory with the practical case study. The faculty was consulted for a solution *super casibus dubiis.*[21] In effect this meant that a great many cases were sent to the faculty because there was always something 'dubious' to be found. Since the cases represented problems from every walk of life, they provide a well-documented cross-section of social conflicts. The six volumes of the *System of Medical Jurisprudence* published by Michael Alberti from 1725 to 1747[22] are in line with the *Consilia* of the law faculty. What makes them particularly attractive are the breadth of the medical problems and – in the nature of the genre – the fact that this necessitated finely-reasoned justifications of the medical judgements involved.

This makes them ideal sources for investigating professional medical ethics. Firstly, the medical *Consilia* are about professional opinions, since they represent the views of the elite of the profession. Indeed, in Alberti's *Consilia* one sees him setting the standards of medical professionalism.[23] In the inquisitional documents, on the other hand, one sees the issues society regarded as problematical.[24] One is therefore in a position to observe how the medical profession applies its ethics to the arbitration of social dilemmas.

Secondly, the role of the 'subjects' or 'objects' of the process of professional judgement becomes clearer: one perceives the behaviour of parties in litigation, their view of the problem, that of guilt or innocence, and how opinions are variously overridden or how the solution of the case leads to changes in cultural perceptions. Many of the cases have to do with women, who are definitely not professionals in the sense here described, and this introduces the question of tension between medical ethics and ethics derived from more general social views.

Thirdly, the close ties of the *System of Medical Jurisprudence* to the juridical *Consilia* of the law faculty let one observe the effect of ideological and epistemological changes from a wider perspective. The faculties of law and medicine in Halle pioneered the integration of natural law theory with everyday life in Protestant society. The *Consilia* are a specifically Protestant genre, not to be found in Catholic countries.[25] This underlines their particular relationship with natural law theory and its ability to impose its views about how life should be lived.

The subtext of professional ethics is the control of passions. *The Jurisconsultus* and the physician are invariably faced with the opposite to their self-discipline, expertise and *decorum:* the fear, love, jealousy, despair, exaltation of those whose cases they judge. It is in this arena that we may best grasp the interaction between professional judgements and shifts in perception in the cultural sphere.

One example must suffice to show how medico-legal authority rationalized an underworld with quite different parameters. In an infanticide case of 1732, printed in vol IV of Alberti's *System of Medical Jurisprudence* (1737)[26], repeated questioning of the accused reveals a desperate world of poverty and sexual misery. The implacable legal inquisition usual in criminal cases in effect deprives both the woman and the man, whose child has died, of all dignity. The empiricism required by law and medicine has no obligation to society other than proof. The decorum of the professional demands the assertion of authority, not his understanding dark human pressures to survive. The case history reveals the following: Casha Catherina Turckowa, a mature woman of 30 and a farm labourer, living with a shepherd of 20, gives birth in a stable 'standing over straw and manure while holding onto the stable-partition ... not able to see the child because of the darkness'. She thinks the child did not breathe and wraps it in a green apron. She asks her lover to bury the child. He testifies he found the earth frozen and takes the body to the river in the hope that the child will be swept away and drowned. He is terrified and rides out of town to escape from the situation. A farmer finds the child and legal proceedings begin. The social misery they establish is not uncommon for the eighteenth century sub-culture of farm labour. Casha is 'deflorata' before her first marriage (one illegitimate child), has further children, but her husband dies and she takes her present lover. She is ambivalent about him (he is much younger). He is dishonest with her to the extent that while willing to marry, he has signed up with a military regiment, and, as the pastor of the village testifies, cannot marry without regimental permission (in most cases not forthcoming). The legal inquisition pries the details of coitus from the pair, and the lovers, whose passion for each other does not bear up under the circumstances, launch into mutual recriminations. Pitiless though this seems, the reason is clear: they face criminal charges and the death sentence. The process of law strips A. S. (the lover) and Casha Turckowa of all vestiges of dignity.

The denuding of the social fabric and personal relationships (formidably miserable as it is) does not, however, constitute the object of criminal proceedings. The aim is to trace paternity (thus sexual inquiries) and the circumstances of the infant's death. The case documentation therefore contains the autopsy reports of the city physician and surgeon and the minute post-mortem explanations of whether this was a live-birth or not. Here medical evidence comes into its own and in its thoroughly passionless form makes its case for 'cause of death': a live birth is predicated and death through suffocation determined. Dispassionate scientific observation leads, in this instance and in others, to the juridical solution (conviction). But, as will be discussed below, precisely such pitiless discrepancy between the social situtation of the accused and the workings of the system, eventually leads to changes. Public opinion will side with the 'victim'. Nonetheless this example shows the social dilemma created by secularized professional ethics as they search out 'objective' criteria, and the consequences of professional authority based primarily on fact-finding. In the next section on the modern introduction of medical expert testimony in Michael Alberti's *System of Medical Jurisprudence*, the insufficiencies of social realities are, again, not part of the professional agenda. Empirical authority legitimizes medical action, but does not necessarily encourage understanding social malaise.

If infanticide became a 'privileged crime' at the end of the eighteenth century it was with due regard to 'loss of control' while in pain and degradation, in stark contrast to the proof then possible through medicine's juridical brief as 'expert witness'.

Medical Expert Witness Testimony

'History is a cabinet, wherein one can see everything that happens; all revolutions, eventus rerum, can be seen in it. One finds the Historiam sapientiae et stultitiae; in it can be seen who ruled wisely and who unwisely'. ('Die Historie ist ein Cabinett, darinnen man alles sehen kan was passiret; alle revolutiones, eventus rerum, kan man da sehen. Man findet die Historiam sapientiae et stultitiae; da siehet man, wer weislich und nicht weislich regiret').[27] Nicolaus Gundling (1671–1729), student of Thomasius and fellow professor of law (after 1712), in this quote from his *Discursus Politicus* thus links history with natural science, claiming that practical knowledge for distinguishing the ineffectual and silly from the wise can be found through the empiricism of examples and cases. The case study or example from nature gains a decisive epistemological role.[28] It is the test case or focus for arguments on right behaviour. The Halle faculties in their running war with orthodoxy pressed for the dismantling of traditional authority. In its stead they placed reasoning from experience. Experience was useful because it combined knowledge with great flexibility and choice in its application. Instead of learning from authoritative texts, the faculties in Halle promoted the substitution of learning for and from, or in relation to, the case. The case study exemplified empiricism par excellence. Thus they could argue the relevance of modern observation as the proper authority for professional knowledge. This emphasis on modern knowledge allowed usefulness to appear as a criterion of judgement. What was useful in grasping the practical explication of the case became the right way to approach how to act and what to teach.

Notker Hammerstein in his book *Jus und Historie* (1971) shows that juridical reform in Halle sought the inclusion of precedent case law because the knowledge of cases would undermine the authoritarian use of codified law. *Historie* does not mean what we mean by history, however. It denotes the study of examples in the past (*historia exemplum*), both in law cases and in the general behaviour of individuals (usually heroic) from which one might draw lessons. Johann Peter von Ludewig (1668–1743), a colleague of Stryck and Thomasius, commended the English practice of law because it was most closely tied to argument from cases.[29] A top-quality *Jurisconsultus* combined knowledge of Roman law, the *Carolina* (German law after 1532), and competence in the territorial law cases with the ability to use them as applied to the particular matter in hand. One of the major duties of the faculty of law in

Halle was to provide binding consultation on particular cases. *Jurisconsultus* is then an exact description of what these law faculty members actually practised, namely to serve as an official body of experts for consultation on cases tried by the courts.[30] Thomasius and Stryck approached jurisprudence in view of precisely this focus on the empirical value of the case; the explication of the case showed how law was subject to proof. This proof rested finally upon empirical evidence clearly established through fact-finding.

It was Thomasius and Stryck who brought down witchcraft cases and the use of torture because both these established practices did not rest on evidence of an empirically proven nature (witchcraft), or did not provide empirical evidence (the use of torture as distortive of evidence).[31] The application of the law alone, that is, judging whether someone was guilty because penal law could be invoked (as in witchcraft prosecutions), was not enough. Evidence became primary in a new way. For example, there seemed to be no empirical evidence that witchcraft existed; therefore one had to question whether there ought even to be court trials of these cases. Eventually this led to the complete demise of witchcraft prosecutions.

Medicine was not only influenced, but closely implicated in these changes. If the notion of *decorum* had given the learned physician new scope for a professional authority all his own, that is, one tied to its own expertise rather than to general moral obligations, then the emphasis on empirical knowledge (the interpretation of case histories) enabled the doctor to show his professional expertise as an arbiter of justice, right knowledge, prudence and right judgement.

The 'science' of medicine derives its professional code not from learned physicians not being surgeons, but from their ability to produce a conclusive argument in terms of medical evidence.[32] That evidence had to stand up to the scrutiny of the *Jurisconsultus* of the Stryck-Thomasius mould, and it did.

Symptomatic for this turn of events are the six volumes of medical (forensic) *Consilia* published by Michael Alberti (1682–1757) between 1725 and 1747. The first volume is prefaced by Thomasius. This is hardly coincidence and Alberti follows the full programme of Thomasian epistemological and legal reform. One of the things Alberti makes quite clear in his prefaces to these volumes is the need for unassailable medical evidence. Time and again one finds the *Consilium* of the medical faculty judging the evidence and train of logic of the city physician and surgeon first called to investigate. Alberti's judgements on his colleagues' performance stress one fundamental connection: justice cannot be done unless the physician has the expertise to provide conclusive medical evidence. This medical expertise does not derive from any preconceived monocausal medical theory or metaphysics or philosophy. It is concerned with empirical observation.

> According to Hippocrates ignorance is a bad resource: thus a doctor neglecting his studies is said by the Casuists to sin mortally. So it is lawful to ask from which resources good knowledge is to be drawn. For this reason the doctor should not embrace dubious opinions and should not be open to grave errors; in applying his knowledge to the civil court he should not try philosophical subtleties or tricks, such as, for example, deciding forensic cases by the principles of Cartesian philosophy, of corpuscular philosophy, or of that asylum, the pre-established harmony, which brings more pain than light (*nihil lucis, plus crucis*) by impeding rational judgements and forensic practice.[33]

Good knowledge which leads to justice is that of all the empirical expertise a learned physician can muster. It is directly related to his practical experience, which calls into question authority (ancient or modern) and looks into every medical detail. From reading the *Consilia* one gets the impression that Alberti, a true workaholic, practises what he preaches. Prior medico-legal literature is reviewed, applied as a case demands, judged as to its empirical value, cited as to its ambiguities.[34] Immediate evidence is dealt with in the same manner. The concluding forensic judgement leaves few unresolved questions, and where these remain they are pointed out. Alberti, in effect, creates the link between professionalism, expertise and justice. He also links professionalism and prudence.

Prudence is a key word of the period because it is attached to the early eighteenth century attempt to create cultural demarcations for the professionalized middle class: those who became writers, doctors, lawyers and clergy, in a word, the educated as arbiters of the Enlightenment.[35]

Medical ethics, in its specificity as an ethics for doctors, and not as a subdivision of moral philosophy, springs from the claim that only the competent professional can judge the facts pertaining to the case. Alberti is therefore writing for doctors who want to be professionals, and is showing them how to do it. He is also writing for the *Jurisconsultus* who can incorporate medical expertise into the models for case rulings. The moral aims of justice are therefore directly dependent on doctors. No one else has the competence and the *Consilia* are popular vindications of this ability before a general public.

There is nothing wrong with specifically defining how an abstraction such as justice can be practically arrived at. In seeming to resolve ambiguities, the experts on medical evidence made their knowledge a criterion of justice and conscience. What remained problematical were social issues. The manner in which medical ethics was perceived as coincidental with professional knowledge created the object or subject of that expertise. The demise of witchcraft prosecutions hinged on fact-finding. It was this which exonerated 'victims' who had been previously subject to prosecution based on due process derived from textual authority. Witchcraft had been real on a non-empirical basis, and was now ridiculed on an empirical basis. Infanticide cases, on the other hand, revealed 'victims' who did not benefit from the methods of empirical proof: on the contrary, infanticide became more provable.

Infanticide and Public Opinion

A typical case from the *Consilia* of the sixth volume, published in 1747, recounts the infanticide of an unwed servant girl of 23 years from a village under the jurisdiction of Magdeburg.[36] The case illustrates the basic tensions at play in legal cases prosecuting for sexual offences. Traditional moral views were codified in law. Fornication, concealment of pregnancy and murder were punishable offences.[37] Thus civic virtue could be coerced where it failed to be applied through individual willpower. The agency of control were the courts and the official testimony of those advising them, here the faculties of law and medicine. Both the inquisition protocols and the findings of medical men decided the case. Both were bound by the civic adherence to duty, that is, to *sum up post factum* all empirical evidence. There was very little leeway in this matter, as there would be in the private doctor-patient relationship, where treatment is open to a degree of trial and error. Medical jurisprudence had no alternative but to use exact empirical findings. The most easily verifiable evidence were autopsy reports and these were the core of medical testimony.

Medical testimony on infanticide cases was usually two-tiered: one, the written report on the original autopsy findings by the city physician and a surgeon called in by the court; two, the review of the evidence by the medical faculty. In the 1743 case (published 1747) the autopsy recorded that the child was perfect in body and mature at birth (*partus perfectus et maturus*).[38] The umbilical cord was cut and tied; a fracture of the skull was evident; a contusion visible; there was very little blood left in the body. The autopsy did not seem to the city physician or the surgeon to give conclusive evidence of cause of death, however. Therefore the medical faculty was called upon to give advice.

The *Consilium* of the medical faculty drew on the legal documentation of the entire case, that is, the autopsy and the inquisition protocols.[39] The inquisition protocol in the 1743 case established the following facts: the 23-year-old servant girl gave birth while on the way to the outhouse. The child 'shot out' onto the stone paving of the courtyard. The woman carried the infant to a manure pile and buried it there, hitting it twice with a manure fork. Under questioning she admitted she wanted the child to die. The inquisition established the father to be a Grenadier soldier who admitted he had sexual intercourse with the woman. The medical faculty summed up these facts and reviewed the autopsy report, deciding that the central legal and medical question to be resolved was whether the child had died as a result of its fall to the cobblestones. This was answered in the negative. The contusion was indeed caused by the fall, but the use of violence, as well as putting the child into the manure heap in very cold weather and leaving the umbilical cord unbound until the child was later retrieved by a midwife, was directly instrumental to death. The fact that the mother admitted to an intention to kill and that she abandoned the child (negligence) is emphasized. The *Consilium* adds that there was no melancholia (depression) evident during or after the birth, even though an unassisted birth could cause mental unbalance. The law faculty *Consilium* concurs and the final judgement is death by beheading.

Noticeably absent from the inquisition protocols and the *Consilia* are any indications of empathy with the plight of the woman. The moral integrity of the legal judgement rests its case on the skeletal reduction of the action and intention of the defendant to the facts as they are ascertained by professional inquisition: that of law in the protocols, that of medicine on evidence. The *decorum* of the professions decreed their supportive role in the legal sanctions of the State. In Alberti's *Consilia* the standards of medical authority and integrity take precedence over any inclinations to use medical ambivalence to rescue the ignorant or those caught up in circumstances beyond their control. The judgement is made on the moral assumption – relevant to those judging and those accused – that choice of 'wrong' is a wilful and knowledgeable choice. It was known that soldiers were not allowed to marry; it was morally irrelevant if the woman was not knowledgeable about sexuality.

The *decorum* evolved from natural law theory pertained to a civic order based on honour: as women were without professional status their honour was intricately bound to sexual virtue; the professional man's honour was not sexually defined, but bound instead to the knowledge he applied for the good of society. That these two forms of dignity bridged an abyss that opened ever more widely to reveal socially defined injustice is the most intriguing ethical tale of the latter half of the eighteenth century.

Natural law theory eventually shifted from the Thomasian concern with the good of the community to a contemplation of the 'natural'.[40] The natural is hard to define, but whatever it came to mean, it implied questioning the moral conservatism codified by the State and strengthened scepticism of traditional moral values. In the case cited, the 'natural' view would presently come to emphasize the social pressures on the servant girl and would question the repression by the State of the soldier's 'natural' desire for marriage. Medicine and its ability to intervene would be judged not on its professional authority, but on what this intervention meant when the general public and not the few judge. The ethical dilemma, newly perceived, would be that between the rationale of the professions and the social plight of the mother. To even conceive of the idea of 'victim' requires a great deal of social deliberation on the impact of traditional morality. In a sense this was the 'progress' achieved by Enlightenment scrutiny of civic virtue in its secularized context, a change possible only when the forum of debate widened. Public opinion found a voice when periodicals and treatises took up social questions, as they increasingly did in mid-century.

The crime of infanticide early in the eighteenth century was defined by the legal extension of traditional, religiously reinforced morality. The Carolingian Code (*Constitutio criminalis carolina*) of 1532 remained the general framework for German law well into the eighteenth century and it specified infanticide as murder, but did not lay down exact criteria for its identification.[41] The constitutive elements of the crime of infanticide therefore had to be established by the *Consilia* and the judges themselves. The *Consilia* were often the true guidelines of what constituted crime, since judges deferred to the written advice of the law faculties.

For infanticide to be legally prosecuted a live birth must have taken place.[42] The infant had to be fully developed in all bodily parts and evidence of premeditation to murder established. The concealment of pregnancy was a criminal act. Before 1700 punishment for infanticide was live burial; after 1700 death by the sword.[43] In Prussia, Frederick William I decreed on 3 August, 1720 that infanticide be punished by the woman being sewn into a sack and then drowned (*poena cullei*).[44] This was reinforced in 1723 by a new edict to the same effect.[45] When Frederick the Great came to the throne in 1740 legal punishment in Prussia was reformed.[46] In that year the *poena cullei* was replaced by the milder punishment of beheading. In 1746 the king abolished church punishments (*Kirchenbusze*), in use for sexual failings, and in 1765 the Crown changed course in trying to prevent rather than punish infanticide.[47] This trend toward milder punishment continued, so that in 1790 only seven sentences were carried out for all crimes punishable by death.[48]

The post 1740 changes in criminal law, or rather in the way the State wished criminal offences to be prosecuted, a change in the relationship between society and penal authority, are a result of Enlightenment redefinitions concerning delinquents.[49] These were argued outside the juridical literature in popular writings, in effect realizing what Christian Thomasius had envisioned when he brought the dilemmas of witchcraft prosecutions before a general audience in the German language periodicals he had written and edited earlier in the century.[50]

The moral and ethical debates and the pressure they exercised on public opinion were a result of the hard-won freedom to publish initiated by Thomasius between 1688 and 1690.[51] Open debate in periodicals and in theatre productions gradually prospered under the polemicists of Enlightenment, not least among them G. E. Lessing. By the *Storm and Stress* period of German social criticism (*c.* 1770) infanticide was a preferred topic in the debate on *Menschenliebe* (love of humanity), a more compassionate idea than that conveyed by the drier term human rights. The *Storm and Stress* plays were especially effective.[52]

These emotionally charged plays were tragedies in which women were usually innocent victims to be pitied for the seductive callousness of irresponsible men, themselves the objects of cruel social pressures and self-inflicted moral misjudgements. In these powerful lachrymose inventions the audience got the point if it went away angry and tearful about the injustice of it all. In one play, Johann Michael Reinhold Lenz' *Zerbin*, a wonderful satirical twist lets the hero – who has just ruined the tragic heroine's life by seducing her, falsely promising marriage and leaving her pregnant – teach a hugely popular lecture course on morals and *jus naturae* in Leipzig.[53]

The discrepancy Lenz emphasizes is a crucial one. The early impact of natural law theory rested on social change engineered through a progressive liberal social elite with considerable power of social intervention through the exercise of their profession. Their considerable feat lay in achieving a social consensus in which professionalism arbitrated right and wrong conduct (*Decorum*). The cool authority of *Consilia* judgements created a mirror for the murky violence inherent in village social and sexual relations, themselves following either harsher rules of justice or a fatalistic forgiveness of culprits.[54] By 1770 (the appearance of the *Storm and Stress* movement) the mirror image of social relations perceivable in *Consilia* cases mutated to a stage version before middle-class audiences, with its idealized victims and unhappy villains (distributed along the lines of gender stereotypes).

The ethics of authority, professionalism and natural law theory (and its Thomasian rationale for the control of the passions) had already been established, but this had actually reinforced the dilemma of women and men living outside 'polite society' – domestic servants, poverty-stricken clergy and teachers, dispossessed merchants, apprentices, labourers. Their staged plight, notably the typological young and beautiful victim driven to infanticide (*die schöne Kindesmörderin*) manufactures the social ideal of sensibility, empathy and mercy, which in turn influenced the judiciary. Infanticide ceased to be punished by death not because it was not considered a crime, or because medical evidence did not suffice, but because the judiciary began to engage in explanatory finesse and reintroduced an ambivalence in medical evidence co-equal to the new status of infanticide as a crime of psychological aberration and social desperation. It achieved the status of a 'privileged crime'[55] because polite society's control of the passions could not be envisioned for the plight of the servant girl. Her heroism was measured in her being driven to murder tragically.

These developments show – and this is my point – that no monolithic code of morals or professional ethics exists or can be applied without the sometimes contrapuntal, and often times sensitive balances, of a social order which begins to think about itself in articulate ways. Alberti was right to demand a professionalization of medical evidence. It made the profession come clean on its premises and reasoning. Thomasius was right in demanding a civil and not a religious basis for judicial process. His interpretation of natural law theory opened a role for expert opinion based on the claims of responsible medical knowledge. Medical ethics thus attained a legitimacy of its own. The social mirror of the *Consilia* metamorphosed into the image-focusing mirror of the pamphlet, play and treatise of the late eighteenth century, the political literature in which the humane and the 'natural' determined new discussions.

But what of the passions of the woman driven to infanticide? The *Consilia* cases in Alberti's *System of Medical Jurisprudence* show the desperate, suffocating world of the dispossessed. The impression is not of grand passion, but of ignorance on sexual matters, sex forced on girls, drunkenness or supreme selfishness by men who could escape the consequences.[56] Concealment was paramount in a society where sexuality outside of marriage was regarded as a crime punishable by law. The inquisition protocols show officialdom extracting horrific truths from the desperate victims.

The sexual honour of women was equivalent to the *decorum* so rationally gained by the professional, and this was stripped down fiercely to an unbearable exposure for the woman who so desperately did not want to be pregnant, as the example of the unwed mothers in the *Consilia* show. The dishonoured had no voice in this scheme of things. But a most illuminating defence emerged for which the great educationalist Johann Heinrich Pestalozzi's 1780 treatise on *Law and Infanticide. Truths and Dreams, Research and Images* (published 1783) can be given as a dramatic example.[57]

Pestalozzi had the wonderful gift of spontaneous emotional reaction and he, a product of a small-town Swiss upbringing, rages against the cold crimes of officialdom. 'Straining at gnats and swallowing camels whole is the spirit of the Law and of our Morality, otherwise we would honour humanity more than forced spinsterhood and childlessness, which we seek to buy through the devastation of human lives.'[58]

In sum this quote gives the essence of what morality should be about and what the long debates of the Enlightenment really accomplished when they secularized moral thinking. Pestalozzi in his heated defence makes the point that sexuality is natural to men and women and this is anything but a crime.[59] The criminal and the immoral lies not in sexuality, but in the irresponsible disregard of its consequences. He argues care by the State, not prosecution.[60] He argues dishonesty on the part of parents who disown daughters or force marriages.[61] He argues irresponsibility on the part of the legal profession and men who codify loopholes in marriage contracts.[62] In effect he takes the social structure to task. Such an approach to the reform of moral values is a difficult one and its very scope made new demands on medical and legal ethics.

The crucial development to which Pestalozzi's writings and the agenda of *Storm and Stress* plays point, that of taking up specific social wrongs, focuses the Enlightenment's achievement. Opinions are argued within the public forum. Public opinion, rather than the opinion of professional expertise, now had a distinct influence. At the latter end of the eighteenth century this provided a countervailing force to those obligations and duties developed by the professions. The *decorum* of the professional sphere is necessarily restricted to its authoritative knowledge, as has been shown in this analysis of the early eighteenth century's break with learned tradition and epistemological reliance on the case history. Its *decorum* is self-legitimizing and hierarchical in the sense that it judges and arbitrates the behaviour of its dependents or clients.

The doctor and the lawyer, as I hope I have shown, worked out the parameters of their own values, those of objectivity and reliable knowledge, and they did this specifically within the debate against traditional authority (moral systems), choosing the casuistic flexibility of judgements related to cases. In this sense they asserted their immediate professional independence. The *Consilia* show precisely where and when the medico-legal alliance was consolidated, to forge its influential position which to all intents and purposes created the power of the professions in adjudicating behaviour through sanctions and the power of professional judgement.

Ethics, in the medico-legal sense, are narrow. They affect judgements from within the parameters they have set. On the other hand, they are open to the pressures of public opinion, a development, however, that specifically began with the Enlightenment. After mid-century, professional conduct was dependent on other debates, no longer able to defend its actions on professional merits alone. The abstract, namely natural law theory and the epistemology of Baconian empiricism, needed to be linked with its very human side, the reevaluation of infanticide prosecutions, based on the perception of 'human devastation' to which Pestalozzi's exemplary liberal writings opened the mind.

Notes

1. On the early history of the University of Halle, see: J. Geyer-Kordesch, 'German medical education in the eighteenth century: the Prussian context and its influence', in W. F. Bynum and R. Porter (eds), *William Hunter and the Eighteenth-Century Medical World* (Cambridge: Cambridge University Press, 1985) 185 ff.
2. Assessment of his influence in N. Hammerstein, *Jus und Historie* (Göttingen: Vandenhoeck & Ruprecht, 1972); M. Stolleis (ed.), *Staatsdenker im 17. und 18. Jht,* (Frankfurt am Main: Metzner, 1977); E. Bloch, *Natural Law and Human Dignity* (London: MIT

Press, 1986); R. Lieberwirth, *Christian Thomasius, Sein wissenschaffliches Lebenswerk, Eine Bibliographie* (Weimar: Hans Bohlaus Nachfolger, 1955).

3. The view that Stahl and Thomasius had close ideological ties in respect to medical reform and anti-materialist views is substantiated in my *Habilitationsschrift:* J. Geyer-Kordesch: *Georg Ernst Stahl: Medizin, Pietismus, und Aufklärung in Brandenburg-Preussen* (MS 1988).
4. There is no good monograph on Alberti. For information on his life and work see W. Kaiser and A. Volker, *Michael Alberti* (1682–1757), (Wissentschaftliche Beiträge der Martin-Luther Universität Halle-Wittenberg, Halle, 1982). The assessment of Alberti's position can be established through his writings. For an overview of law and medicine see E. Fischer-Homberger, *Medizin vor Gericht, Gerichtsmedizin von der Renaissance bis zur Aufklärung* (Bern: H. Huber, 1983).
5. N. Hammerstein, *Jus und Historie, Ein Beitrag zur Geschichte des historischen Denkens an den Deutschen Universitäten im späten 17. und im 18. Jahrhundert* (Göttingen, 1972) 156 ff. Herein also the information on the juridical faculty.
6. J. Geyer-Kordesch, 'German Medical Education' 181 ff. Therein comparisons of faculty size and student numbers at German universities. Literature given in notes, *passim.*
7. *Ibid.*, 186 ff.
8. N. Hammerstein, *Jus und Historie* 167.
9. C. Thomasius, *Einleitung zur Vernunfft=Lehre* (Halle, 1691); *Ausübung der Vernunfft=Lehre* (Halle, 1691); *Enleitung zur Sittenlehre* (Halle, 1692); *Ausübung der Sittenlehre* (Halle, 1696); see also: N. Hammerstein, *Jus und Historie,* 72 ff.
10. N. Hammerstein, *Jus und Historie,* 72 ff; also Karl-Heinz Ilting, 'Naturrecht', in O. Brunner, W. Conze, R. Koselleck, *Geschichtlich Grundbegriffe, Historisches Lexikon zur politisch-sozialen Sprache in Deutschland,* (Stuttgart: Klett-Cotta, 1987) Bd. 4, 293.
11. See under: 'Eudaimonia', J. M. Baldwin (ed) *Dictionary of Philosophy and Psychology* (Gloucester, Mass., 1960) vol I 350.
12. On the importance of the concept of 'usefulness' see: W. Schmidt-Biggemann, *Topica Universalis, Eine Modellgeschichte humanistischer und barocker Wissenschaft* (Hamburg: Meiner, 1983) 275 ff; N. Hammerstein, *Jus und Historie,* 73 ff.
13. Most famously in C. Thomasius, *Freymüthige, Lustige und Ernsthaffte, iedoch Vernunfft - und Gesetz-Mäszige Gedancken, oder Monats-Gespräche, über allerhand, fürnehmlich aber Neue Bücher* (Halle, 1690).
14. Schmidt-Biggemann, *Topica Universalis,* 274.
15. N. Hammerstein, *Jus und Historie,* 20.
16. 'Usefulness' is indeed a central concept of secularized ethics, crucial to the Enlightenment recasting of virtue. See: W. Schmidt-

Biggemann, *Topica Universalis* (Hamburg, 1983), 274 ff.

17. Background to this in N. Hammerstein, *Jus und Historie*, 59 ff.
18. *Ibid.*, 67 ff.
19. Schubart-Fikentscher, *Hallesche Spruchpraxis, Consiliensammlungen Hallescher Gelehrter aus dem Anfang des 18. Jahrhunderts* (Weimar: Hermann Bohlaus Nachfolger, 1960). The information on the *Consilia* is taken from Chapter I 'Allgemeine Fragen' of this book.
20. *Ibid.*, 1.
21. *Ibid.*, 4.
22. M. Alberti, *Systema jurisprudentiae medicae, quo casus forenses, a Jctis et medicis decidendi, explicantur omniumque facultatum sententiis confirmatur, in partem dogmaticam et practicam partitum, casibus relationibus, judicis, responsis et defensionibus juridicis et medicis forensibus specialibus illustratum. Halae,* (1725) vol I; vol II, Fulda, (1729); vol III, Schneeberg, (1733); vol IV, Leipzig (1737); vol V, Leipzig (1740); vol VI, Leipzig (1747).
23. See the more detailed treatment of this theme in J. Geyer-Kordesch, 'Natural Law and Medical Ethics in the Eighteenth Century', in B. Baker, D. Porter and R. Porter, *The Codification of Medical Morality*, Vol One: Medical Ethics and Etiquette in the Eighteenth Century, (Dordrecht, Kluwer Academic Publishers, 1993) 123–39.
24. 'Inquisition' here means the written protocols of answers given to questions put to the suspect and the witnesses. These are usually included in the *Consilia* documents which Alberti publishes, although they are not reproduced in full.
25. Schubert-Fikentscher, *Hallesche Spruchpraxis*, 9.
26. M. Alberti, *Jurisprudentia Medicae*, vol IV, (Leipzig: 1737), Casus I: Infanticidum ob neglectum regimen ex frigore, squalore et sufficatione commissum, 1–70.
27. N. Hammerstein *Jus und Historie*, 277; quotes the *Discursus Politicus*, 4; The translation is mine.
28. See my article on: 'Medizinische Fallbeschreibungen und ihre Bedeutung in der Wissensreform des 17. und 18. Jahrhunderts' (Medical case studies and their epistemological role in 17th and 18th century science) in: *Medizin, Gesellschaft und Geschichte*, (Heft 9, 1991), 7–19.
29. N. Hammerstein, *Jus und Historie*, 173.
30. Schubart-Fikentscher, *Hallesche Spruchpraxis*, 16 ff.
31. The Stryck-Thomasius alliance against witchcraft trials is discussed in N. Hammerstein, *Jus und Historie*, 158; the medical side to this is not, and there is still much to be said. The seminal text was *De criminae magiae* in its various editions from 1703 onwards (Halle).
32. See especially the preface to M. Alberti, *Systema jurisprudentiae medicae*, (Tomus III, Schneeberg, 1733).
33. The translation from the Latin was provided by R. French; M. Alberti, *Systema jurisprudentiae medicae*, (Tomus II, Schneeberg, 1733).

34. See, for example Alberti, *Systema jurisprudentiae medicae,* (Halle, 1725), *Praefatio authoris,* but also, in comparison, the *Praefatio* by Thomasius in the same volume.
35. Prudence translates to *Klugheit,* and there is an immense literature in this particular period on wordly behaviour, a sure indication of a shift in behavioural norms. The Thomasian publications already influence this. For example: C. Thomasius, *Kurzer Entwurff der politischen Klugheit, sich selbst und andern in allen menschlichen Gesellschaften wohl zu rathen und zu einer gescheiden conduite zu gelangen* (Frankfurt am Main und Leipzig, 1713).
36. M. Alberti, *Systema completa peractio jurisprudentiae medicae,* (Tomus VI, Leipzig, 1747), 7–14.
37. On the legal side to infanticide prosecutions see: Chapter III: 'Die Rechtsprechung', in W. Wächtershäuser, *Das Verbrechen des Kindesmordes im Zeitalter der Aufklärung,* (Lengerich: Erich Schmidt Verlag, 1973).
38. M. Alberti, *Systema jurisprudentiae medica,* Tomus VI, 8. The following information *passim.*
39. *Ibid.*, 7 ff.
40. The argument 'from nature', is, for example, used substantially by Johann Heinrich Pestalozzi, *Über Gesetzgebung und Kindermord, Wahrheiten und Träume,* (Frankfurt, 1783), especially 31–3 ff.
41. Wächtershäuser, *Das Verbrechen des Kindesmordes,* 59 ff.
42. *Ibid.*, 63 ff.
43. *Ibid.*, 68.
44. *Ibid.*, 69.
45. *Ibid.*, 70.
46. *Ibid.*
47. On the whole issue of penal reform, see: G. Kleinheyer, 'Wandlungen des Deliquentenbildes in den Strafrechtsordnungen des 18. Jahrhunderts', in: B. Fabian, W. Schmidt-Biggemann, R. Vierhaus, *Deutschlands Kulturelle Entfaltung, Die Neubestimmung des Menschen* (München: Kraus International Publications, 1980).
48. *Ibid.*, 238.
49. *Ibid.*, *passim.*
50. See, for example, the selection of Thomasian writings, P. von Düffel (ed.), *Deutsche Schriften* (Stuttgart: Reclam, 1970).
51 *Ibid.*, *Nachwort,* 195 ff.
52. J. M. Ramecker, *Der Kindesmord in der Literatur der Sturm und Drang Periode, Ein Beitrag zur Kultur-und Literaturgeschichte des 18. Jahrhunderts* (Rotterdam: Nijgh & van Ditmar, 1927). This contains a bibliography on the *Storm and Stress* period.
53. *Ibid.*, 186.
54. See, for example, R. Schulte, 'Kindesmörderinnen auf dem Lande', in H. Medick and D. Sabean, *Emotionen und Materielle Interessen* (Göttingen: Vandenhoeck & Ruprecht, 1984). Schulte's article,

however, deals only with the late nineteenth century. One would have to assume that things did not change much.

55. W. Wächtershäuser, *Das Verbrechen des Kindesmordes,* 146 ff.
56. M. Alberti, *Systema jurisprudentiae medicae,* (1727–47): All volumes contain infanticide cases. They are amongst the predominant subject matter treated. In reading through them, one is impressed by the unedifying lack of responsiblity on the part of the male seducer and the lack of any prosecution under the criminal offence of fornication.
57. J. H. Pestalozzi, *Über Gesetzgebung und Kindermord, Wahrheiten und Träume, Nachforschungen und Bilder,* (written 1780; published 1783), in: A. Buchenau, E. Spranger, H. Stettbacher (eds), J. H. Pestalozzi, *Samtliche Werke* (Berlin 1927–52) Bd. 9, Zürich, 1956.
58. *Ibid.,* 53.
59. *Ibid.,* 29 ff.
60. *Ibid.,* 28 ff.
61. *Ibid.,* 18 ff.
62. *Ibid.,* 15.

8

The Ethical Discourse on Animal Experimentation, 1650–1900

Andreas-Holger Maehle

Introduction

The current interest in the ethics of animal experimentation has obviously stimulated historical research on this subject. Following the pioneer studies of Hubert Bretschneider (1962) and Richard D. French (1975)[1], historians have mainly focused on the emergence of anti-vivisection movements in Western countries during the late nineteenth and early twentieth centuries. Britain, in particular, which in 1876 enacted the world's first law regulating experiments on living animals, has been studied in considerable detail in this respect.[2] By way of contrast, publications on moral attitudes towards animal experimentation before about 1850 have been limited to selected groups or single persons, such as to the first Fellows of the Royal Society[3] and the Schaffhausen school of physicians[4] in the seventeenth century, or to British men of letters, such as Pope and Johnson[5], and the German writer Christlob Mylius[6] in the eighteenth century. Due to these different states of research it has hitherto been difficult to reconstruct the general development of the 'vivisection controversy' from its very beginnings in the seventeenth up to its culmination in the last decades of the nineteenth century. This chapter chiefly summarizes the main results of a more comprehensive study on scientific and ethical debates about animal experimentation before 1800.[7] Proceeding from the first controversies, continuity and change of ideas in the ethical discourse on animal experimentation are traced to the end of the nineteenth century. Special attention is paid to the influence of theological and philosophical concepts and of social connotations.

Vivisection and Cruelty: the Birth of a Moral Issue

As it is well-known, the history of modern animal experimentation began with a revival of Galenic vivisection[8] in the Renaissance. It was particularly Galen's *On Anatomical Procedures,* which had become available in Greek through the *Editio Aldina* of his works in 1525 and in a Latin translation by Winther von Andernach in 1531, that served as a source of descriptions of vivisectional techniques. Andreas Vesalius (1514–64) and Realdo Colombo (1516–59) both included protocols of their repetitions of Galen's animal vivisections in their own anatomical works.[9] Only the cutting of a *living* animal, they stressed, could show the *functions* of the body and its single organs.[10] This notion of the specific advantage of studying living animals – originally pointed out by Galen himself [11] – soon found its way into anatomical and medical text books of the seventeenth century, becoming a scientific standard argument in favour of vivisection. Frequently it was accompanied by a strong condemnation of *human* vivisection: the ancient Alexandrian physicians Herophilos and Erasistratus (both 3rd century BC) were supposed to have actually performed vivisections on convicted criminals. Moreover, there were persistent rumours that Vesalius and Berengario da Carpi (*c.* 1460–1530) had dissected patients who had still been alive. From the sixteenth century onwards a lot of medical authors, for example Colombo, Jean Riolan jr. (1580–1657), Marco Aurelio Severino (1580–1656), Francis Glisson (1597–1677), Hermann Conring (1606–81), Ysbrand van Diemerbroeck (1609–74) and Philippe Verheyen (1648–1710), unanimously rejected these vivisections of human beings as a horrible crime and deadly sin. But simultaneously they advocated or practised *animal* vivisection as a morally acceptable alternative in order to study the bodily functions according to 'Galen's example'.[12]

Thus with regard to the ethics of vivisection, animals were assigned to the part of a less valuable substitute of man, which might be sacrificed for the sake of physiological knowledge. One has not to look far to find the theological and philosophical basis for this early attitude towards animal experimentation. As Keith Thomas has shown in detail, many contemporary theologians confirmed man's right to make use of the animal world. Irrespective of their denomination, they chiefly pointed to God's grant of dominion to man according to *Genesis* 1:26,28 and to its renewal after the Flood – now including the right to kill animals for food –

according to *Genesis* 9:2–3. The use of animals in scientific experiments could well be justified with this God-given right of dominion, all the more since science was generally expected to strengthen man's control of nature for his benefit.[13] This Judaeo-Christian anthropocentrism was furthermore supported by the very similar Aristotelian view of man's relationship to animals as expressed in the *Politics* and *Physics*. The Neapolitan anatomist and surgeon Severino, for instance, in 1645 justified his animal vivisections with the authority of Aristotle's statement that animals existed for the sake of man.[14] Finally, the seventeenth-century school of natural right, represented by Hugo Grotius (1583–1645), Samuel von Pufendorf (1632–94) and Christian Thomasius (1655–1728), enforced such anthropocentrism. It was a doctrine of this school that law had developed within a community of *rational* beings. Animals, being regarded as irrational creatures, did not fall within the system of natural right. Pufendorf, especially, elaborated this view in his influential *De jure naturae et gentium* (1672), teaching that man had no legal or contractual obligations towards animals and lived in a natural, permanent state of war with them. Therefore it was allowed to hurt or kill animals – just as an enemy – in one's own interest.[15] Against this general background Isaac Barrow's often-quoted verdict on animal vivisection, pronounced in an academic speech at Cambridge in the 1650s, may well be taken as emblematic for contemporary attitudes:

> O innocentissimam crudelitatem, et feritatem facile excusandam![16]

Yet, the belief in the scientific value and moral admissibility of vivisection occasionally contrasted with utterances of compassion by the experimentalists themselves. Colombo for example, in describing his vivisections, spoke of the 'poor' or 'unhappy dog', correcting himself in one breath, 'or rather the happy dog, because he affords to us a sight suitable for acquiring knowledge of the most beautiful things'.[17] Or, Thomas Bartholinus (1616–80), in a defence of his discovery of the lymphatic vessels, asserted that vivisection was the only way to study the highly important flow of the body fluids, admitting in the same context that he was 'prone to compassion' and therefore used strangled animals whenever possible.[18] Similar signs of ambivalence to animal experiments have been traced in letters or published writings of other contemporary scientists, such as Robert Boyle (1627–91), Robert Hooke (1635–1703), and Niels Stensen (1638–86).[19] They must not be interpreted, however, as expressions of very serious moral concern. Remarks of this kind were dropped rather incidentally, and the extent of the experimental work of the quoted scientists makes clear that their compassion with suffering animals cannot have been a major obstacle to them. One has to consider here, too, that sufficiently effective anaesthetics were unknown until the middle of the nineteenth century and that signs of intense pain of vivisected animals could hardly be overlooked.[20] Still, in the middle of the seventeenth century the first indications for actual moral criticism of animal vivisection can be found. In his work *Zootomia Democritaea* (1645) Severino vaguely referred to critics of vivisection who agreed with the teachings of Pythagoras (6th century BC) and his follower Porphyrios (*c.* 232–304) that it was a sin to cut any living brute. Moreover it was regarded as 'impious to destroy what God has created'.[21] Similar allusions to Pythagorean or neo-Platonist views on man's right treatment of animals can be discerned in later comments on vivisection by Bartholinus[22] and by the Helmstedt anatomist and surgeon Lorenz Heister (1683–1758). The latter suspected, in 1728, that the 'calumniators' (i. e. critics) were 'disciples of the Pythagorean school' who feared to torture the soul of a relative or friend 'because of some kind of metempsychosis'.[23] Obviously, an early moral argument against animal vivisection was based on a belief in the transmigration of souls: a reincarnated human soul might be affected. This finding matches with the observations of Narhar K. Gharpure and K. Thomas that vegetarian sects in seventeenth-century Britain, such as the Tryonists, were influenced by Pythagorean thought, and that the doctrine of metempsychosis is traceable both in the writings of contemporary English Platonists and in popular superstitions.[24] To the educated public Pythagoras' objections to the slaughtering of animals – based on his belief in transmigration of souls – became widely known through respective passages in Ovid's *Metamorphoses*.[25] Alexander Pope (1688–1744), for instance, quoted them in an essay against cruelty to animals, which he published in the *Guardian* in 1713.[26] Moreover, attention to the topic of metempsychosis was evoked by reports of travellers to India, who described the corresponding doctrine in Brahmanism.[27] Still, serious belief in transmigration of souls seems to have been uncommon in Western Europe.[28] As a German philosophical commentator wrote in 1709, objections to animal vivisection because of the Pythagorean or Brahman doctrines of metempsychosis were 'based on a false presupposition, the absurdity of which everyone with clear understanding easily grasps'.[29]

Another moral argument against vivisection, which also appeared in the middle of the seventeenth century, was derived from a much more widely held belief. It was formulated in 1653 by the Paris anatomist Jean Riolan jr., who in his old age had become an adversary of animal vivisection both for scientific and moral reasons. His scientific objections referred to the problem of transferability from animal to man and to artificial conditions produced in vivisected animals by the severe woundings.[30] His moral criticism is evident from a polemic against Bartholinus' animal vivisections:

> Believe me, this anatomy of living animals is similar to the slaughtering of living animals as it is performed by the butchers. Encouraged through this kind of work, they do not hesitate to cut the throat of living human beings for an unimportant reason. In the same way anatomists who are accustomed to dissections of living animals will be ready to open secietly moribund, but still living, human beings – as if they were dead – in order to find those things in man which they had looked for in living animals. For this reason I hate this far too curious anatomy and its researchers and followers.[31]

Riolan's apprehension that animal experiments would result in human experimentation was obviously based on the idea that cruelty to animals would lead to cruelty to human beings. In his time this general idea was already an old one. As has been demonstrated by John Passmore, in the history of Christian attitudes to animals it can be traced back at least to the teachings of Thomas Aquinas (*c.* 1225–74).[32] Moreover, the belief that the killing of animals brutalizes man had already been expressed in the vegetarian writings of Plutarch (*c.* 50–125) and Porphyrios[33] as well as in the passages on Pythagoras in Ovid's *Metamorphoses.*[34] In the seventeenth and eighteenth centuries the butcher was frequently quoted as a typical example of a brutalized person.[35] The idea that physicians experimenting on animals – the so-called 'vivisectors' – were a potential danger to their patients was to pervade the ethical discourse on vivisection in the whole eighteenth and nineteenth centuries.[36]

Both seventeenth-century arguments against animal experimentation – that based on the belief in metempsychosis and that resulting from a fear of brutalization – were essentially anthropocentric. It was not the suffering of experimental animals as such that gave rise to concern, but the possible torments of a reincarnated human soul or the supposed negative effects on the moral standards of the experimenting physician. Anthropocentrism, of course, was also a characteristic of moral justifications by 'vivisectors', which too can be found for the first time around 1650.

Severino, for example, pointed to the acquisition of scientific knowledge by means of vivisection. Simultaneously taking advantage of the authority of classical authors, he appealed to Democritus, who (as the legend told) had explained to Hippocrates that he dissected animals not because he hated the works of God, but because he inquired into the nature and seat of the bile. In Severino's eyes, animal vivisection was, therefore, both an honourable and a useful work.[37] Both the argument of gaining knowledge and the argument of authority, were frequently used by seventeenth-century experimentalists. As for the former, Gaspare Aselli's discovery of the mesenteric chyle vessels (1627), William Harvey's demonstration of the circulation of the blood (1628), Jean Pecquet's finding of the thoracic duct (1651) and the first descriptions of the lymphatic vessels by Bartholinus and Olof Rudbeck (1653)[38] became examples of the success of animal vivisection, which were quoted in the second half of the seventeenth century in an almost stereotyped manner.[39] As for the latter argument, besides Democritus and Hippocrates, Aristotle and Galen were often referred to as pioneers of animal dissection and vivisection, respectively.[40] Yet it cannot always be discerned clearly, whether these two arguments were intended as scientific or as *moral* justifications. An unmistakable early moral justification of animal experimentation can be traced in the toxicological writings of the Schaffhausen physician Johann Jakob Wepfer (1620–95). Having poisoned and vivisected animals in order to study the effects of various drugs and minerals[41], Wepfer was confronted with the charge of cruelty. Responding to this he pointed to the importance of his experimental results for the diagnosis and treatment of poisonings in man, i.e., he used the argument of *medical utility*.[42] Moreover, he employed a so-called *tu quoque*-argument: The critics themselves, he stated, were not reluctant to 'fill their stomach with beef, veal, lamb, fish and the like almost every day'.[43] In other words, if slaughtering was seen as morally acceptable, animal experimentation had to be permitted, too.

These two seventeenth-century arguments in defence of animal experiments – medical utility and the accepted use of animals for other purposes, such as food production – were frequently repeated by scientists throughout the next two centuries.[44] In contrast to this, a third argument in favour, which also emerged before 1700, proved to be less persistent, for it grew out of a passing intellectual movement: the *physicotheological argument*. Malcolm R. Oster has recently shown that Robert Boyle regarded his animal experiments as ethically sanctioned, since this sort of scientific activity 'necessitated, in return, respect for the created order as a "Holy Book"'.[45] As an explicit moral justification the physicotheological argument was employed by Boyle's contemporary Thomas Willis (1621–75). In the dedication of his *Cerebri anatome* (1664), addressed to Gilbert Sheldon (1598–1677), the Archbishop of Canterbury, Willis expressed his hope that he had 'justly sacrificed' some 'hecatombs of almost every sort of animals' for his zootomical studies. The study of the laws of nature, he asserted, was like reading God's words 'from another tablet and larger bibles': there was no page which did not preach power, grace, wisdom, and faithfulness of its author, i.e. the Creator.[46]

It seems to have been customary among anatomists of the later seventeenth and early eighteenth centuries to justify the dissection of *human corpses* by referring to its theological value. Using the design argument, they emphasized that the appropriate structures of the body were a strong proof for the existence and wisdom of God.[47] Obviously, the physicotheological justification of animal vivisection was an extension of this line of reasoning. This is particularly substantiated by an hitherto neglected early-eighteenth-century disputation, which – very probably for the first time – *exclusively* dealt with the morality of vivisection. It was presented to the Leipzig philosophical faculty in 1709.[48] Defending the current practice of vivisecting animals, its author Christian Sigismund Wolff, a medical student and Master of Arts, used two basic arguments: medical utility and theological value. With regard to the former he quoted contemporary examples from physiological animal experimentation in the fields of blood circulation and lymphatic absorption.[49] As for the latter, he referred to physicotheological writings by Friedrich Hoffmann (1660–1742), Georg Albrecht Hamberger (1662–1716) and Johann Friedrich Wucherer (1682–1737), which demonstrated the existence and attributes of God from the anatomy of the human body. If the dissection of *corpses* revealed 'God's power and wisdom', Wolff argued, vivisection of animals could surely accomplish the same or even more, since it disclosed the wonders of the *living* body.[50] Though this physicotheological argument in favour of animal vivisection seems to have still been popular in the 1740s[51], it was already attacked at that time.[52] Due to the general decline of physicotheology in the nineteenth century this kind of argument finally sank into oblivion. At the height of the 'vivisection controversy' in the 1870s and 1880s only weak reminiscences to it are traceable, such as when the Breslau physiologist Rudolf Heidenhain (1834–97) spoke of 'religious' feelings which overcame scientists in recognizing the perfect functions of an organ.[53]

If one surveys the attitudes and arguments described above with respect to animal experimentation from the sixteenth to the early eighteenth century, one can say that vivisection started to become a moral issue around 1650. The first controversial statements concerning the morality of animal vivisection chiefly occurred within medical circles. This is hardly surprising, for in this period vivisections were often carried out by anatomists at the universities.[54] Yet, those animal experiments which were performed at the Royal Society in London, and published in its *Philosophical Transactions,* became known to a wider educated public, as is evident from literary responses to these experiments. Writers such as Samuel Butler (1612–80), Thomas Shadwell (*c.* 1641–92), Thomas Brown (1663–1704), and Jonathan Swift (1667–1745) established and kept up a literary genre which may be called 'virtuoso-satire'. It generally derided all scientific endeavours of the early Fellows of the Royal Society (the so-called virtuosi) including their physiological and toxicological experiments on animals. A closer look at these satires reveals a remarkable change in their content. In the beginning, i.e. from about 1660 until 1700, only the alleged uselessness of animal experiments was the target of criticism: the experimenting virtuosi were described as debasing their talents in useless trivialities instead of applying themselves to acquire practical and useful knowledge. After 1700, however, this criticism enlarged. Some of the satirists, such as Susanna Centlivre (1669–1723), Joseph Addison (1672–1719), and Mark Akenside (1721–70), in addition 'discovered' the aspect of cruelty in animal experimentation. Also the apprehension that vivisection of animals would result in human vivisection now became a theme of satire.[55] Thus, compared to medical men, there seems to have been a time lag of roughly fifty years in the general educated public, until animal experiments were recognized as a morally relevant issue. Obviously, the method of experimenting on animals needed a certain level of dissemination, before the public became aware of its inherent ethical problems. Yet, changes in the general view of the man-animal relationship have to be considered here, too. Such changes and their reflection in further comments on the ethics of animal experimentation will be discussed in the following section.

Man's Relationship to Animals and the Ethics of Animal Experimentation: Changing Views

During the eighteenth century theological and philosophical views of the man-animal relationship underwent some important changes. There was still a broad consensus that man – being God's steward on earth – was allowed to kill animals for food and clothes, to destroy them if they were harmful or dangerous, and to make use of their capacity for work. Yet, wanton killing of animals and any sort of cruelty to them increasingly came under attack.[56] The reasons which were given here belonged to such different fields as biblical exegesis and Christian morals, animal psychology, and the theory of natural rights.

From the later seventeenth century onwards roughness and cruelty to animals were censured on the basis of scriptural passages which obviously demanded a considerate treatment of the 'brute creation'. Though this kind of argument is particularly prominent in writings of Protestant clergymen, it can also be found among authors dealing with natural right or moral philosophy. The most frequently quoted text was *Proverbs* 12:10, which teaches that 'a righteous man regardeth the life of his beast'. Several other passages from the Old Testament were interpreted in the same sense, for example, the command to rest on the Sabbath for both man and his cattle (*Exodus* 20:10 and 23:12, *Deuteronomy* 5:14) or the precept not to muzzle the ox that treads out the corn (*Deuteronomy* 22:6–7). The censure of Balaam, who had beaten his ass (*Numbers* 22:28–30), was seen as an unmistakable sign of God's care for animals. On these grounds callousness towards animal suffering was also regarded as contradictory to the divine principle of grace and mercy. Finally, based on the old belief that cruelty to animals would lead to cruelty to man, the maltreatment of animals was taken as an indirect offence against Christian morals, because it might prepare the way for a violation of the command of charity.[57] In the second half of the eighteenth century these thoughts were also preached from the pulpit, for instance by the Leipzig theologian Christian Gottlieb Jöcher (1694–1758) and by James Granger (1723–76), the vicar of Shiplake, Oxfordshire.[58] Towards the end of the century Thomas Young (1772–1835), a Fellow of Trinity College Cambridge, brought this theologically based argument against cruelty to its perfection: in his *Essay on Humanity to Animals* (1798) he cited and interpreted at length no less than nine pertinent scriptural passages in order to censure about fifteen common sorts of cruelty to animals.[59]

Another argument for the careful treatment of animals arose, after the middle of the eighteenth century, from debates on the problem of animal souls. Discussions on this subject had above all been provoked by the radical Cartesian doctrine that animals were soulless, unfeeling machines or automata.[60] A crucial point here was the question of pain. Though René Descartes (1596–1650) himself had *not* held the view that animals were absolutely insensitive to pain[61], some of his followers, such as the Oratorian Father Nicolas Malebranche (1638–1715) and the Jansenist Antoine Arnauld (1612–94), had propagated this opinion.[62] Several eighteenth-century critics, such as the Leipzig professor of philosophy and physics Johann Heinrich Winkler (1703–70) or the British clergymen John Hildrop (d. 1756) and Richard Dean (*c.* 1727–78), did not only try to refute the Cartesian 'beast-machine' theory and to find proofs for the existence of sensitive, more or less rational, and even immortal souls in animals.[63] Going beyond this chiefly theoretical level of dispute, they also drew ethical conclusions. Winkler argued that, since animals owned sensitive souls, no reason could be given why it should be allowed to torment them. Pain was imperfection *per se.* Only the aspect of perfection, however, would lead to real pleasure and happiness.[64] Hildrop, believing in rational, immaterial and immortal animal souls, thought that a rough treatment of the 'innocent unhappy Creatures' would mean 'a Breach of natural Justice'.[65] And Dean, taking the same view on animal souls, emphasized that sensibility and intelligence entitled animals to considerate treatment by man, just as their miseries gave them a claim 'to some Returns from a just and benevolent Being, in another State'.[66] As in the case of the biblical argument against cruelty to animals, the argument based on the existence of animal souls was fully developed in the last decade of the eighteenth century. In 1791, the Danish Protestant clergyman Lauritz Smith (1754–94) published a comprehensive book on the *Nature and Destination of Animals and Man's Duties towards Animals.*[67] For the most part it dealt with the mental faculties of animals, although its declared purpose was not an exhaustive discussion of the question of animal souls, but to bring 'alleviation to the brute creation which is groaning in its sufferings'.[68] Similarly, in 1799, the German lawyer Johann Friedrich Ludwig Volckmann (1757–1815), who knew and cited Smith's work, tried to demonstrate in detail that animals owned 'memory, phantasy, moral sense', and some degree of 'rationality', in order to convince his readers that such creatures had to be treated carefully. Volckmann clearly expressed the idea behind this argument. If man took less pride in himself and showed a higher esteem for the talents of animals, he would abstain from cruelty towards them.[69]

The argument that the souls of animals were similar to those of human beings was supported by the philosophical concept of the Great Chain of Being, which was popular and widely accepted in the eighteenth century.[70] The idea that all creatures were closely linked with each other – like the segments of a chain – challenged the view particularly held by the Roman Catholic Church[71] that there was a gap between man as the only being with a rational soul and the realm of irrational animals. Moreover, the metaphor of a chain was often used in exchange with that of a 'scale' of all beings, which ascended from the lower to the higher animals and, via man, up to the angels. Though hierarchically structured and thus essentially anthropocentric, it implied that there were only gradual differences between the creatures, which might be very small in neighbouring species. Several authors, in the second half of the eighteenth century, such as Hildrop and his colleague Reverend Humphrey Primatt, or the English writer and politician Soame Jenyns (1704–87), applied the concept of a chain or scale of beings to the problem of animal souls. Following the principle of continuity inherent in this concept, they emphasized that animals were also sensitive to pain and owned certain degrees of intellect. These faculties, in turn, entitled animals to considerate treatment by man.[72]

Finally, the doctrine of the school of natural right that a legal relationship between human beings and animals did not exist was qualified or even abandoned in the course of the eighteenth century. In principle, this happened in two ways. Either *indirect* obligations towards animals were constructed on the basis of direct duties to God, to other human beings or to oneself; or animal rights – by analogy to human rights – were conceded, the consequence being *direct* obligations towards animals. Whereas the latter development took place mainly in the 1770s and 1780s, the former had already started in the early eighteenth century.

In 1722, Siegmund Jakob Apinus (1693–1732), professor of logic and metaphysics at the Nuremberg Gymnasium, published his Altdorf dissertation on a problem of natural right, discussing the question *whether it is allowed to mutilate the bodies of animals.* Though he chiefly dealt with the moral admissibility of docking in dogs (which he denied), he also introduced some important ideas concerning man's general rights over animals. Apinus agreed with the doctrine of natural right that there was no contractual relationship, which might involve direct human obligations to animals. But he stressed that animals were objects of man's duties to God. These duties included the 'conservation of animals' ('brutorum conservatio') and respect for God's 'direction of animals to their purposes' ('directio brutorum ad suos fines'). According to the first principle it was man's duty to care for domestic animals and to abstain from killing or hurting animals without necessity; and according to the second one, it was forbidden to mutilate an animal, for this would mean a disregard for its God-given design.[73] Apinus thus constructed indirect obligations to animals which resulted from direct obligations to God. About thirty years later David Hume (1711–76), in his *Essay Concerning the Principles of Morals* (1751), brought forward another concept of indirect obligation. He too denied that man and animals could form a 'society', because this would presuppose 'a degree of equality'. Animals, however, were far inferior to human beings, both physically and mentally. Yet, man 'should be bound by, the laws of humanity, to give gentle usage to these creatures'.[74] Thus Hume advanced an obligation to animals which was essentially a consequence of direct duties within the human community. Following a similar line of reasoning Immanuel Kant (1724–1804) finally stated in his *Metaphysics of Morals* (1797) that a considerate treatment of animals was nothing else but 'man's duty to himself'. In Kant's view, a legal relationship involving direct mutual obligations could exist only between rational, i.e. human, beings. There was, however, an indirect obligation to abstain from violence and cruelty to animals, because man's compassion for suffering human beings might be weakened and gradually obliterated.[75] Evidently, Kant's concept of human duties to animals was determined by the old, anthropocentric idea that cruelty to animals would result in cruelty to men. Animal suffering *as such* was not morally relevant here, but only the effects of cruelty on human morality.

The hitherto described concepts of indirect obligation more or less restricted human rights over animals compared to Pufendorf's 'state of war'-view[76] of the man-animal relationship. Still, the basic doctrine of the school of natural right that animals were creatures without rights remained undisputed or was even confirmed in these concepts. Yet, towards the end of the eighteenth century some thinkers broke with this doctrine and stated the existence of animal rights.

A first step in this direction was made by Charles Bonnet (1720–93) in his *La palingénésie philosophique* (1769). He based his considerations on the view that a divine order existed in nature and that the purpose of this order was the greatest possible happiness 'of sentient and of thinking beings'. Because of this, moral behaviour had to aim at a maximum of conformity with this order. It was, therefore, an offence against the laws of morality, Bonnet stated, if man treated 'a sentient being as if it was insensible' or 'an animal like a pebble-stone'. Accordingly, he demanded that the 'natural laws' should not only rule the interrelations between human beings, as the school of natural right had taught, but man's relationship to *all* beings. Though Bonnet did not speak of animal rights, he expressed his conviction that every sentient being had some sort of claim to happiness: a moral man would not even kill a gnat without reason, because it was 'a sensitive being, which enjoys in its manner the sweets of existence'.[77] Only seven years later, in 1776, Humphrey Primatt made the decisive second step by asserting that animals had 'a right to happiness'. He argued that the suffering of animals was worse than that of man, because they had no hope for a Future Life. Furthermore, being creatures without the faculty of speech, they could not accuse their tormentors; and, being irrational, they were also unable to sin and to endure pain as a punishment. According to Primatt, all this meant that 'present pain' was the only evil for animals and 'present happiness' their only good.[78]

It already appeared in outline in Primatt's considerations that rationality as the old criterion for the possession of rights was going to be replaced by the new criterion of the capacity to feel pain. Correspondingly he also attacked the old criterion, using an argument which was based on an analogy to the reprehensibleness of racism and slavery: since both physical characteristics and mental faculties were given by God, they could neither be an object of pride nor of contempt. Just as the white man was not authorized through the colour of his skin to oppress the black as a slave, so an intelligent man was not allowed to tyrannize over a fool. Accordingly, intellectual superiority gave human beings no right to maltreat or torment animals.[79] Another criticism of the old criterion of rationality came in 1787 from Wilhelm Dietler (d. 1797), later professor of logic and metaphysics at the university of Mainz. In this year Dietler – who knew Primatt's comments on the subject – published a booklet on *Justice to Animals*. He argued here that the lack of rationality in animals and their incapability to lodge claims were insufficient reasons to deny the existence of 'animal rights': an under-age child showed the same characteristics in this respect, yet nobody would deny that it was 'illegal' and 'unjust' to hurt or kill the child, in other words, that the child had certain rights. Hence animals had certain rights as well.[80] Two years later Jeremy Bentham (1748–1832) used virtually the same argument in his *Introduction to the Principles of Morals and Legislation* (1789) by pointing out that 'a full-grown horse or dog, is beyond comparison a more rational, as well as a more conversible animal, than an infant of a day, or a week, or even a month, old'. With his famous dictum 'the question is not, Can they *reason?* nor, Can they *talk?* but, Can they *suffer?*' he epitomized the new view on the criteria for the possession of rights.[81]

Thus in the writings of Primatt, Dietler and Bentham an alternative to the elder concept of indirect obligation to animals can be discerned: animals have a right to considerate treatment, and man has immediate duties towards them. Yet, the practical demands derived from these two concepts of obligation did not differ much. If we compare for example the conclusions of Kant and Bentham as exponents of these concepts, an almost complete consensus appears: both Kant and Bentham accepted a speedy killing of animals in slaughtering or in the eradication of vermin; and they both repudiated cruelty to animals.[82]

Seen as a whole, the described changes in theological and philosophical views of man's relationship to the animal world seem to reflect the development of a more 'friendly climate' for animals in the eighteenth century. Obviously, a number of contemporary intellectuals was prepared to assume a somewhat less anthropocentric attitude than had prevailed in the seventeenth century. It has to be emphasized, however, that such kindness to animals was still confined to an educated élite. Though it had become increasingly popular during the seventeenth and eighteenth centuries to keep pets for purely emotional reasons (particularly in the towns)[83], still a very rough treatment of animals dominated everyday life.

Maltreatment of horses, cattle and other domesticated animals and cruelties in slaughtering seem to have been common. Blood-sports, such as bull-baiting, badger-baiting, cock-throwing, cock- and dog-fighting, were still popular among the lower classes, especially in Britain, as was hunting among the upper classes.[84] It was this background of common 'cruelties' against which eighteenth-century authors developed their ideas on the man-animal relationship and on man's duties to animals.[85] The general acceptance of their pleas for a more considerate treatment of animals must not be overestimated. When James Granger preached kindness to animals in 1772, he produced 'almost universal disgust to two considerable congregations', because his mention of dogs and horses was regarded as 'a prostitution of the dignity of the pulpit'.[86] Dietler, in 1787, remarked that many people could not understand at all how it occurred to an author to write about justice for animals.[87] And Young, in 1798, still feared to expose himself to ridicule by publishing a book on 'Humanity to Animals'. To many this subject would appear 'whimsical and uninteresting' and its particulars 'ludicrous and mean'.[88] Yet, it was the new theological and philosophical conceptions of man's relationship to animals which underlay the eighteenth-century discourse on the ethics of animal experimentation.

In 1742, the Leipzig philosopher Johann Heinrich Winkler attacked the hitherto uncontested physicotheological argument in favour of vivisection. He particularly criticized Christian Sigismund Wolff here, who (as mentioned above) had put forward this argument in his disputation.[89] Winkler reproached Wolff with having omitted the aspect of God's grace towards all sentient creatures: if animal vivisections were necessary in order to promote man's insight into divine magnificence and to amplify the glory of the Creator, all human beings would have to vivisect, despite the infliction of very severe pain. Accordingly, God would have created animals and endowed them with sensitivity in order to increase man's knowledge about divine perfection through their torments. This, however, was certainly contradictory to God's grace.[90] At least three of the ideas described above concerning the man-animal relationship formed the basis of this criticism. Firstly, there was the idea of God's care for animals and concern for animal suffering, as substantiated by respective passages in the Bible. Censuring cruelty to animals in general, Winkler listed nine of them.[91] Secondly, a decidedly anti-Cartesian position on the question of animal souls came into play. Winkler was convinced that animals owned sensitive, more or less rational, immaterial and immortal souls. From 1741 until 1743 he even gave four seminars, which exclusively dealt with the existence and faculties of animal souls in opposition to the Cartesian doctrine of a 'beast-machine'.[92] Thirdly, the concept of moral obligations to animals took effect. In Winkler's view, both man's direct duties to God and to other human beings implied an indirect obligation to refrain from the cruelty involved in vivisection. A man who renounced animal vivisection fulfilled his duty to God by imitating His grace as well as his duty to other men by avoiding the danger of brutalization (which might result in human vivisection).[93] According to that, Winkler also disagreed with Pufendorf's doctrines of a natural, permanent war and the absence of a pact between human beings and animals. Even if these doctrines were true (the Leipzig philosopher argued), they could not serve as a justification for vivisection of animals, because in this way vivisection of enemies during a war, and vivisection of any person with whom no contract has been concluded, might equally be justified.[94]

In analyzing further critical comments on the morality of animal experimentation, one finds remarkably similar patterns of underlying general ideas. In the criticism of the next fifty years merely variations of emphasis on certain ideas can be discerned. When Alexander

Pope, in 1744, during one of his well-known conversations with Joseph Spence (1699–1768), questioned the moral admissibility of Stephen Hales' (1677–1761) animal vivisections, the poet's opinion on animal souls came into play. Pope was inclined to attribute immortal, thinking souls to higher animals, such as dogs (which were the most frequently used species in animal experiments at this time). Obviously for this reason he felt moral concern for the fate of experimental animals.[95] Moreover, the concept of the Great Chain of Being seems to have exerted some influence here. Via his famous *Essay on Man* (1733) Pope was one of its leading advocates, and he belonged to those who applied it also to mental faculties.[96] Correspondingly, he doubted, in the conversation on vivisection, that one could have a right 'to kill creatures that we are so little above as dogs, for our curiosity, or even for some use to us'.[97] So, in the case of Pope the argument from animal souls seems to have been especially important. Yet, it has to be remembered, too, that in his earlier years the poet had censured cruelty to animals by adducing Pythagoras' condemnation of slaughtering according to Ovid and Plutarch's notion that humanity may be extended to the meanest animals. In addition he had cited pertinent scriptural passages, such as *Deuteronomy* 22:6–7 and *Jonah* 4:11.[98] Therefore the authority of the Old Testament and of classical authors may have influenced Pope's view of vivisection as well.

The aspect of brutalization – and thus of an indirect obligation to exempt animals from vivisection – was expressed most clearly in two essays by Alexander Adam von Sinclair (*c.* 1713–78) and Samuel Johnson (1709–84), which were published in 1751 and 1758, respectively. Sinclair, a private tutor at the court of Prince Victor of Schaumburg, warned emphatically that vivisection of animals would lead medical students 'from compassion to cruelty, and from a Christian tenderness of their conscience to blood-shed'.[99] Similarly, Johnson expressed his apprehension that a future physician, trained in vivisection, would 'extend his arts of torture, and continue those experiments upon infancy and age, which he has hitherto tried upon cats and dogs'. Animal vivisections would 'tend to harden the heart, extinguish those sensations which give man confidence in man, and make the physician more dreadful than the gout or stone'.[100] Sinclair even thought to have something like an empirical proof for his fear that cruelty to animals would lead to cruelty to human beings: the English – he maintained – treated their 'black slaves in America' much worse than the French, because they were more accustomed to cruelty through their 'hunting and baiting, manifold anatomical inquiries, cock- and man-fighting, and customary races'.[101] Besides this fear of brutalization, however, both in Sinclair and Johnson an anti-Cartesian position in the debate on animal souls can be demonstrated. The former called the Cartesian belief that animals were mere machines a 'delusion', from which people were gradually freed by 'experience and reason'.[102] And the latter thought that the 'Cartesian, who denies that his horse feels the spur, or that the hare is afraid when the hounds approach her' was 'deceived by fallacies not easily detected'.[103] In the 1760s anti-Cartesianism was still a crucial point in moral criticism of animal experimentation. In 1764 no less a man than Voltaire denounced vivisection of dogs on the basis of an anti-Cartesian view of the question of animal pain, arguing against the 'mechanist' that the canine sense organs and nerves – laid open in the very process of vivisection – were the same as in man.[104] And Bonnet, in 1769, spoke of the doctrine of animal automatism as 'a kind of philosophical heresy', admonishing not to dissect living animals as if they were 'slates'.[105]

Finally, in the last decade of the eighteenth century also the new idea of animal rights took effect among critics of animal experimentation. The Danish clergyman Lauritz Smith as well as the British writer and farmer John Lawrence (1753–1839) rejected animal experiments as immoral and simultaneously propagated the 'Rights of Beasts'. Smith had obviously been influenced by Dietler, whose booklet on justice to animals he cited.[106] Like the Mainz philosopher, the clergyman did not accept the argument that animals could not possess rights because of their incapability to understand the ideas of right and duty. If this argument was correct, the fetus, children, and mentally disordered persons could not have rights either. In a similar way as Humphrey Primatt, Smith therefore stated that animals had a 'right to happiness'.[107] Lawrence substantiated the existence of animal rights somewhat differently. He asserted that animals had feeling and more or less rational souls and took this as a sufficient reason to concede rights to them. As for domestic animals, these rights consisted in 'good and sufficient nourishment, comfortable shelter, and merciful treatment; to commit no wanton outrage upon their feelings, whilst alive, and to put them to the speediest and least painful death, when it shall be necessary to deprive them of life'.[108] If one considers this philosophical background, the bitterness of Lawrence's and Smith's censure of vivisection becomes understandable. The former complained that a surgeon might keep a vivisected animal 'in a continued state of the most exquisite and agonizing torture, even for whole days and nights, under the pretext of making an experiment for *the profit* of science'[109]; and the latter called vivisection for the sake of scientific knowledge 'the most cruel injustice towards the animal'.[110] In addition to their concept of direct duties to animals based on the new idea of animal rights, both Smith and Lawrence, however, continued to use the older concept of an indirect obligation because of the danger of brutalization. Smith warned that future generations – accustomed to the practice of animal vivisection – would perhaps feel authorized 'to anatomize living human beings', and Lawrence substantiated his similar fears with the familiar example of human vivisection by Herophilos.[111]

Thus, taken as a whole, the ethical discourse on animal experimentation in the second half of the eighteenth century reflects virtually every contemporary development within the general view of the man-animal relationship. The number of critical comments on the morality of animal experiments is still too small in this period, however, to discern specific changes in argument. Also, older ideas were carried along with newer ones. Yet, one can say that there seems to have been a trend from religiously motivated arguments against vivisection, based on the conception of divine grace, towards more philosophically orientated arguments on the basis of the concept of moral duty and justice. In this way secularization evidently made itself felt here.

A rather constant point of eighteenth-century criticism of animal experimentation was the apparent lack of therapeutical consequences. Johann Heinrich Winkler, for instance, admitted that anatomical science had capitalized on vivisection, but he doubted that an increase of knowledge in this field was a precondition to human happiness.[112] Johnson simply stated in 1758: 'I know not, that by living dissections any discovery has been made by which a single malady is more easily cured.'[113] And as late as 1800 one could read in a sarcastic short essay on vivisection by the Göttingen mathematician and poet Abraham Gotthelf Kästner (1719–1800) that someone who 'has the heart to torment dogs' did not furnish proof of his ability to cure human beings.[114] For the most part this kind of criticism was directed against physiological animal experiments. Yet, the area of pharmacological or toxicological experimentation was also included[115], and here even medical experts agreed. The central problem with tests of drugs and poisons was that of the transferability of observed effects from animals to human beings. Contemporary physicians dealing with the improvement of the *materia medica* through experimental research therefore advocated additional trials on human beings, which should be carried out first on convicted criminals or on the researcher himself, and in a second step on patients.[116]

Such low esteem for the medical utility of animal experimentation contrasted, of course, with statements by defenders of this practice. The argument of medical benefit – already established in the seventeenth century[117] – remained crucial for physicians and scientists who gave moral justifications of their animal experiments. As one would expect, it was used by researchers who devoted themselves to the solution of practical problems in medicine. Henri-Louis Duhamel Dumonceau (1700–82), for example, who studied the healing of fractures in doves, pointed out that such work aimed at the 'preservation of our health and the treatment of diseases'.[118] Similarly Richard Brocklesby (1722–97), having tested on dogs the effects of a 'poisonous Root lately found mixed among the Gentian', assured: '... when good Purposes are answer'd in the Whole of Things by inferior Natures yielding to superior ones, Man may, without just Imputation to his moral Character, sacrifice the Interest of a baser Order to the Happiness of one superior.'[119] But also in the field of basic physiological research animal experiments were justified with the argument of medical benefit. When Albrecht von Haller (1708–77), in 1752, presented his findings concerning sensibility and irritability to the Göttingen Royal Society of the Sciences, he spoke of the 'utility for the human race and the necessity', which would excuse the 'cruelties' involved in his vivisectional experiments.[120]

So, in the eighteenth century, there was evidently a marked disagreement over the question of benefit derived from animal experiments. In fact, examples of important consequences of animal experimentation for therapeutics or prophylaxis can hardly be found in this period.[121] Contemporary defenders of vivisection promised medical benefit[122], but they were still unable to furnish really striking proofs. Not surprisingly therefore, the legal admissibility of vivisection began to be challenged in the second half of the eighteenth century. The Leipzig jurist Karl Ferdinand Hommel (1722–81), who was influenced by Winkler's ideas, argued that it was illegal to do something *certainly wrong,* namely the infliction of pain on animals, in the hope of acquiring an *uncertain good,* i.e. the health of human beings. Accordingly, he suggested cautioning medical students or surgeons in case a charge was brought against them because of animal vivisection.[123] The effect of such a suggestion must not be overestimated, however. An eighteenth-century prosecution, or even conviction, because of vivisection of animals has not been handed down, whereas severe maltreatment of horses and cattle was already occasionally punished in Germany with fines and detention. In the absence of legal provisions a judge of the eighteenth century could punish cruelty to animals as a so-called *crimen extraordinarium*.[124] One has to bear in mind in this context, too, that vivisection of human beings was still seriously taken into consideration. In 1709 Christian Sigismund Wolff, in his disputation at the university of Leipzig, had not only advocated animal experiments. On the grounds that society would 'profit medically as well as politically', he had also recommended the vivisection of criminals who have been sentenced to death.[125] In 1745, the writer Christlob Mylius (1722–54), a cousin and friend of Gotthold Ephraim Lessing, published an ethical calculus[126], in which he compared the morality of animal vivisection with that of human vivisection. His result was that in the former the good outweighed the evil, whereas the latter remained a crime, even if its conceivable medical utility was taken into account.[127] But seven years later Pierre-Louis Moreau de Maupertuis (1698–1759), the President of the Berlin Academy of Sciences, suggested in an open letter to King Frederick the Great that physicians should make use of convicted criminals for the testing of drugs and poisons, for trying out new surgical techniques and even for vivisectional experiments in physiology in order to accelerate medical progress.[128] Thus, as in the seventeenth century, animal vivisection was still something like a rather harmless and acceptable alternative to human vivisection. Anthropocentrism continued to be the prevalent attitude in the issue of animal experimentation. This is also reflected by the meanwhile customary use of the *tu quoque*-argument by eighteenth-century scientists. For instance Heister, Haller, Duhamel and Brocklesby all justified their animal experiments in this way, arguing that the slaughtering of animals for food was accepted by most people and that, therefore, vivisection for the sake of medical knowledge had to be permitted as well.[129]

Nevertheless, the doubts about the medical value and the moral, respectively legal, admissibility of animal experimentation, which had been aroused in the course of the eighteenth century, carried on the ethical discourse. As a new stage of this discourse the formulation of ethical principles for research on living animals set in towards the end of the century. A pioneer in this respect was the Manchester physician and writer Thomas Percival (1740–1804). His ideas about animal experimentation cannot be found in his famous *Medical Ethics* (1803)[130], but in his much less well known collection of moralizing children's stories, entitled *A Father's Instructions*, which was first published in 1775. Among tales that were directed against various cruelties to animals he also included one about 'Cruelty in Experiments'.[131] The moral of this story (which was about father and son experimenting on fishes with 'mephitic water')[132] ran as follows:

> 'Beware, my son ... of observing spectacles of pain and misery with delight. Cruelty by insensible degrees, will steal into your heart; and every generous principle of your nature will then be subverted. The philosopher, who has in contemplation the establishment of some important truth, or the discovery of what will tend to the advancement of *real science*, and to the good and happiness of mankind, may perhaps be justified, if he sacrifice to his persuits the life and enjoyment of an inferior animal. But the emotions of humanity should never be stifled in his breast; his trials should be made with tenderness, repeated with reluctance, and carried no farther than the object in view unavoidably requires. Wanton experiments on living creatures, and even those, which are merely subservient to the gratification of curiosity, merit the severest censure. They degrade the man of letters into a brute; and are fit amusements only for the cannibals of New-Zealand.'[133]

Evidently, Percival's considerations went beyond the old idea of brutalization through animal experiments: careful treatment of experimental animals, limitation of repetitions, concentration on the immediate aim of an inquiry, and renunciation of trials without a well-definded scientific or medical purpose can be identified as ethical principles, which he wished the researcher to respect. In this way Percival anticipated corresponding ethical demands which were formulated by theological commentators only around 1800. Dealing with the morality of experimentation on living animals in the general context of human cruelties towards the 'brute creation', Thomas Young from Trinity College Cambridge and the vicar of Buckingham, Henry Crowe (1778–1851), as well as the German Protestant clergymen Franz Volkmar Reinhard (1753–1812) and Christian Adam Dann (1758–1837), came virtually to the same conclusions as Percival.[134] An additional principle, set up by Dann and Reinhard, was to renounce vivisection, if the same result could be attained by anatomical studies on corpses.[135] Obviously, this point reflected the criticism of adversaries of animal experimentation, such as Sinclair, Smith and Lawrence, who had taken the view that many vivisections were superfluous, because they were replaceable by pure anatomy.[136]

The first fully elaborated ethical code for research on living animals, containing seven principles, was published in 1831 by the London physician and experimental physiologist Marshall Hall (1790–1857) in the introduction to his *Critical and Experimental Essay on the Circulation of the Blood.* The majority of his principles corresponded to those listed above. A new demand, however, was to choose for experimentation 'the lowest order of animals' which was appropriate to the purpose 'as the least sentient'. Hall particularly recommended batrachians here. Moreover, he gave concrete advice how to avoid unnecessary repetitions of an experiment. If possible, every trial should be performed under the eyes of competent witnesses, so that it was 'duly attested'. The results should then be published 'in the simplest, plainest terms', and results of other researchers – especially if they deviated from one's own – should be quoted literally.[137] In order to translate his demands into reality Hall wished the establishment of a 'society for physiological research'. Its members should assist each other, discuss and improve the design of a proposed series of experiments, and decide about the actual performance.[138] A rather similar suggestion had been made only two years before in Germany by the Württemberg public-health officer Christian Gottlob Hopf (1765–1842), formerly a senior lecturer of medicine at Tübingen. Though not an adversary of animal experimentation as such, Hopf was upset about the lack of method and design in many toxicological tests on animals as described in Mathieu Orfila's *Toxicologie générale* (1826), a fact, which in his opinion turned these tests into useless cruelties. In order to avoid such reprehensible experimentation, he suggested the enactment of a law according to which every researcher would have to apply for a permit to conduct a series of animal experiments. These applications should be directed to the *Collegia medica* (i.e. the Boards of Health), and they should contain details about the plan and method of the proposed trials as well as a testimony about a sufficient number of experimental animals (in order to prevent multiple experimentation on the same animal).[139]

Until the British *Cruelty to Animals Act* in 1876 neither Hopf's nor Hall's suggestions were realized. Yet, their historical significance must not be underestimated. They did not only reflect a growing concern for experimental animals among physicians. Evidently, they were also reactions to an increasing antipathy towards animal experimentation in the public. With respect to Hall's own animal experiments Diana Manuel has recently described this hostile environment in detail.[140] In fact, Hall himself had explicitly stated that a physiologist who neglected his ethical code would 'scarcely escape from the imputation of cruelty'.[141] Thus the stage of setting up ethical principles in the discourse on animal experimentation – in the late eighteenth and early nineteenth centuries – must again be seen against the general background of the man-animal relationship.

Pro- and Anti-vivisection: their Ethical Basis and Social Context

Generally, one can say that in the course of the nineteenth century the man-animal relationship became more and more emotional. This is particularly true for those two species which were still preferred for experimentation: dogs and cats. Already in the eighteenth century the fashion of pet-keeping does not seem to have been without influence on the ethical debate about animal experimentation and man's right treatment of animals in general. Several of the authors cited above, such as Pope, Johnson, Bentham and Smith, can be identified as dog- or cat-fanciers in their private lives.[142] In the first half of the nineteenth century the keeping of pets became common, particularly in early industrialized and urbanized countries, such as Britain. Richard D. French and James Turner have tried to explain this phenomenon with the thesis that inhabitants of towns kept pets as surrogates for the lost rural way of life, i.e. because of nostalgia.[143] Moreover, Harriet Ritvo has recently suggested that the keeping of pedigree dogs and cats soon became a symbol of social status and order. Dog shows and cat shows, especially, which started in Britain in the late 1850s and early 1870s respectively, seem to reflect this aspect.[144] Whatever the deeper motives were, the relationship to pets was loaded with emotions and this obviously influenced contemporary attitudes towards animal experimentation. Another factor was the increasing anthropomorphization of animals. The academic eighteenth-century dispute on the problem of animal souls was superseded in the nineteenth century by an enormously popular and often naive literature on animal psychology.[145] The tendency to anthropomorphize animals was reflected, too, in contemporary art, particulary in the highly esteemed animal paintings by Edwin Landseer (1802–73).[146] Also, in the early nineteenth century the first laws against cruelty to horses, cattle and other domestic animals were enacted in Britain and Germany. The very first of this kind was the British *Martin's Act* of 1822.[147] In Germany several states soon passed analogous laws: Saxony in 1838, Württemberg in 1839, Hanover and Hesse-Darmstadt in 1847, Prussia in 1851, and Bavaria in 1861. In contrast to Britain, in some German states, for example, Württemberg, Hanover and Prussia, maltreatment of animals was punishable only if it had occurred in public and had violated the feelings of spectators. Evidently, the old anthropocentric idea of the need to protect human morality against brutalization came to bearing here. This unilateral view still featured in the penal code of the new German Empire (1871), which then uniformly regulated animal protection. Yet, despite such differences in legislation, the degree of punishment did not vary much, consisting in fines and several weeks of detention.[148] Although these early laws for animal protection, did *not* yet contain any provisions concerning experimentation on animals, they clearly reflected the developed sensitivity for animal suffering, at least in the educated public. Finally, the first animal protection societies were founded in the 1820s and 1830s: the world's first one was the Society for the Prevention of Cruelty to Animals, established in London in 1824 (since 1840 Royal S.P.C.A.)[149]; in Germany the pioneers were the animal protection societies of Stuttgart (1837), Dresden and Nuremberg (both 1839).[150] The two declared main tasks of such societies were the enforcement of the respective laws or police orders and education of the general public.[151] As a consequence of the latter, a new genre of literature emerged in the early nineteenth century: rather popularly written, sometimes inflammatory treatises against cruelty to animals. It is in these writings where the ethical discourse on animal experimentation was now chiefly carried on.

The authors of such treatises were simultaneously protagonists of organized animal protection: William Youatt (1776–1847), Honorary Veterinary Surgeon of the S.P.C.A., Thomas Ignatius Maria Forster (1789–1860), co-founder of the Animals' Friend Society (A.F.S., split off from the S.P.C.A. in 1832), Lewis Gompertz (d. 1861), co-founder of the S.P.C.A. and founder and President of the A.F.S., H. W. von Ehrenstein, one of the first members of the Dresden Society against Cruelty to Animals. Their obvious aim was to shake the public into action. Accordingly, all the old arguments for a more careful treatment of animals – based on the Bible, on animal souls, on the idea of moral obligations to animals, on the fear of brutalization through cruelty to animals – were repeated and specified. Also, common cruelties in various areas, such as field-sports, fishing, animal fights, everyday treatment of horses and cattle, slaughtering, cookery etc., were extensively described and censured. Animal experimentation was included as one of these many issues.[152] The quite emotional, exalted style of this early animal protection literature somewhat clouds the underlying ethical principles. Yet, two central ideas can be discerned. Firstly, the utilitarian principle that the propriety or impropriety of human conduct with regard to animals should be decided by its increasing or diminishing the 'general sum of enjoyment'[153]; and secondly, the idea going back to Rousseau that compassion is the sole inborn basis of human morality, and that it should be extended to all fellow-creatures, i.e. to animals as well.[154] A feature common to all of those early animal protectionists was their low opinion of possible medical benefits arising from animal experimentation. As they saw it, many or even most animal experiments were useless cruelties, partly because of the old problems of artificial conditions in vivisection and the lack of transferability from animal to man, partly because these experiments were merely repetitions for the purposes of verification or demonstration.[155] On these grounds authors such as Youatt and Gompertz inaugurated a strategy that was to become very common among anti-vivisectionists of the next decades: scrutinizing the medical literature of their time, they listed examples of allegedly senseless and shockingly cruel animal experimentation. Not surprisingly, François Magendie (1783–1855) was singled out here as a first 'black sheep'.[156] Evidently, experiments which could not be recognized as immediately contributing to the alleviation of human (or animal) suffering in diseases violated the utilitarian principle. Medical men defending animal experimentation quickly adjusted their own argument to these tactics. In 1842 the anatomist Friedrich Wilhelm Theile (1801–79) published his annual oration as rector of the university of Berne *On the usefulness of physiological experiments with animals for medicine and on the preconceived ideas against such experiments.* His whole address was built on the single argument of medical benefit, which he tried to substantiate by adducing numerous examples of useful animal experimentation in the fields of nutritional physiology, surgery, and toxicology. He also defended the repetition of experiments as a means of scientific verification and medical teaching. Moreover, he argued that in the context of new questions the same experiment might give new information.[157]

Besides this utilitarian line of reasoning, the idea of compassion to animals also took effect in the issue of animal experimentation. Influenced by Rousseau, Arthur Schopenhauer (1788–1860), in his *Basis of Morality* (1840), elevated compassion to the central moral principle, which he held to be the source of the cardinal virtues 'justice' and 'philanthropy', and which in his view had to be extended to animals as well.[158] In the same work he sharply criticized Kant's concept of a merely indirect obligation to animals (based on man's direct duty to himself to avoid brutalization)[159], because it meant that animals were only 'the pathological phantom for exercising compassion with human beings'.[160] In Schopenhauer's eyes this concept illustrated that animals were regarded as mere means which might be used to 'any ends, such as vivisections, hunting, bull-fights, races, whipping to death in front of an immovable cart loaded with stones'. In this way he indentified Kant's ideas about the man-animal relationship as those of traditional Judaeo-Christian anthropocentrism.[161] This view, however, was abhorred by Schopenhauer, as it is particularly clear from his comments on the subject in his *Parerga and Paralipomena* (1851). His main argument here against anthropocentrism was that it ignored the metaphysical identity of human beings and animals based on their common will to exist. Respect for this identity rather than the fear of brutalization should be the basis of animal protection.[162] As for the specific problem of animal experimentation, this would mean that 'it would no longer be open to every quack to test each phantastic whim of his ignorance by inflicting the most horrible torment upon numberless animals'.[163] Schopenhauer strongly condemned animal experimentation which was carried out to decide about 'purely theoretical, often very futile questions'. Yet, he agreed with the Göttingen professor of medicine Johann Friedrich Blumenbach (1752–1840), whose lectures he had attended earlier in the century, that this method might occasionally be employed 'in very important and immediately useful studies'.[164] Thus ultimately utilitarian thinking also entered Schopenhauer's concept of the man-animal relationship, when it was applied to the issue of animal experimentation. Paradoxically, he did not much differ from Kant here, who stated that 'painful physical experiments for the mere sake of speculation are to be abhorred, if the end may be achieved without them'.[165]

When Schopenhauer put down his thoughts about animal experimentation in *Parerga and Paralipomena,* chloroform had already been introduced both in the clinic and in the physiological laboratory. As early as 1847 the French physiologist Pierre Flourens (1794–1867) had tested the anaesthetic properties of the new compound in vivisected animals.[166] In the early 1850s chloroformisation was employed in most animal vivisections, as Schopenhauer observed, yet it had to be dispensed with in the (then frequently conducted) studies in the functions and sensibility of the nervous system.[167] This methodically necessary renunciation of analgesia or narcosis in certain fields of animal experimentation (for example, in toxicology), was one of the reasons why the event of anaesthesia did *not* essentially change the ethical debate: adversaries of vivisection could still adduce enough examples of painful experimentation without the use of anaesthetics. Moreover, they suspected that many experimental animals were only paralized by application of curare, i.e. rendered motionless while still fully conscious of pain.[168] Thus the public antipathy towards animal experimentation grew without hindrance. In 1863 the British journalist Frances Power Cobbe (1822–1904) started the world's first full-fledged anti-vivisectionist campaign against an experimental physiologist, Moritz Schiff (1823–96) in Florence.[169]

The emergence of anti-vivisection movements during the next five decades, first in Britain and soon afterwards in other Western countries, such as Germany, Switzerland, Sweden and the United States, has been described and analyzed in detail by several historians and, therefore, does not need to be reconstructed here again.[170] Remarkable practical consequences of contemporary anti-vivisectionist agitation were the British *Cruelty to Animals Act* of 1876 and the decree concerning animal experimentation at Prussian universities, issued in 1885 by the Minister of Education Gustav von Gossler (1838–1902), which was adopted by the other states of the German Empire before the turn of the century. Their provisions clearly reflected the ethical principles which had been set up at the beginning of the century[171]: animal experiments should only be performed for the acquisition of new physiological or medical knowledge. As an illustration of lectures they were only permitted, if they were regarded as absolutely necessary for the understanding of the subject matter. Whenever possible, experimental animals should be anaesthetized, and lower species should be prefered to higher ones. In Germany, the professors and lecturers of the medical faculties were entitled to animal experimentation *ex officio*. In Britain, every researcher who wished to carry out experiments on living vertebrate animals had to submit an application to the Home Secretary, endorsed both by a president of one of the country's eleven leading scientific or medical bodies and by a medical professor. If a licence was granted, the researcher could perform the permitted experiments at registered places, which were subject to controls by inspectors of the Home Secretary. The British Act also contained penalties (fines and imprisonment up to three months), which were not included, however, in the Prussian decree.[172]

The fact that the ethical principles concerning animal experiments had attained a legal status in Britain, and a bureaucratic one in Germany, did not calm anti-vivisectionist agitation. Quite on the contrary, the 'vivisection controversy' became sharper. Anti-vivisection societies, which had first been founded in England (in 1875) and in Germany (in 1879), changed their policy from demanding restriction to one of total abolition of animal experimentation.[173] In order to understand this radicalization one has to consider the social forces underlying the ethical debate. Above all one has to realize that experimental physiology was institutionalized in the course of the nineteenth century (first on the Continent and afterwards in Britain as well)[174], which meant that the general public was more and more confronted with the actual practice of animal experimentation.

The deeper motives for anti-vivisectionist responses in the public from the later nineteenth to the early twentieth century have been a subject of recent scholarship, and some main interpretations may be mentioned here: Richard D. French has argued, in 1975, that at the heart of the Victorian anti-vivisection movement was public concern over the fact that modern science and medicine were becoming leading institutions in society.[175] More recently, Nicolaas A. Rupke has elaborated this view, taking into account the social composition of the late-nineteenth-century opposition to animal experimentation. According to him, the aristocracy, the clergy and the judiciary were prominent in the anti-vivisection movement, because they saw their cultural authority waning as that of scientists grew.[176] Similarly, Ulrich Tröhler and Roland Neff – referring mainly to the contemporary Continental debates – have interpreted anti-vivisection as an expression of general hostility towards modern science (which was regarded as materialistic), but also of fear of the future in the age of industrialization and mechanization.[177] Carol Lansbury has tried to explain the strong engagement of women in the anti-vivisectionist movement as well as the striking solidarization of suffragettes and workers with respect to anti-vivisection, which happened in Edwardian England. She argues that women – exposed to sexual violence and degrading gynaecological examination – subconsciously identified with the vivisected animal, as did workers who felt a kind of kinship with their 'fellow beasts of burden' and who saw themselves as potential subjects of experimentation in hospitals.[178] A less psychological, more sociological, explanation for the high female membership in Victorian anti-vivisection societies (about 70 per cent in the 1880s) has finally been suggested by Mary Ann Elston. She sees animal protection and anti-vivisection as an aspect of contemporary philanthropy and moral reform, i.e. of fields of activity for which women were then regarded as especially well suited.[179] Certainly these theories about underlying social forces help us to understand the intensity of the 'vivisection controversy' and the style of agitation at the turn of the last century. Yet, the influence of these forces on the *ethical arguments* as such seems to have been comparatively small. In analyzing the pertinent publications of the period between 1870 and 1900 one still finds the old pros and cons and the familiar lines of reasoning.

In the last decades of the nineteenth century one 'main line' of the ethical discourse accompanied by two 'secondary lines' can be discerned. The 'main debate' still centered around the medical utility – and here particularly the therapeutical consequences - of animal experiments. Exponents of contemporary medicine and natural science, such as James Paget, Richard Owen, Rudolf Virchow, Rudolf Heidenhain, and Ivan Petrovic Pavlov, publicly defended animal experimentation by adducing examples of its medical importance. Paget, for instance, referred to experimental studies in surgical ligatures of arteries, Virchow pointed to the historical role of animal experimentation for the development of the concept of localization both in pathology and therapy, Pavlov summarized some of his animal experiments concerning the physiology of digestion.[180] At von Gossler's request, Heidenhain, in 1884, even produced a whole book on the subject. Written for the educated general public it demonstrated the utility of animal experimentation in six selected fields of physiology and in eighteen areas of practical medicine.[181] The more or less outspoken idea behind these apologies was basically utilitarian: the amount of pain inflicted on experimental animals was regarded as acceptable in view of the large sum of pain in human (and animal) diseases, which might be prevented or alleviated on the basis of experimentally gained knowledge. The counterpart of this argument was of course the contention of anti-vivisectionists that animal experiments were useless cruelties. Following the example of the early-nineteenth-century animal protectionists, the leaders of organized anti-vivisection, such as Miss Cobbe in Britain and Ernst von Weber (1830–1902) and Hermann Stenz (d. 1922) in Germany, compiled 'catalogues', so to speak, of seemingly senseless and cruel experiments, which they extracted (in words and pictures) from scientific publications.[182] Another aspect of this 'main line' in the ethical discourse was anthropocentrism. It can be found on both sides. The advocates of animal experimentation expressed it by their incessant use of the *tu quoque*-argument that slaughtering, shooting, or castration of animals was widely accepted and that it was therefore unjust to single out the vivisecting scientist for moral criticism.[183] The adversaries revealed their anthropocentrism by their continuous warning of brutalization through vivisection, i.e. by their emphasis on the moral consequences for man. In 1877, Marie-Espérance von Schwartz (1818–99) alias Elpis Melena, one of the leading German anti-vivisectionists, even wrote a whole novel around this old argument of brutalization: it featured a wicked and cynical 'vivisector' who eventually causes the death of his own virtuous – and anti-vivisectionist – daughter.[184]

Only a few contributors to this 'main debate' assumed a critical attitude towards the central issue of medical utility. On the side of the apologists particularly Ludimar Hermann (1838–1914), professor of physiology in Zurich, has to be mentioned. Though he also strongly defended vivisection, warning that by reducing it 'one would save the life of a number of animals ... only by paying in human lives', he felt that the sole argument of diminishing human suffering might be considered ignoble and egoistic. Accordingly, he elevated the acquisition of knowledge to the only adequate justification of animal experimentation.[185] Of course this presupposed an anthropocentric world view, which was in fact very evident in Hermann's argument. He actually carried the *tu quoque*-argument to its extreme, annexing to his booklet *Die Vivisectionsfrage* (1877) – in which those thoughts were published – recent statistics on the extent of castrations of cattle in the German Empire. Yet, he was cautious enough to comment that he did not thereby intend 'to justify little sins by the impunity of greater ones'. His declared idea behind this strategy was to put vivisection in a proper perspective to the general use of animals in society.[186] A similarly critical attitude towards the argument of medical utility was later assumed, too, by Bernhard Rawitz (b. 1857), lecturer in comparative anatomy at the university of Berlin, in an address to the local German Society for Ethical Culture, published in 1898. He explicitly acknowledged Heidenhain's argument of medical benefit, but stressed that science was an end in itself. For Rawitz, serious scientific work was a kind of moral exercise, and progress in the natural sciences meant moral progress. Thus, in Rawitz' opinion, the anti-vivisectionists (and not the 'vivisectors') were truly immoral.[187]

On the side of the adversaries of animal experimentation it was Ernst Grysanowski (1824–88) who dealt with the question of medical utility in a more differentiated way. Grysanowski, physician and 'medical authority', so to speak, of the early German anti-vivisection movement[188], admitted that in surgery and toxicology animal experiments had provided some useful results and ought to be tolerated for this reason.[189] Yet, his essential point did not concern practical utility (which he denied to physiological experimentation), but the necessity of animal experimentation. In his view most animal experiments were superfluous – and therefore immoral – because hygiene would prevent most diseases.[190] As for therapy, Grysanowski was ready to rely solely on the old 'vis medicatrix naturae', i.e. the healing force of nature.[191]

The two 'secondary lines' of argument within the late-nineteenth-century debate did not accept the aspect of medical utility at all. Here solely the ideas of compassion to animals and of animal rights, respectively, were decisive. The exponent of the first of these two 'lines' was the composer Richard Wagner (1813–83), who joined the German anti-vivisection movement in 1879. Influenced partly by the non-anthropocentric view of the man-animal relationship in Brahmanism, partly by the corresponding thoughts of Schopenhauer, Wagner developed a 'cosmology of compassion': not only the interrelations between human beings, but also man's relationship to animals and to the whole of nature should be ruled by compassion. In this way he hoped to overcome the predominant 'cult of utility', which he abhorred as the cause of man's alienation from nature and as the principle of modern industrialized, mechanized, and militarized society. For Wagner, animal experimentation was the 'demon' of contemporary utilitarian thinking. On these grounds he demanded the total abolition of this practice.[192] Wagner's criticism most clearly reflected the general hostility towards modern science as a characteristic of anti-vivisectionism. Yet, his ideas about animal experimentation did not exert great influence beyond the circle of his devoted admirers, the 'Bayreuther Kreis'. The organized anti-vivisection movement merely used Wagner's prominent name for propaganda purposes.[193]

Similarly, the other of the two 'secondary lines' within the ethical debate of the late nineteenth century was formulated by an exponent of a comparatively small group. In 1891, the former Eton master Henry Salt (1851–1939), a 'rationalist, socialist, pacifist and humanitarian' (as he described himself), founded the Humanitarian League in London. Though prominent intellectuals, such as Salt's socialist friends George Bernard Shaw and Edward Carpenter, committed themselves to the League, it never gained the importance of the R.S.P.C.A. or of the Victoria Street Society for the Protection of Animals liable to Vivisection (founded in 1875).[194] The League's aims were particularly set down in Salt's book *Animals' Rights Considered in Relation to Social Progress,* which was first published in 1892. Quoting directly from Primatt, Bentham, and Lawrence, Salt here took up again the late-eighteenth-century concept of animal rights. In his view, animals should have a right to live a natural life, which permits their individual development and is subject only to 'limitations imposed by the permanent needs and interests of the community'. His central principle was that all practices inflicting unnecessary pain on any sentient being were incompatible with humanity.[195] On this basis Salt and his League did not only campaign for the abolition of animal experimentation, but also for the abandonment of private slaughtering, for general protection of domestic and wild animals, and – in order to alleviate human suffering as well – for the discontinuance of the death penalty and of corporal punishment, for the gradual reduction of armaments, and for a more considerate treatment of 'subject races in our colonies'.[196] Disillusioned by the First World War the Humanitarian League disbanded in 1919.[197] Its significance for the contemporary discourse on the ethics of animal experimentation, however, lay in its uncompromising rejection of the argument of benefit, or as Salt put it:

> Nothing is necessary which is abhorrent, revolting, intolerable, to the general instincts of humanity. Better a thousand times that science should forego or postpone the questionable advantage of certain problematical discoveries, than that the moral conscience of the community should be unmistakably outraged by the confusion of right and wrong. The short cut is not always the right path; and to perpetrate a cruel injustice on the lower animals, and then attempt to excuse it on the ground that it will benefit posterity, is an argument which is as irrelevant as it is immoral.[198]

Epilogue

Any reader who is familiar with the present-day discussions on the ethics of animal experimentation will certainly have noticed the striking parallels between current arguments and the historical discourse outlined in this chapter. Now as then the question of medical benefit resulting from experiments on animals is a major issue. During the last ten years prominent medical scientists both in Britain and on the Continent have again publicly defended the practice by presenting numerous examples of its utility in human and veterinary medicine.[199] Although the recent examples of medical benefit are much more convincing than their nineteenth-century forerunners (particularly in the fields of pharmacotherapy and surgery), obstinate anti-vivisectionists – even scientifically trained ones – still generally deny the usefulness of animal experimentation and continue to list seemingly futile and painful experiments.[200] The putative brutalizing effect of experimenting with animals is still an additional argument among the adversaries. The most radical of them have even characterized experimenting scientists as persons with sadistic tendencies.[201] Modern apologists of animal experimentation, on the other side, have not stopped using the argument in support of their position of pointing to man's general custom of keeping and breeding animals for diverse purposes, such as production of food and clothes, for work, or simply for fun (such as equestrian sport, training of dogs)[202], which means that the anthropocentric *tu quoque*-argument, known since the seventeenth century, has not lost its significance. In the current philosophical debates on man's relationship to animals a remarkable revival of historical concepts can be observed. Peter Singer and Tom Regan have followed in Bentham's footsteps by making sentiency the criterion which gives a moral status to animals. On these grounds they condemn animal experimentation as an expression of unwarranted 'speciesism' and a violation of animal rights, respectively. In many respects their often-quoted books on this subject, *Animal Liberation* (1975) and *The Case for Animal Rights* (1984), also read like modern supplements to Henry Salt's *Animals' Rights*.[203] In fact both Singer and Regan quote Salt as one of their intellectual forefathers.[204] And most recently, Schopenhauer's concept of elevating compassion to the central principle determining the ethics of the man-animal relationship has been taken up again, too, by the Berlin philosopher Ursula Wolf.[205]

Yet, in view of the continuing influence of historical concepts and strategies of argument, the changes of context must not be overlooked. The enormous amount of present-day animal experimentation can hardly be compared with its limited extent in the period from 1650 to 1900. Correspondingly, anti-vivisectionism is now not only directed against the work of individual researchers (as in the seventeenth and eighteenth centuries) or of certain university laboratories (as in the nineteenth century), but also against the many millions of animal experiments carried out world-wide each year in pharmaceutical and chemical companies. Animal experimentation has therefore become a problem both of medical ethics and of the ethics of economy. Moreover, anti-vivisectionist sentiment has seized more and more professional groups and social strata over the last 350 years or so. In the seventeenth century animal experimentation seems to have been discussed as a moral problem merely within medical circles. In the course of the eighteenth century the whole contemporary range of academics (i.e., besides physicians, also theologians, philosophers, and jurists) as well as men of letters became involved in the debate. The nineteenth century witnessed the emergence of anti-vivisection societies, which were principally open to everyone, but initially showed an upper class orientation with the aristocracy being strongly represented.[206] An extension of anti-vivisection societies to the working class can be observed at the turn of the last century.[207] And nowadays animal experimentation belongs to those ethical topics which are most widely and passionately discussed by the general public. A new qualitative element has also been brought into the debate during the last years by the development of alternative methods, such as cell and tissue culture, work on isolated organs, and computer simulation, which can replace animal experiments in certain scientific questions and tests.[208]

Seen from the philosophical point of view, the present ethical discourse on animal experimentation seems to be a specific expression of a general tendency to redefine man's relationship to the animal world and to the whole of nature.[209] Modern anti-vivisectionists have now begun to campaign against animal experimentation as one of several forms of the 'exploitation' of nature.[210] It will be interesting to observe in the future if this association with ecological thinking will ultimately lead to a severe erosion of traditional Judaeo-Christian anthropocentrism. If this happened, the consequences for the practice of animal experimentation would undoubtedly be very serious.

Notes

1. H. Bretschneider, *Der Streit um die Vivisektion im 19. Jahrhundert. Verlauf - Argumente - Ergebnisse* (Stuttgart: G. Fischer, 1962); R. D. French, *Antivivisection and Medical Science in Victorian Society* (Princeton-London: Princeton University Press, 1975).
2. J. Turner, *Reckoning with the Beast: Animals, Pain, and Humanity in Victorian Mind* (Baltimore-London: Johns Hopkins University Press, 1980); C. Lansbury, *The Old Brown Dog: Women, Workers, and Vivisection in Edwardian England* (Madison-London: University of Wisconsin Press, 1985); H. Ritvo, *The Animal Estate: The English and Other Creatures in the Victorian Age* (Cambridge, Mass.-London: Harvard University Press, 1987), ch. 3; N. A. Rupke (ed.), *Vivisection in Historical Perspective* (London-New York: Routledge, 2nd ed. 1990); R. Neff, *Der Streit um den wissenschaftlichen Tierversuch in der Schweiz des 19. Jahrhunderts* (Basle: Schwabe, 1989).

3. W. Shugg, 'Humanitarian Attitudes in the Early Animal Experiments of the Royal Society', *Annals of Science*, xxiv (1968), 227–38; A. Guerrini, 'The Ethics of Animal Experimentation in Seventeenth-Century England', *Journal of the History of Ideas*, l (1989), 391–407; M. R. Oster, 'The "Beame of Diuinity": Animal Suffering in the Early Thought of Robert Boyle', *British Journal for the History of Science*, xxii (1989), 151–79.
4. A.-H. Maehle, 'Zur wissenschaftlichen und moralischen Rechtfertigung toxikologischer Tierversuche im 17. Jahrhundert: Johann Jakob Wepfer und Johann Jakob Harder', *Gesnerus*, xliii (1986), 213–21.
5. M. Daly, 'Quasi-Anti-Vivisection in the Eighteenth Century', *Durham University Journal*, n.s. li (1990), 187–90; A.-H. Maehle, 'Literary Responses to Animal Experimentation in Seventeenth- and Eighteenth-Century Britain', *Medical History*, xxxiv (1990), 27–51.
6. *Idem*, 'Der Literat Christlob Mylius und seine Verteidigung des medizinischen Tierversuchs im 18. und 19. Jahrhundert', *Medizinhistorisches Journal*, xxi (1986), 269–87. See also *idem* and U. Tröhler, 'Animal Experimentation from Antiquity to the End of the Eighteenth Century: Attitudes and Arguments', in Rupke, *Vivisection*, 14–47.
7. A.-H. Maehle, *Kritik und Verteidigung des Tierversuchs: Die Anfänge der Diskussion im 17. und 18. Jahrhundert* (Stuttgart: F. Steiner, 1992).
8. In this paper the single term 'vivisection' is used in its original narrow sense, i.e. only if the *cutting* of a *living* animal (or human being) is actually involved. In compounded terms, such as 'anti-vivisection' or 'vivisection controversy', it is understood in its current broad sense including any kind of animal experimentation.
9. See N. Mani, 'Die Editio Princeps des Galen und die anatomisch-physiologische Forschung im 16. Jahrhundert', in F. Krafft and D. Wuttke (eds), *Das Verhältnis der Humanisten zum Buch* (Boppard: Boldt, 1977), 209–26; *idem*, 'Physiologische Konzepte von Galen bis Haller', *Gesnerus*, xlv (1988), 165–90; J. J. Bylebyl, 'Disputation and description in the renaissance pulse controversy', in A. Wear, R. K. French and I. M. Lonie (eds), *The medical renaissance of the sixteenth century* (Cambridge: Cambridge University Press, 1985), 223–45.
10. Cf. A. Vesalius, *De humani corporis fabrica libri septem* (Basle: J. Oporinus, 1543 - reprint Brussels: Culture et Civilisation, 1964), 658; R. Colombo, *De re anatomica libri* XV (Venice: N. Beuilacqua, 1559 - reprint Brussels: Culture et Civilisation, 1983), 256.
11. See Ch. Singer (ed.), *Galen on Anatomical Procedures* (London-New York-Toronto: Oxford University Press, 1956), 226 (De anatomicis administrationibus IX.1).
12. Cf. Colombo, *De re anatomica*, 256; J. Riolan jr., *Schola anatomica novis et raris observationibus illustrata* (Paris: A. Perier, 1608), 20–3; *idem*, *Anthropographia, et osteologia* (Paris: D. Moreau, 1626), 69–72;

M. A. Severino, *Zootomia Democritaea: id est, anatome generalis totius animantium opificii* (Nuremberg: Endter, 1645), 150–3; F. Glisson, *Anatomia hepatis* (London: Du-Gardian and O. Pullein, 1654), 4–5; H. Conring, *Introductio in universam artem medicam* (Helmstedt: H. Müller, 1654), 88–90, 93–4; Y. van Diemerbroeck, *Opera omnia, anatomica et medica* (Utrecht: M. v. Dreunen and W. v. Walcheren, 1685), 2; Ph. Verheyen, *Corporis humani liber primus* (Brussels: T'Serstevens, 2nd ed. 1710), 1. For the possibility of actual human vivisection in Hellenistic Alexandria see J. Longrigg, 'Anatomy in Alexandria in the Third Century B. C.', *British Journal for the History of Science*, xxi (1988), 455–88, and H. von Staden, *Herophilus. The Art of Medicine in Early Alexandria* (Cambridge: Cambridge University Press, 1989), 138–53. For the same in the Renaissance see M. Roth, *Andreas Vesalius Bruxellensis* (Berlin: G. Reimer, 1892), 473–85, and R. K. French, 'Berengario da Carpi and the use of commentary in anatomical teaching', in Wear *et al.*, *The medical renaissance*, 42–74.

13. Cf. K. Thomas, *Man and the Natural World. A History of the Modern Sensibility* (New York: Pantheon, 1983), 17–30. *Genesis* 2:4b–25, which represents an earlier, more archaic and less anthropocentric account of the creation, was neglected by early modern theologians in this context. According to this version animals had been created as man's helpers, and man had only been empowered to name all animals – not to reign over them. See also J. Passmore, *Man's Responsibility for Nature. Ecological Problems and Western Traditions* (London: Duckworth, 1974), 8, 13.
14. Cf. Aristotle, *Physics* 194 a 34–6, and *Politics* 1256 b 15–20; Severino, *Zootomia*, 152.
15. Cf. S. von Pufendorf, *De jure naturae et gentium*, G. Mascovius (ed.) (Frankfurt-Leipzig: Knoch, 1744), i, 509–10; Th. H. Juchem, *Die Entwicklung des Tierschutzes von der Mitte des 18. Jahrhunderts bis zum Reichsstrafgesetzbuch von 1871* (jur. thesis, Universität Bonn, 1940), 14.
16. 'Oh what a most innocent cruelty and easily excusable ferocity!'; cf. A. Napier (ed.), *The Theological Works of Isaac Barrow* (Cambridge: University Press, 1859), ix, 46.
17. Cf. Colombo, *De re anatomica*, 259–61.
18. Cf. Th. Bartholinus, *Defensio vasorum lacteorum et lymphaticorum adversus Joannem Riolanum* (Copenhagen: G. Holst, 1655), 96. See also N. Mani, 'Darmresorption und Blutbildung im Lichte der experimentellen Physiologie des 17. Jahrhunderts', *Gesnerus*, xviii (1961), 85–146, at 125–6.
19. See Shugg, 'Humanitarian Attitudes'; Oster, '"Beame of Diuitiy"'; A. Faller, 'Niels Stensen und der Cartesianismus', in G. Scherz (ed.), *Nicolaus Steno and his Indice* (Copenhagen: Munksgaard, 1958), 140–66.

20. Bartholinus, *Defensio,* 95, and Conring, *Introductio,* 89, for example, explicitly point to the disturbing struggle of vivisected animals.
21. Cf. Severino, *Zootomia,* 152.
22. See Bartholinus, *Defensio,* 96–7.
23. Cf. L. Heister, *De anatomes subtilioris utilitate* (Helmstedt: P. D. Schnorr, 1728), 8, 12. For a summary of the Pythagorean and neo-Platonist doctrines of metempsychosis see U. Dierauer, *Tier und Mensch im Denken der Antike. Studien zur Tierpsychologie, Anthropologie und Ethik* (Amsterdam: B. R. Grüner, 1977), 18–24, 80–9.
24. See N. K. Gharpure, *Tierschutz, Vegetarismus und Konfession (eine religions-soziologische Untersuchung zum englischen 17. und 18. Jahrhundert)* (Munich: E. Hohenhaus, 1935), 37–47, 102–6; Thomas, *Man and the Natural World,* 138, 291–2.
25. Cf. *ibid.*, 292; Ovid, *Metamorphoses,* xv, 106–7, 116–24, 459–78.
26. See N. Ault (ed.), *The Prose Works of Alexander Pope* (Oxford: B. Blackwell, 1936), i, 107–14.
27. For example A. Olearius (ed.), *Des Hoch-Edelgebornen Johan Albrechts von Mandelslo Morgenländische Reisebeschreibung* (Schleswig: J. Holwein, 1658), 26, 112–13; see also Pufendorf, *De jure,* i, 509.
28. See also J. Passmore, 'The Treatment of Animals', *Journal of the History of Ideas,* xxxvi (1975), 195–218.
29. Cf. Ch. S. Wolff, *Disputatio philosophica de moralitate anatomes circa animalia viva occupatae* (Leipzig: J. S. Fleischer, 1709), 24–5.
30. See Mani, 'Darmresorption', 121–5; *idem,* 'Jean Riolan II (1580–1657) and Medical Research', *Bulletin of the History of Medicine,* xlii (1968), 121–44; K. E. Rothschuh, 'Jean Riolan jun. (1580–1657) im Streit mit Paul Marquart Schlegel (1605–1653) um die Blutbewegungslehre Harvey's', *Gesnerus,* xxi (1964), 72–82; A.-H. Maehle, 'Diskussionen um die Berechtigung des medizinischen Tierversuchs im 17. und 18. Jahrhundert', *Würzburger medizinhistorische Mitteilungen,* v (1987), 65–84.
31. J. Riolan jr., 'Animadversiones secundae ad Anatomia Reformatam Thomae Bartholini', in *idem, Opuscula nova anatomica* [2nd part] (Paris: M. Dupuis, 1653), preface, [5–6]:
    'Crede mihi, haec Anatome viventium Animalium similis est Lanienae viventium animalium, qualem exercent Lanij; Istis operationibus audaciores facti, non dubitant Viventes homines levi de causa iugulare; sic Anatomici viventium animalium dissectionibus assuefacti facile viventes adhuc Homines moribundos clanculum, tanquam mortuos aperirent, ut ea, quae in animalibus viventibus quaerunt, in hominibus inveniant. Propterea istam Anatomem nimis curiosam odi, et eius scrutatores et sectatores.'
32. See Passmore, 'Treatment of Animals', 201.
33. See Dierauer, *Tier und Mensch,* 292–3.
34. Ovid, *Metamorphoses,* xv, 463–9.
35. See D. Harwood, *Love for Animals and how it Developed in Great*

Britain (Ph.D. thesis, Columbia University New York, 1928), 73–4; H. Hastings, *Man and Beast in French Thought of the Eighteenth Century* (Baltimore: Johns Hopkins Press, 1936), 247–8; L. G. Stevenson, 'On the Supposed Exclusion of Butchers and Surgeons from Jury Duty', *Journal of the History of Medicine*, ix (1954), 235–8.

36. See below, 218–20, 232.
37. Cf. Severino, *Zootomia,* 153; E. Littré (ed.), *Oeuvres complètes d'Hippocrate* (Paris, 1839–61 – reprint Amsterdam: Hakkert, 1962), ix, 354–5 (Pseudoepigrapha 17).
38. The years in brackets signify the dates of publication. See G. Aselli, *De lactibus sive lacteis venis quarto vasorum mesaraicorum genere novo invento* (Milan: J. B. Bidellius, 1627); W. Harvey, *Exercitatio anatomica de motu cordis et sanguinis in animalibus* (Frankfurt: W. Fitzer, 1628); J. Pecquet, *Experimenta nova anatomica, quibus incognitum hactenus chyli receptaculum, et ab eo per thoracem in ramos usque subclavios vasa lactea deteguntur* (Paris: S. and G. Cramoisy, 1651); Th. Bartholinus, *Vasa lymphatica, nuper Hafniae in animantibus inventa, et hepatis exsequiae* (Copenhagen: G. Holst, 1653); O. Rudbeck, *Nova exercitatio anatomica, exhibens ductus hepaticos aquosos, et vasa glandularum serosa, nunc primum inventa* (Västerås: E. Lauringer, 1653).
39. See, for instance, J. van Horne, *Novus ductus chyliferus* (Leyden: F. Hack, 1652), [2–3]; Bartholin, *Defensio,* 95–6; W. Rolfinck, *Dissertationes anatomicae methodo synthetica exaratae* (Nuremberg: M. Endter, 1656), 31; R. Boyle, *The Works* (London: A. Millar, 1744), i, 465; F. Hoffmann sen., *Cardianastrophe admiranda seu cordis inversio memorabilis* (Leipzig: Ch. Kirchner, 1671), preface, [3].
40. See, for instance, Riolan, *Anthropographia,* 66–7; Severino, *Zootomia,* 162; Conring, *Introductio,* 87–8, 90, 94; Rolfinck, *Dissertationes,* 30–4; Th. Bartholinus, *Anatomia, ex Caspari Bartholini parentis Institutionibus ... reformata* (Leyden-Rotterdam: Hack, 1669), preface, 1.
41. See A.-H. Maehle, *Johann Jakob Wepfer (1620–1695) als Toxikologe. Die Fallstudien und Tierexperimente aus seiner Abhandlung über den Wasserschierling (1679)* (Aarau-Frankfurt a. M.-Salzburg: Sauerländer, 1987).
42. Cf. J. J. Wepfer, *Cicutae aquaticae historia et noxae* (Basle: J. R. König, 1679), 132, 134. See also Maehle, *Wepfer,* 125–6.
43. Cf. Wepfer, *Cicutae aquaticae historia,* 132; Maehle, *Wepfer,* 124.
44. See below, 221–2, 231–2.
45. Oster, 'Beame of Diuinity', 172.
46. Cf. Th. Willis, *Cerebri anatome: cui accessit nervorum descriptio et usus* (London: J. Martyn and J. Allestry, 1664), dedication, [3–4]; see also W. F. Bynum, 'The Anatomical Method, Natural Theology, and the Functions of the Brain', *Isis,* lxiv (1973), 445–68.
47. See A.-H. Maehle, '"Est Deus ossa probant" – Human Anatomy and

Physicotheology in 17th and 18th Century Germany', in Ä. Bäumer and M. Büttner (eds), *Science and Religion / Wissenschaft und Religion* (Bochum: Brockmeyer, 1989), 60–6.

48. Wolff, *Disputatio.*
49. *Ibid.*, 18–24.
50. *Ibid.*, 16–18. Cf. F. Hoffmann, *De atheo convincendo ex artificiosissima machinae humanae structura oratio* [Halle, 1693] (no place, Ch. A. Zeitler, 1705); G. A. Hamberger, 'De Deo ex inspectione cordis demonstrato' [1692], in *idem, Fasciculus dissertationum academicarum physico-mathematicarum* (Jena: Gollner, 1708), 1–36; J. F. Wucherer, *Dissertatio academica de atheo ex structura tou egkephalou convincendo* (Jena: Müller, 1708).
51. See Ch. Mylius, 'Untersuchung, ob man die Thiere, um physiologischer Versuche willen, lebendig eröffnen dürfe?', *Belustigungen des Verstandes und des Witzes,* April 1745, 325–40; Maehle, 'Der Literat Christlob Mylius', 272, 278.
52. See below, 217.
53. Cf. R. Heidenhain, *Die Vivisection im Dienste der Heilkunde* (Leipzig: Breitkopf and Härtel, 1879), 51
54. Cf. J. C. C. Rupp, 'Matters of Life and Death: The Social and Cultural Conditions of the Rise of Anatomical Theatres, with Special Reference to Seventeenth Century Holland', *History of Science,* xxviii (1990), 263–87.
55. For details and references to particular works of the quoted writers see Maehle, 'Literary Responses'.
56. See also Thomas, *Man and the Natural World,* 143–90.
57. Cf. Pufendorf, *De jure,* i, 511; Ch. Gerber, *Unerkannte Sünden der Welt* (Dresden-Frankfurt: Ch. Hekels and J. J. Winckler, 5th ed. 1705–12), i, 266–74; J. H. Winkler, *Institutiones philosophiae universae usibus academicis accomodatae* (Leipzig: Fritsch, 3rd ed. 1762), iii, 133–9; J. Hildrop, 'Free Thoughts upon the Brute-Creation', in *idem, The Miscellaneous Works* (London: J. and J. Rivington, 1754), i, 159–294, on 230–2; H. Primatt, *Ueber Barmherzigkeit und Grausamkeit gegen die thierische Schöpfung* [transl. of *A Dissertation on the Duty of Mercy and Sin of Cruelty to Brute Animals* (London, 1776)] (Halle: J. J. Gebauer, 1778); L. Smith, *Versuch eines vollständigen Lehrgebäudes der Natur und Bestimmung der Thiere und der Pflichten des Menschen gegen die Thiere* (Copenhagen: Ch. G. Proft, 1793), 473–85; F. V. Reinhard, *System der Christlichen Moral* (Vienna: C. Grässer and Härter, 1816), v, 122–34.
58. Cf. Ch. G. Jöcher, [sermon on Lucas 14:5, Paulinerkirche Leipzig, Dominica XVII. post Festum Trinitatis, 1752], quoted in Winkler, *Institutiones,* iii, 134–6; J. Granger, *An Apology for the Brute Creation or Abuse of Animals censured* (London: T. Davies, 1772).
59. Cf. Th. Young, *An Essay on Humanity to Animals* (London: T. Cadwell, Jun. and W. Davies, 1798).

60. See L. Cohen Rosenfield, *From Beast-Machine to Man-Machine. The Theme of Animal Soul in French Letters from Descartes to La Mettrie* (New York: Oxford University Press, 1940); Hastings, *Man and Beast;* H. Kirkinen, *Les Origines de la Conception Moderne de l'Homme-Machine. Le Problème de l'Ame en France a la Fin du Regne de Louis XIV (1670–1715)* (Helsinki: Suomalainen Tiedeakatemia, 1960).
61. See J. Cottingham, '"A Brute to the Brutes?": Descartes' Treatment of Animals', *Philosophy,* liii (1978), 551–9.
62. Cf. N. Fontaine, *Mémoires pour servir à l'Histoire de Port-Royal* (Cologne: Aux dépens de la Compagnie, 1738), ii, 52–3; Ch.-A. Sainte-Beuve, *Port-Royal* (Paris: E. Renduel, 1840–59), ii, 306; Ch. Beard, *Port Royal. A Contribution to the History of Religion and Literature in France* (London: Longman, Green, Longman, and Roberts, 1861), ii, 68–9.
63. See [J. H. Winkler (ed.)], *Die verschiedenen Meynungen einiger Weltweisen von der Existenz der Seelen der Thiere in einer Gesellschaft guter Freunde untersucht* (Leipzig: B. Ch. Breitkopf, 3rd ed. 1743); [*idem*], *Die Frage, ob die Seelen der Thiere Verstand haben?* (*ibid.*,1742); [*idem*], *Philosophische Untersuchung der Frage, Ob die Seelen einiger Thiere einen gewissen Grad der Vernunft haben* (*ibid.*, 1742); [*idem*], *Philosophische Untersuchung der Frage, Ob die Seelen der Thiere mit ihren Leibern sterben?* (*ibid.*,1743); *idem, Institutiones,* i, 569–608; Hildrop, 'Free Thoughts'; R. Dean, *An Essay on the Future Life of Brute Creatures* (London: G. Kearsly, 1768), ii, 49–104.
64. Winkler, *Institutiones,* iii, 132.
65. Hildrop, 'Free Thoughts', 230.
66. Dean, *Essay,* ii, 104–9.
67. L. Smith, *Forsig til en Fuldstaendig Laerebygning om Dyrenes Natur og Bestemmelse og Menneskets Pligter mod Dyrene* (Copenhagen: J. F. Schultz, 1791). I have used the German edition, *Versuch eines vollständigen Lehrgebäudes.*
68. Cf. *ibid.*, preface, xxi–xxii.
69. Cf. J. F. L. Volckmann, *Menschenstolz und Thierqualen - eine Vertheidigung der seufzenden Creatur vor dem Richterstuhle der Menschlichkeit* (Helmstedt: C. G. Fleckeisen, 1799), 3–24, 81, 135, 146.
70. See A. O. Lovejoy, *The Great Chain of Being. A Study of the History of an Idea* (Cambridge, Mass.- London: Harvard University Press, 1964).
71. See Passmore, 'Treatment of Animals'; Ch. W. Hume, *The Status of Animals in the Christian Religion* (London: The Universities Federation for Animal Welfare, 1957), 28–30.
72. Cf. Hildrop, 'Free Thoughts', 272–5; Primatt, *Barmherzigkeit und Grausamkeit,* 13–14; S. Jenyns, *The Works,* Ch. N. Cole (ed.) (London: T. Cadell, 1790), iii, 56–80, 179–95.
73. Cf. S. J. Apinus, *Dissertatio ex iure naturae an liceat brutorum corpora*

mutilare et speciatim Ob es recht sey dass man den Hunden die Ohren abschneide (Altdorf: J. W. Kohlesius, 1722), 12–17.
74. Cf. D. Hume, *The Philosophical Works*, Th. Hill Green and Th. Hodge Grose (eds) (London, 1882–86 - reprint Aalen: Scientia, 1964), iv, 185–6.
75. Cf. I. Kant, *Werke*, W. Weischedel (ed.) (Darmstadt: Wiss. Buchgesellschaft, 1956), iv, 349, 577–9.
76. See above, 205.
77. Cf. Ch. Bonnet, *Oeuvres d'histoire naturelle et de philosophie* (Neuchâtel: S. Fauche, 1779–83), vii, 405–8.
78. Cf. Primatt, *Barmherzigkeit und Grausamkeit*, 34–40.
79. Cf. *ibid.*, 16–17.
80. Cf. W. Dietler, *Gerechtigkeit gegen Thiere* (Mainz: Schiller, 1787), 28–9.
81. Cf. J. Bentham, *An Introduction to the Principles of Morals and Legislation*, J. H. Burns and H. L. A. Hart (eds) (London: Athlone, 1970), 282–3.
82. Cf. *ibid.*, and Kant, *Werke*, iv, 578–9.
83. See Thomas, *Man and the Natural World*, 107–20.
84. See *ibid.*, 100–1, 143–50; Harwood, *Love for Animals*, 47–75; R. W. Malcolmson, *Popular Recreations in English Society 1700–1850* (Cambridge: Cambridge University Press, 1973), 45–51.
85. Cf. e.g. Apinus, *Dissertatio*, 9–10; Jöcher, [sermon on Lucas 14:5], 134–5; Dean, *Essay*, ii, 108; Granger, *Apology*, dedication, 10–15; Primatt, *Barmherzigkeit und Grausamkeit*, 51–2, 158–9; Dietler, *Gerechtigkeit*, 42–70; Reinhard, *System*, v, 133–4; Young, *Essay*, 40–186; Volckmann, *Menschenstolz*, 29–30, 33, 220.
86. Cf. Granger, *Apology*, postscript.
87. Cf. Dietler, *Gerechtigkeit*, iii.
88. Cf. Young, *Essay*, 1. See also Passmore, 'Treatment of Animals', 209.
89. See above, 209.
90. Cf. Winkler, *Institutiones*, iii, 137–9.
91. See *ibid.*, 133.
92. See note 63 above.
93. Cf. Winkler, *Institutiones*, iii, 137.
94. Cf. *ibid.*, 136. Here Winkler evidently followed Wolff, who had used the same argument before in his *Disputatio*, 12–13.
95. Cf. J. Spence, *Observations, anecdotes, and characters of books and men collected from conversation*, J. M. Osborn (ed.) (Oxford: Clarendon, 1966), i, 118–19. See also Maehle, 'Literary Responses', 41–2.
96. See A. Pope, *An Essay on Man*, M. Mack (ed.) (London: Methuen, 1950), 41–5; see also Lovejoy, *Great Chain of Being*, 183–207.
97. Cf. Spence, *Observations*, 118.
98. Cf. Ault, *Prose Works of Alexander Pope*, i, 107–14. See also Maehle, 'Literary Responses', 36.
99. Cf. A. A. von Sinclair, *Vermischte Abhandlungen und Anmerkungen aus*

den Geschichten, dem Staatsrechte, der Sittenlehre und den schönen Wissenschaften (Frankfurt-Leipzig: Knoch and Esslinger, 1751), 291–428 [328], particularly 408 [308]. Sinclair's criticism of vivisection had been provoked by an article by H. F. Delius, 'Schreiben an Herrn K* Ob es auch anatomische Belustigungen gäbe', *Belustigungen des Verstandes und des Witzes*, October 1743, 360–5. Delius, later professor of medicine in Erlangen, had recommended vivisection of frogs as a convenient method for the study of the blood circulation. See also A.-H. Maehle, '"Ob es auch anatomische Belustigungen gäbe" – Ein Disput über die Ästhetik der Leichenpräparation im 18. Jahrhundert', *Würzburger medizinhistorische Mitteilungen*, vi (1988), 89–109.

100. Cf. S. Johnson, *The Idler and the Adventurer*, W. J. Bate, J. M. Bullitt and L. F. Powell (eds) (New Haven-London: Yale University Press, 1963), 53–6 (Idler No. 17). Johnson mainly seems to have been scandalized at vivisections performed by Richard Brocklesby, who had repeated some of Albrecht von Haller's experiments on sensibility and irritability. See Maehle, 'Literary Responses', 44–5; J. Wiltshire, *Samuel Johnson in the Medical World: the Doctor and the Patient* (Cambridge-New York-Port Chester: Cambridge University Press, 1991), 135–7.
101. Cf. Sinclair, *Vermischte Abhandlungen*, 410–11 [310–11].
102. Cf. *ibid.*, 416 [316].
103. Cf. Johnson, *Idler*, 33 (Idler No. 10).
104. Cf. Voltaire, *Dictionnaire philosophique*, J. Benda and R. Naves (eds) (Paris: Garnier, 1961), 51 (article 'Bêtes').
105. Cf. Bonnet, *Oeuvres*, vii, 410–12.
106. See Smith, *Versuch eines vollständigen Lehrgebäudes*, xvii–xviii.
107. Cf. *ibid.*, 392–6.
108. Cf. J. Lawrence, *A Philosophical and Practical Treatise on Horses, and on the Moral Duties of Man towards the Brute Creation* (London: Sherwood, Neely, and Jones, 3rd ed. 1810), i, 127–9.
109. Cf. *ibid.*, 138.
110. Cf. Smith, *Versuch eines vollständigen Lehrgebäudes*, 463.
111. Cf. *ibid.*, 462; Lawrence, *Treatise on Horses*, i, 140.
112. Cf. Winkler, *Institutiones*, iii, 138.
113. Johnson, *Idler*, 56.
114. Cf. A. G. Kästner, *Sinngedichte und Einfälle* (Frankfurt-Leipzig: L. Schellenberg, 1800), 221–2. For similar statements questioning the medical utility of vivisection see also *idem*, *Epigramme*, C. Becker (ed.) (Halle: M. Niemeyer, 1911), 204; Sinclair, *Vermischte Abhandlungen*, 415–16 [315–16]; Smith, *Versuch eines vollständigen Lehrgebäudes*, 459–60.
115. See Johnson, *Idler*, 55–6.
116. See e. g. B. Langrish, *Physical Experiments upon Brutes* (London: C. Hitch, 1746), ix–x, xvii, xx–xxi, 56–7; W. Lewis, *An Experimental*

History of the Materia medica (London: H. Baldwin and R. Willock, 1761), viii–ix; J. A. Murray, 'De observationibus et experimentis apud bruta captis caute ad corpus humanun applicandis' [1772], in *idem*, *Opuscula* (Göttingen: J. Ch. Dieterich, 1785–86), i, 227–52; J. F. Gmelin, *Allgemeine Geschichte der Gifte, Erster Theil* (Leipzig: Weygand, 1776), 30–42; G. F. Hildebrandt, *Versuch einer philosophischen Pharmakologie* (Braunschweig: Waisenhausbuchhandlung, 1786), 70–83. See also M. P. Earles, 'Experiments with Drugs and Poisons in the Seventeenth and Eighteenth Centuries', *Annals of Science*, xix (1963), 241–54; R. Winau, 'Experimentelle Pharmakologie an der Universität Göttingen im 18. Jahrhundert', *Medizinhistorisches Journal*, vii (1972), 135–45; *idem*, 'Vom kasuistischen Behandlungsversuch zum kontrollierten klinischen Versuch', in H. Helmchen and R. Winau (eds), *Versuche mit Menschen in Medizin, Humanwissenschaft und Politik* (Berlin-New York: W. de Gruyter, 1986), 83–107.

117. See above, 208
118. Cf. H.-L. Duhamel Dumonceau, 'Observations sur la réunion des fractures des os. Premier mémoire', *Histoire de l'Académie Royale des Sciences*, 1741, 97–112, at 98.
119. R. Brocklesby, 'An Account of the poisonous Root lately found mixed among the Gentian', *Philosophical Transactions*, xlv (1748), 240–3, at 242.
120. Cf. A. von Haller, 'De partibus corporis humani sensilibus et irritabilibus', *Commentarii Societatis Regiae Scientiarum Gottingensis*, ii (1752), 114–158, at 114.
121. See also K. E. Rothschuh, *Physiologie. Der Wandel ihrer Konzepte, Probleme und Methoden vom 16. bis 19. Jahrhundert* (Freiburg i. Brsg.-Munich: K. Alber, 1968), 28, and recently M. Daly, 'Vivisection in Eighteenth-Century Britain', *British Journal for Eighteenth-Century Studies*, xii (1989), 57–67, who points to 'dead-end vivisection' in the 18th century.
122. See Wolff, *Disputatio*, 18–19; Heister, *De anatomes ... utilitate*, 12; Mylius, 'Untersuchung ob man die Thiere ... eröffnen dürfe?'
123. Cf. K. F. Hommel, *Rhapsodia quaestionum in foro quotidie obvenientium neque tamen legibus decisarum*, K. G. Roessig (ed.) (Bayreuth: J. A. Lubeck, 1782–87), ii, 46–7 and iv, 84–5. In the early 18th century the killing of dogs for scientific purposes had still been regarded as a prescriptive right of doctors, medical students and surgeons; see H. Klüver, *Electa de jure canum Vom Hunderecht ubi praecipuae controversiae quae circa canes accidere possunt explicantur et dissolvuntur* (Stade: H. Brummer, 1711), 21.
124. Cf. Hommel, *Rhapsodia*, ii, 38–41; see also W. Sellert, 'Das Tier in der abendländischen Rechtsauffassung', in *Studium generale. Vorträge zum Thema: Mensch und Tier*, Tierärztliche Hochschule Hannover (ed.) (Hanover: M. and H. Schaper, 1984), 66–84.
125. Cf. Wolff, *Disputatio*, 28–40.

126. For the history of ethical calculi see L. I. Bredvold, 'The invention of the ethical calculus', in R. Foster Jones (ed.), *The Seventeenth Century* (Stanford: Stanford University Press, 1951), 165–80.
127. Cf. Mylius, 'Untersuchung ... ob man die Thiere eröffnen dürfe?'. See also Maehle, 'Der Literat Christlob Mylius'.
128. Cf. P.-L. M. de Maupertuis, *Lettres* (Dresden: G. C. Walther, 1752), 198–205.
129. Cf. Heister, *De anatomes ... utilitate*, 12–14; Haller, 'De partibus', 114; Duhamel, 'Observations', 98; R. Brocklesby, 'An Account of some Experiments on the Sensibility and Irritability of the several Parts of Animals', *Philosophical Transactions*, il (1755), 240–5.
130. See Ch. D. Leake (ed.), *Percival's Medical Ethics* (Huntington, New York: R. E. Krieger, 1975).
131. Th. Percival, 'A Father's Instructions', in *idem*, *The Works, Literary, Moral, and Philosophical* (London: J. Johnson, 1807), i, 1–377, at 50–1.
132. For details and the real scientific background see Maehle, 'Literary Responses', 48–9.
133. Percival, 'Father's Instructions', 51.
134. See Young, *Essay*, 170–5; H. Crowe, *Zoophilos; or, Considerations on the Moral Treatment of Inferior Animals* (Bath-London: Cruttwell and Longman etc., 2nd ed. 1820), 78–95; Reinhard, *System*, v, 134–5; Ch. A. Dann, *Bitte der armen Thiere, der unvernünftigen Geschöpfe, an ihre vernünftigen Mitgeschöpfe und Herrn die Menschen* (Tübingen: L. F. Fues, 2nd ed. 1838), 22–5.
135. Cf. *ibid.*, 24; Reinhard, *System*, v, 134.
136. Cf. Sinclair, *Vermischte Abhandlungen*, 416 [316]; Smith, *Versuch eines vollständigen Lehrgebäudes*, 459, 463; Lawrence, *Treatise on Horses*, i, 142–3. Reinhard was evidently influenced by Smith, whose *Versuch eines vollständigen Lehrgebäudes* he cited in his *System*, v, 134. For the general idea of gaining physiological knowledge through anatomical methods see L. G. Stevenson, 'Anatomical Reasoning in Physiological Thought', in Ch. McC. Brooks and P. F. Cranefield (eds), *The Historical Development of Physiological Thought* (New York: Hafner, 1959), 27–38.
137. Cf. M. Hall, *A Critical and Experimental Essay on the Circulation of the Blood; Especially as Observed in the Minute and Capillary Vessels of the Batrachia and of Fishes* (London: R. B. Seeley and W. Burnside, 1831), 1–11.
138. Cf. *ibid.*, 7.
139. Cf. Ch. G. Hopf, 'Haben die in der neuern Zeit beinahe zur grausamen Mode gewordenen Versuche an Thieren, zumal an Katzen und Hunden, um die Wirkungsart der Arzneimittel und Gifte zu erforschen, zu irgend einem haltbaren Resultate geführt?', *Zeitschrift für die Staatsarzneikunde*, xviii (1829), 465–74.
140. See D. Manuel, 'Marshall Hall (1790–1857): Vivisection and the

Development of Experimental Physiology', in Rupke, *Vivisection,* 78–104.

141. Cf. Hall, *Essay on the Circulation,* 1–2. Despite his code Hall was subsequently accused of cruelty to his experimental animals; see Manuel, 'Marshall Hall', 97–100.
142. See Maehle, 'Literary Responses', 41, 46; Thomas, *Man and the Natural World,* 115 , 119; Smith, *Versuch eines vollständigen Lehrgebäudes,* 17–22. Also Lawrence, who was a horse-fancier, may be mentioned here; see his *Treatise on Horses.*
143. See French, *Antivivisection,* 373–4; Turner, *Reckoning with the Beast.* 30–3.
144. See Ritvo, *Animal Estate,* ch. 2.
145. Cf. French, *Antivivisection,* 375–9.
146. See *ibid.,* 379–85.
147. For a discussion of *Martin's Act,* its amendments and consequences see B. Harrison, *Peaceable Kingdom. Stability and Change in Modern Britain* (Oxford: Clarendon, 1982), 82–122; Turner, *Reckoning with the Beast,* ch. 3; Ritvo, *Animal Estate,* ch. 3.
148. Cf. Juchem, *Entwicklung des Tierschutzes,* 46–57; U. Hahn, *Die Entwicklung des Tierschutzgedankens in Religion und Geistesgeschichte* (Diss. med. vet., Tierärztliche Hochschule Hannover, Hanover, 1980), 120–6.
149. See the references in note 147 above.
150. See U. Tröhler and A.-H. Maehle, 'Anti-vivisection in Nineteenth-century Germany and Switzerland: Motives and Methods', in Rupke, *Vivisection,* 149–87, on 149–50.
151. Cf. Harrison, *Peaceable Kingdom,* 91–103; H. W. von Ehrenstein, *Schild und Waffen gegen Thierquälerei. Ein Beitrag zu allgemeiner Förderung der Menschlichkeit* (Leipzig: B. G. Teubner, 1840), iv, 154–90.
152. Cf. W. Youatt, *The Obligation and Extent of Humanity to Brutes, principally considered with reference to Domesticated Animals* (London: Longman, Orme, Brown etc., 1839); Th. I. M. Forster, *Philozoia; or Moral Reflections on the Actual Condition of the Animal Kingdom, and on the Means of Improving the same* (Brussels: Deltombe and W. Todd, 1839); L. Gompertz, *Fragments in Defence of Animals, and Essays on Morals, Soul, and Future State* (London: W. Horsell, 1852); Ehrenstein, *Schild und Waffen.*
153. Cf. Youatt, *Obligation and Extent of Humanity,* 195.
154. Cf. Ehrenstein, *Schild und Waffen,* 1–7; J. J. Rousseau, 'Discours sur l'Origine et les Fondements de l'Inégalité parmi les Hommes', in *idem, Oeuvres Complètes,* V. D. Musset-Pathay (ed.) (Paris: Dupont, 1823–4), i, 221–356, on 259–62.
155. Cf. Youatt, *Obligation and Extent of Humanity,* 194–7, 201; Forster, *Philozoia,* 33–4, 75–6; Gompertz, *Fragments,* 119; Ehrenstein, *Schild und Waffen,* 24, 59–60.

156. Cf. Youatt, *Obligation and Extent of Humanity,* 197–204; Gompertz, *Fragments,* 120–1. Forster explicitly recommended this strategy to the Animals' Friend Society; see his *Philozoia,* 34.
157. Cf. F. W. Theile, *Ueber den Nutzen physiologischer Versuche an Thieren für die Heilkunde und über die Vorurtheile gegen solche Versuche* (Berne: Weingart, 1842).
158. Cf. A. Schopenhauer, *Sämtliche Werke,* A. Hübscher (ed.) (Wiesbaden: Brockhaus, 2nd ed. 1947–50), iv, 205–49.
159. See above, 214.
160. Cf. Schopenhauer, *Werke,* iv, 161–2.
161. Cf. *ibid.,* 162.
162. Cf. *ibid.,* vi, 393–401.
163. *Ibid.,* 400.
164. Cf. *ibid.,* 396–7.
165. Cf. Kant, *Werke,* iv, 579.
166. See B. M. Duncum, *The Development of Inhalation Anaesthesia with Special Reference to the Years 1846–1900* (London-New York-Toronto: Oxford University Press, 1947), 170.
167. Cf. Schopenhauer, *Werke,* vi, 400.
168. See for example G. Hoggan, *Morning Post,* 2 February, 1875, partly reprinted in French, *Antivivisection,* 414–15; H. Stenz, *Die Vivisektion in ihrer wahren Gestalt. Unwiderlegliche Thatsachen aus der Fachlitteratur* (Berlin: Weltbund zur Bekämpfung der Vivisektion, c. 1899), 1–30.
169. See P. Guarnieri, 'Moritz Schiff (1823–96): Experimental Physiology and Noble Sentiment in Florence', in Rupke, *Vivisection,* 105–24; J. J. Dreifuss, 'Moritz Schiff et la vivisection', *Gesnerus,* xlii (1985), 289–303.
170. See the works quoted in notes 1 and 2 above.
171. Cf. above, 222–4.
172. Cf. French, *Antivivisection,* 143–4; Bretschneider, *Streit um die Vivisektion,* 157.
173. Cf. French, *Antivivisection,* 160–3. Tröhler and Maehle, 'Anti-vivisection', 178; and for Switzerland, Neff, *Streit um den wissenschaftlichen Tierversuch,* 116–18.
174. See W. Coleman and F. L. Holmes (eds), *The Investigative Enterprise. Experimental Physiology in Nineteenth-Century Medicine* (Berkeley-Los Angeles-London: University of California Press, 1988); P. Elliott, 'Vivisection and the Emergence of Experimental Physiology in Nineteenth-century France', in Rupke, *Vivisection,* 48–77.
175. Cf. French, *Antivivisection,* 371–2.
176. Cf. Rupke, *Vivisection,* 8.
177. Cf. U. Tröhler, 'Was ist neu? – Der medizinische Tierversuch im Meinungsstreit', *Swiss Pharma,* vii (1985), 7–16; Neff, *Streit um den wissenschaftlichen Tierversuch,* viii, 69–71.
178. Cf. Lansbury, *Old Brown Dog; eadem,* 'Gynaecology, Pornography,

and the Antivivisection Movement', *Victorian Studies*, xxviii (1985), 413–37.

179. Cf. M. A. Elston, 'Women and Anti-vivisection in Victorian England, 1870–1900', in Rupke, *Vivisection*, 259–94. In German and Swiss anti-vivisection societies, in the same period, about 40 per cent of the members were women. Cf. Tröhler and Maehle, 'Anti-vivisection', 174; Neff, *Streit um den wissenschaftlichen Tierversuch*, 50.

180. Cf. J. Paget, R. Owen and S. Wilks, 'Vivisection: Its Pains and Its Uses'(part I–III), *The Nineteenth Century*, x (1881), 920–48; R. Virchow, 'Ueber den Werth des pathologischen Experiments' in W. Mac Cormac and G. H. Makins (eds), *Transactions of the International Medical Congress ... London, August 2nd to 9th, 1881* (London: J. W. Kolckmann, 1881), i, 22–37; Heidenhain, *Vivisection im Dienste der Heilkunde;* I. P. Pavlov, *Das Experiment als zeitgemässe und einheitliche Methode medizinischer Forschung. Dargestellt am Beispiel der Verdauungslehre*, transl. by A. Walther (Wiesbaden: J. F. Bergmann, 1900). For the context of these contributions see N. Rupke, 'Pro-vivisection in England in the Early 1880s: Arguments and Motives', in *idem, Vivisection*, 188–208; A.-H. Maehle, 'Tierversuchsdiskussion und Naturverständnis vor 100 Jahren: Die Kontroverse Grysanowski-Heidenhain', *Niedersächsisches Ärzteblatt*, lxi (1988), No. 6, 36–40; M.P. Mul'tanowskij, 'Die Äusserungen I.P. Pavlovs zu Fragen der Geschichte der Naturwissenschaft und der Medizin', *Medizinhistorisches Journal*, ii (1967), 208–30.

181. R. Heidenhain, *Die Vivisection* (Leipzig: Breitkopf and Härtel, 1884).

182. See F. P. Cobbe, *Licht an dunklen Stätten*, transl. by Agnes Gräfin Egloffstein (Hanover: Schmorl and von Seefeld, 1883); E. von Weber, *Die Folterkammern der Wissenschaft. Eine Sammlung von Thatsachen für das Laien-Publikum* (Berlin-Leipzig: Voigt, 1879); Stenz, *Vivisektion in ihrer wahren Gestalt.*

183. See particularly Paget, Owen and Wilks, 'Vivisection'. Only strict vegetarians were consistent in this respect, as Virchow pointed out in his 'Werth des pathologischen Experiments', 35.

184. E. Melena, *Gemma oder Tugend und Laster* (Munich: Franz, 1877). The fact that violence to animals develops into violence to a woman in this story seems to confirm the theses of Lansbury, see above 230.

185. Cf. L. Hermann, *Die Vivisectionsfrage. Für das grössere Publicum beleuchtet* (Leipzig: F. C. W. Vogel, 1877), 17, 40–1, 50. See also the corresponding standpoint of Wilks, 'Vivisection' (part III), 945–6.

186. Cf. Hermann, *Vivisectionsfrage*, 14–18, 59–64.

187. Cf. B. Rawitz, *Für die Vivisection. Eine Streitschrift* (Greifswald: J. Abel, 1898), 14, 44–5.

188. For details concerning Grysanowski's role in German anti-vivisectionism see Tröhler and Maehle, 'Anti-vivisection'.

189. Cf. E. Grysanowski, *Gesammelte antivivisectionistische Schriften* (Münster: J. Basch, 1897), 49–60.

190. *Ibid.*, 45, 62. Actually the idea of a healthy way of life making much of experimental research in medicine superfluous had already been formulated in the early 1790s by L. Smith, yet without recognizable resonance; cf. his *Versuch eines vollständigen Lehrgebäudes*, 460–2.
191. Grysanowski, *Schriften*, 78. For the history of this – originally Hippocratic – idea see M. Neuburger, *Die Lehre von der Heilkraft der Natur im Wandel der Zeiten* (Stuttgart: F. Enke, 1926).
192. Cf. R. Wagner, *Offener Brief an Ernst von Weber Verfasser der 'Folterkammern der Wissenschaft'. Ueber die Vivisection* (Berlin-Leipzig: Voigt, 1880), and J. Thiery and U. Tröhler, 'Doubt about Progress, but Trust in Compassion. Wagner the Antivivisectionist: His Motives and His Contemporaries' Reactions', in W. Wagner (ed.), *'Parsifal' Programmheft* II (Bayreuth: Bayreuther Festspiele, 1987), 65–101, who give further details and backgrounds of Wagner's comment.
193. Cf. *ibid.*, 33–44.
194. Cf. G. Hendrick, *Henry Salt, Humanitarian Reformer and Man of Letters* (Urbana-Chicago-London: University of Illinois Press, 1977), 1–6, 56–62. It was evidently Salt who furnished Shaw with anti-vivisectionist ideas for the 'Preface on Doctors', added to *The Doctor's Dilemma* in 1911 (see Hendrick, l.c., 73–7).
195. Cf. H. Salt, *Animals' Rights Considered in Relation to Social Progress* (New York-London: Macmillan, 1894), v–vi, 1–23.
196. See *ibid.*, chs 2–7, and Hendrick, *Henry Salt*, ch. 3.
197. Cf. *ibid.*, 83–4.
198. Salt, *Animals' Rights*, 78.
199. See W. Paton, *Man and Mouse. Animals in Medical Research* (Oxford-New York: Oxford University Press, 1984), ch. 5; K. J. Ullrich and O. D. Creutzfeldt (eds), *Gesundheit und Tierschutz. Wissenschaftler melden sich zu Wort* (Düsseldorf-Vienna: Econ, 1985), part II; Fred Lembeck (ed.), *Alternativen zum Tierversuch* (Stuttgart-New York: Thieme, 1988).
200. See e. g. R. D. Ryder, *Victims of Science. The Use of Animals in Research* (London-Fontwell, Sussex: Centaur Press, 2nd ed. 1983); B. Rambeck, *Mythos Tierversuch. Eine wissenschaftskritische Untersuchung* (Frankfurt a. M.: Zweitausendeins, 1990).
201. See H. Stiller and M. Stiller, *Tierversuch und Tierexperimentator* (Munich: F. Hirthammer, 4th ed. 1979), 47, 68–99.
202. Cf. O. D. Creutzfeldt, 'Ethik, Wissenschaft und Tierversuche', in Ullrich and Creutzfeldt, *Gesundheit und Tierschutz*, 11–43, on 21–2.
203. Cf. P. Singer, *Animal Liberation. A new Ethics for Our Treatment of Animals* (New York: The New York Review, 1975); T. Regan, *The Case for Animal Rights* (London-Melbourne-Henley: Routledge and Kegan Paul, 1984).
204. See Singer, *Animal Liberation*, 227–8, 274, 295–6; Regan, *Animal Rights*, 400.

205. See U. Wolf, 'Haben wir moralische Verpflichtungen gegen Tiere?', *Zeitschrift für philosophische Forschung*, xlii (1988), 222–46.
206. See Tröhler and Maehle, 'Anti-vivisection', 174.
207. See *ibid.*, 175; Lansbury, *Old Brown Dog*, ch. 2.
208. See D. H. Smyth, *Alternatives to Animal Experiments* (London: Scolar Press, 1978); Paton, *Man and Mouse*, ch. 8; Lembeck, *Alternativen.*
209. See also W. Paton, 'Epilogue', in Rupke, *Vivisection*, 361–4.
210. Cf. Rambeck, *Mythos Tierversuch*, 11, 250–1.

9

Thomas Gisborne: Physicians, Christians and Gentlemen

Roy Porter

Occupational groups display codes of behaviour special to themselves. By creating identity, and distinguishing themselves from other lines of work considered less dignified, such codes stake claims for privileges designed to confer moral, social, and even legal status. Modern medicine has typically claimed, like the other so-called liberal professions, to be both learned and ethical, in ways meant to elevate it above mere trade, to entitle it to respectful deference from its clients (patients), to exempt it from various external legal and political controls, and to legitimize rights of self-government and self-policing.[1]

Modern medical ethics are understood as having evolved to meet the desire of an emergent medical profession to become more tightly-organized and monopolistic, and thereby to achieve a higher degree of public authority and hegemony. John Gregory's *Observations on the Duties of a Physician* (1770) and Thomas Percival's *Medical Ethics; or, A Code of Institutes and Precepts Adapted to the Professional Conduct of Physicians and Surgeons* (1803) are routinely regarded as seminal texts in the British case, laying down rules of proper conduct for medical men, and thereby establishing claims upon the public.[2] It is not hard to locate the points of tension – the rise of the Edinburgh medical school, the development of the infirmary, competition within provincial, free market medical practice – which presumably triggered works such as these.[3]

We remain surprisingly ignorant, however, of the backgrounds against which Gregory and Percival were writing, in terms of both ethical theory and the informal rules of medical practice. How far did late eighteenth century practitioners habitually see themselves as bound by codes, implicit or explicit, of *professional* ethics? Or was, perhaps, their conduct unregulated by any norms, other than the laws of the land and the time-honoured consumer warning, *caveat emptor,* governing all crafts and commercial transactions? Or did doctors subscribe (or, at least, pay lip service) to other precepts – ones not unique to their *calling,* but to their (putative) social status, their religious affiliation, or even the demands of personal and family honour?

In a recent paper, Mary Fissell has argued that it might broadly be said that physicians traditionally liked to represent themselves as bound by gentlemanly manners and honour; that such an 'honour code' suffered a crisis in the second half of the eighteenth century, in part as a result of hostile public reaction to the deeply cynical account of aristocratic *moeurs* advanced in Lord Chesterfield's *Letters to his Son;* and that, through a kind of face-saving operation, new and self-ratifying bodies of professional *medical ethics,* such as Percival's, then had to be formulated, to rescue the good faith of the occupation, and re-establish the credit of medicine upon a sound footing.[4]

Fissell's arguments accord well with a very common reading of Percival's *Medical Ethics.* From the medical reformer, Chauncey Leake, over half a century ago, to more recent sociologists of the medical profession such as Jeffrey Berlant and Ivan Waddington, it has been contended that Percival did not advance a code of medical *ethics,* properly so-called, but rather a body of *etiquette,* that is, prudential precepts of behaviour. Percival's aim (the argument runs) was not to set the profession and practice of medicine upon an objective moral footing, but rather to provide a body of trade-union rules, as it were, to forestall or resolve intra-professional demarcation disputes, and thereby enhance the *esprit de corps* of practitioners, and their muscle-power with respect to their clients. The subsequent incorporation of Percival's *Medical Ethics* into later codes, particularly those of the various American state medical associations in the first half of the nineteenth century, has been regarded, in this interpretation, as symptomatic of the development of medicine as an aggressive, exclusive profession, using its expertise, its monopolistic position, and its idealistic pretensions, to control its clients, and giving support to the Shavian view that all professions are conspiracies against the laity.[5]

It would be utterly beyond the scope of this paper to offer a full assessment of this critical reading of Percival: this would, in any case, be quite redundant, in view of extensive reassessments of Percival by Robert Baker and J. V. Pickstone.[6] Rather I want to indicate that, at the same time as Percival, other influential prescriptions for guiding medical practice were being formulated, from rather different viewpoints, prominencing not the enlightened self-interest of the profession but higher sets of values, ones expressing not just *etiquette* but *ethics*, or, put another way, ones expressing the values appropriate to social rather than narrowly professional groups. This paper will analyse in detail one such directive, Thomas Gisborne's *An Enquiry into the Duties of Men in the Higher and Middle Classes of Society in Great Britain, Resulting from their Respective Stations, Professions and Employments.*

How are we to understand the relationship between the internal regulatory rules of some professional group, and broader codes endorsed by whole social classes or cadres? It is a difficult interpretative issue. Harold Perkin has spoken of the generations around the turn of the nineteenth century as constituting the 'emergence of professional society'.[7] Was the medical profession, from the late eighteenth century onwards, attempting to create specifically *professional* (i.e., not merely gentlemanly) norms for itself, designed to demarcate itself equally from discredited aristocratic privilege, and from a bourgeois, 'beggar-my-neighbour', shop-counter mentality, and to forestall state-regulation? Before we can begin to answer such questions, we obviously need to know much more about the attitudes and actions of medical men when faced with ethico-legal dilemmas, a task begun by Catherine Crawford and David Harley with their illuminating case-studies of Georgian disputes.[8] We also need to be better informed about a wider spectrum of attempts to codify professional ethical value-systems. It is to one of these that I wish to turn.

Thomas Gisborne's *An Enquiry into the Duties of Men* was first published in 1794, and went through six editions, the last appearing in 1811.[9] It was perhaps the age's most popular guide to professional ethical behaviour. Volume I explored the general rights and duties of subjects and citizens, before devoting specific chapters to the duties of the upper orders and members of the Establishment: the sovereign, peers, MPs, civil servants, naval and military officers, members of the legal profession, and magistrates. Volume II surveyed the moral obligations of the clerical profession, physicians, gentlemen engaged in trade and business, and, finally, men of private means.

Thomas Gisborne (1758–1846) – no relation to the contemporary President of the Royal College of Physicians of the same name – was a graduate of St John's College, Cambridge, who became a noteworthy divine of the Church of England, passing his life quietly, first as perpetual curate at Yoxall in Staffordshire, and later as a prebend at Durham Cathedral. He was a close friend of the leading Anglican Evangelicals of his day, especially William Wilberforce, and was conspicuous enough, while still a young man, to have a fine portrait painted of himself and his wife by Joseph Wright of Derby. He wrote extensively on public and ecclesiastical topics, championing an anti-Paleyan, anti-utilitarian rigorism in moral theology. He published sermons, volumes of verse, works on moral philosophy, and attacks on the slave trade. Not least, he was personally acquainted with Thomas Percival, to whom he refers as 'my excellent friend'. Percival apparently sent Gisborne a copy of his *Medical Ethics* while it was still in manuscript.[10]

I propose to offer an exegesis of Gisborne's views about the duties of physicians, contextualizing them against some of his other writings, and against other more or less contemporary formulations of medical ethics. On this basis, I shall finally offer a few wider suggestions about the constitution of medical ethics around the turn of the 19th-century.

In respect to the gentlemanly avocations, the professional classes, and the British State, Gisborne was a thorough-going conservative. He was a warm advocate of the Constitution, of the perpetuation of a social scale differentiated by rank, and of hierarchical values. His account of the various corporations of the State sings the perfections of the *status quo*, seeing its faults as, at worst, Popean 'partial evils':[11]

> The medical profession enjoys in Great Britain that degree of estimation and credit, which a science, conferring on mankind the greatest of all comforts except those of religion, justly deserves. Hence Physicians in this kingdom are almost invariably men of liberal education and cultivated minds. Hence too the art of medicine is carried among us to a singular height of excellence.

Not all contemporaries could have brought themselves in candour to pen such a panegyric.[12] Even the inferiority of physic in the rank-order of the learned professions seemed to spoil the sunny picture hardly at all in Gisborne's judgement. He was prepared to admit that 'In Great Britain, though the Medical Profession does not possess so many splendid prizes as the Church and the Bar':[13]

> and on that account perhaps is rarely if ever pursued by young men of noble families; [yet] it is by no means barren of honours and attractions: it opens the way to reputation and wealth; and raises the Physician to a level, in the intercourse of common life, with the highest classes of society.

Gisborne unfolds the career decisions, stage by stage, to be faced by the aspirant physician. Consistently with his broad commitment to explaining to genteel families the aims and ideals of the professions – and it must be emphasized that only the upper crust of the medical profession falls within his view – Gisborne devoted considerable platitudes to the subject of medical education. Where should one study? London or Edinburgh? Leiden or Göttingen? In such pairings, the choice should not go to the former merely because they were the more fashionable. Rather, in confronting the choice of life, 'Let [the student] sacrifice inferior views and personal gratifications to the prospect of greater proficiency in medical science'.[14]

Once installed, the young gentleman, while chiefly studying anatomy and the principles and practice of physic, ought not to neglect surgical knowledge; not, of course, because he would ever personally practice the cutting art, but so 'as may fully enable him to form a proper judgement, when hereafter he shall meet Surgeons in consultation respecting patients requiring both physical and surgical aid'.[15] Perhaps to show he was up with the times, Gisborne emphasized that 'Chemistry ... must be deemed a fundamental part of medical knowledge', to ensure that prescribing habits will be sound.[16] A solid grounding was further essential in a spectrum of subjects ranging from botany to law – this last because:[17]

> The testimony ... which a Physician may be called upon to give in cases of lunacy, of sudden deaths, of suicide, and of duelling, may be rendered more pertinent and impressive by an acquaintance with the laws of the land relating to those subjects.

Linguistic skills were likewise essential, especially in the Greek and Latin tongues ('with which the medical Student may be supposed to have been rendered familiar by a classical education');[18] both of these were 'requisite for understanding the ancient writers on the art of medicine', and, Gisborne stressed, equally because 'treatises on that science are still composed in Latin by foreigners'.[19] French was no less *de rigueur,* 'not merely for the reasons common to men of all professions who are placed in the upper ranks of society, but likewise that he may peruse with facility the valuable tracts on medical subjects occasionally published in that tongue'.[20] Professional studies must be followed with assiduity, but naturally not 'so far to encroach on higher duties, as to lead a young man into the habit of neglecting public worship, and the private perusal and investigation of the Scriptures'.[21]

This reminder points to a topic of no minor anxiety to Gisborne: the fear that medical attainments, pursued exclusively for their own sake, would undermine higher religious and moral dispositions. In a standard manner, Gisborne saw fit to warn the novice against the tempting excesses of the medical student's life, for instance lest 'by acting the part of a noisy and ostentatious declaimer at medical debating societies, [he should] contribute to transform an institution capable of being turned to the promotion of science, into a scene of theatrical rant, and of senseless, bold, and tumultuous disputation'.[22] But, while not repeating hoary gibes about the atheism of doctors, Gisborne was no less afraid of the possibly perverting, dehumanizing effects of the medical gaze itself. 'Let him beware', Gisborne warned the stripling medical student:[23]

> lest his heart be rendered hard, and his deportment unfeeling, by attendance on dissections of the dead and painful operations on the living; and by being accustomed in his daily visits at an hospital to see and hear multitudes labouring in every stage and under every variety of disease.

Medical professionalism seemed in danger of subverting common fellowship and Christian charity. Proceeding to examine medical practice, Gisborne paid close attention to questions of class and conduct, and the difficult ethical decisions encountered in the necessarily self-promoting business of career-building. Noting that the novice physician 'will find that the great families in the neighbourhood are pre-occupied by some established competitor; and that even if they are not, instead of having recourse in cases of sickness to a young stranger, they will generally prefer sending even to a much greater distance, and at an increased expence, for a Physician of known experience and skill', he confessed that the neophyte must therefore initially be satisfied to acquire as patients 'those persons in the middle classes of society, who are the least opulent; as clergymen [a nice self-deprecatory touch], tradesmen, shopkeepers, and people of similar descriptions'.[24] He must, therefore, trim his expectations to the ways of surrounding bourgeois society, and come to terms with the fact that 'persons in the lines of life mentioned above, are seldom in haste to consult any medical adviser but their apothecary; and rarely apply for further aid until their disorder, be it what it may, has made an alarming progress'.[25]

Naturally, the young physician must set his sights high and aspire to honour in the world; but it was vital that ambition should always be governed by strict propriety:[26]

> The most obvious and the most dangerous temptation to which a young Physician is exposed, when he has actually fixed on a place of residence, and presented himself to the public as a candidate for employment, is that of taking improper methods of introducing himself into practice.

Evidently no stranger to the kinds of subterfuges of market-place infighting amongst medicos discussed at length by Percival, Gisborne was stern in his warnings against all such shady and shabby conduct:[27]

> From every method tinctured with deceit, or involving proceedings in any degree reprehensible, let him turn aside without hesitation, whatever prospects of success it may afford. Let him not seek to obtain, from the mistaken good-humour of his medical friends, exaggerated panegyrics on his abilities; nor urge persons of weight and credit, though not of the faculty, to address importunate and unmerited solicitations in his favour to their acquaintance who live in his vicinity. Let him not lie in wait for opportunities of making an artful parade of his attainments, and of imposing on the unwary by a solemn, pompous, and consequential deportment, or by the sound of technical terms and learned trifling.

But if, in the ways stipulated above, the junior physician must shun the vulgar pomp and self-promotion, which critics saw as all too evident,[28] he must equally guard against reducing himself to toadying:[29]

> Let him not become a supple, cringing, and servile attendant on the Great; ready at all times, like the chameleon, to take the colour of surrounding objects; and catching, like an humble mimic on the stage, the habits and sentiments of his superior. Let him not become an officious instrument in the hands of some wealthy or noble patron, furthering his secret schemes, ministering to his personal or political antipathies, and flattering his religious or irreligious prejudices. Let him not pretend an attachment to a wealthy and numerous sect or party with a view to gain support.

Gisborne names no names, but one may surmise that he is scoring palpable hits against the great politician-courtier physicians of his time, such as Richard Warren and, not least, his own namesake.[30] Furthermore, true to his evangelical convictions, Gisborne instructed the young practitioner to avoid 'addicting himself to field sports, or becoming a frequenter of gambling clubs, an attendant on riotous and drunken meetings, or a partaker of any extravagant or vicious practice which the fashion of the times or the custom of the neighbourhood may have established'.[31]

If suchlike rules defined the self-fashioning of the young physician knocking on the door of the *beau monde,* what of his moral conduct towards individual sick people? It was, of course, paramount that:[32]

> Towards all patients, and towards female patients in particular, the utmost delicacy ought studiously to be observed; and every possible degree of care taken to avoid needlessly exciting a blush on the cheek of the modest, or a painful sensation in the breast of the virtuous.

As this sentiment implies, Gisborne believed that the clinician had a cardinal obligation to be more than technically expert: sincerity and humanity were essential, since 'it is frequently of much importance, not to the comfort only, but to the recovery of the patient, that he should be enabled to look on his Physician as a friend':[33]

> And how can the latter be looked upon as a friend, unless his manners are characterised by kindness and compassion; not the delusive appearance of a concern which he does not feel, assumed as a professional garb through decorum, or for the purpose of ensnaring flattery; not that unmanly pity which clouds the judgement, and incapacitates it from forming a prompt, steady, and rational opinion respecting the measures to be pursued; but that genuine and sober tenderness, springing from the cultivation of habitual benevolence, which, while it wins the affection and cheers the spirits of the patient, stimulates his adviser to exert every faculty of the mind for his relief? And what but this equable mildness of disposition will teach the Physician to bear with patience the wayward humours, and to treat with gentleness the groundless prejudices which he must continually encounter in a sick chamber?

Emphasizing, in a manner notably different from Percival, that the physician must never stray from the straight-and-narrow of strict veracity, Gisborne was perturbed at the growth of a deceptive, almost hypocritical 'professional garb'. One of the evils masked by this was mercenariness. Gisborne arraigned the profession of love of lucre:[34]

> There have been Physicians, the disgrace of their profession, who seem to have considered themselves, in studying medicine, as studying not a liberal science, but a mere art for the acquisition of money; and have thence been solicitous to acquire an insight rather into the humours than into the diseases of mankind.

In comporting himself towards his patients, the young physician must soar above such worldly considerations; for 'an independent and generous man will show himself on every occasion free from the least tincture of sordid avarice'. Not least will he 'exercise particular forbearance in the article of fees towards those who are least able to afford them'.[35] Above all, 'a Physician', he explained, 'ought to be extremely watchful against covetousness; for it is a vice imputed, justly or unjustly, to his profession'.[36]

Broadly a defender of the *status quo,* Gisborne naturally had to tread with some circumspection when faced with the implications of such a possibility ('that it is imputed with justice I am far from meaning to affirm or to intimate').[37] Nevertheless, in a rather roundabout way, he conceded that it might in truth be a 'fact' that 'more avaricious men are found in the medical profession, in proportion to its numbers, than in others equally liberal' – though proceeding to provide the graciously diplomatic exoneration, that such a deplorable state of affairs should properly be blamed upon 'the conduct of its employers'.[38] How was that? It was because 'so capriciously is a Physician treated on many occasions by his patients and their connections; such frequently is the dissatisfaction with which his best exertions are received; that eagerness to be exempted from the necessity of practising may sometimes render him too intent on accumulating an independent fortune'.[39]

No less than greed, the physician must renounce vanity, and all the pomp, circumstance, and egoistic tricks of the trade:[40]

> In attending upon a patient, the Physician, while he omits not the reserve which prudence dictates, will shun all affectation of mystery. He will not alarm the sick man, by discussing his case openly and unguardedly before him; nor will he put on a countenance of profound thought, and gestures of much seeming sagacity, either to augment his importance, or to conceal his ignorance.

The physician must not put on a show of omniscient superiority. Nor must he, out of vainglory or snobbery, belittle the 'intelligence to be obtained from the apothecary, who may have known the constitution of the patient for years, and in his present illness sees him once or twice a day; nor even the information to be procured from nurses, who have seen him every hour'. That was not to imply that the physician must 'implicitly adopt the opinions of the one, nor yield to the absurd fancies and prepossessions of the other'. Rather, his duty was to listen, and form an independent judgement on what was 'valuable in their several recitals', and thereby 'consider the whole as a mass of premises from which he is to deduce his conclusions'.[41]

Overall, bedside relations must be governed by the exercise of a certain tact and paternalist authority. 'The Physician may not be bound, unless expressly called upon, invariably to divulge at any specific time his opinion concerning the uncertainty or danger of the case', he emphasized:[42]

> but he is invariably bound never to represent the uncertainty or danger as less than he actually believes it to be; and whenever he conveys, directly or indirectly, to the patient or to his family, any impression to that effect, though he may be misled by mistaken tenderness, he is guilty of positive falsehood. He is at liberty to say little; but let that little be true.

In thus exercising clinical judgement, it was the physician's duty to judge wisely the interests of the patient and, no less, of the patient's family:[43]

> The state of the malady, when critical or hazardous, ought to be plainly declared without delay to some at least of the patient's near relations; and, except under extraordinary circumstances, to the nearest. On many occasions it may be the duty of the Physician spontaneously to reveal it to the patient himself. It may sometimes also be incumbent on him to suggest to the sick man, or to his friends, the propriety of adjusting all unfinished temporal concerns. And conscience will frequently prompt him discreetly to turn the thoughts of the former towards religion.

As is obvious, Gisborne, like Percival and most progressive medical opinion of the age, believed that, ancient custom notwithstanding, the physician's rightful place was at the dying man's bedside, for it would be wrong to 'desert his patient when there are no longer any remaining hopes of recovery':[44]

> Though life cannot be retained, pain may be mitigated. Even if the patient seems beyond the reach of medicine, the presence of the Physician will compose the minds and alleviate the sorrow of friends and relations.

Naturally, however, at the deathbed, as on all other occasions, no taint of personal ambition must be permitted to intrude:[45]

> The conduct of a Physician whose solicitude for the recovery of his patient is founded on pure and laudable motives, will be free from the influence of private and personal considerations in the application of his art. He will neither be too fond of novelties, nor too fearful of deviating on proper occasions and on solid grounds from the beaten track: he will not obtrude some mysterious nostrum illiberally concealed from the knowledge of his brethren: he will not cherish prepossessions against remedies and modes of proceeding introduced by others, nor partiality for those discovered by himself.

In short, in all that had to be transacted, the interests of the sick must be paramount, and not personal glory, expediency or careerism. This must be the golden rule of treatment. Thus the physician 'will not indulge a lurking wish to persevere in a dubious or unsuccessful system of medical treatment, from the apprehension that a change will argue ignorance in himself, or redound to the credit of another person who may have suggested it'. Likewise:[46]

> He will never recommend as a probable method of cure what he does not actually believe likely to prove so. He will not advise a journey to a public watering-place apparently from anxiety for the sick man, but in reality from a desire to please his wife and daughters by sending them to a scene of fashionable amusement; or in dangerous or hopeless maladies merely to remove the sufferer to a distance, instead of having him continue at home to die under his immediate care. He will not prescribe a medicine, the propriety of which he distrusts, because it is proposed by the patient or recommended by his friends, without explicitly declaring his own opinion of it.

As the drift of the preceding discussion will make clear, the physician's bedside conduct was constantly to be guided by strict moral laws, deontological rather than utilitarian in nature. But what about the penumbral domain of etiquette, in which the physician's own preferences and dispositions might generally be thought to be allowed a greater latitude? Gisborne conceded that many of the desiderata he listed were obviously 'applicable to the Physician only when attending on patients in the upper and middle ranks of society'.[47] Nevertheless the responsibilities of the physician were not confined to succouring 'Quality' patients alone – indeed, with an eye to universal moral laws, he judged that the 'greater number' of the guidelines set out 'have likewise an obvious reference to his duty when visiting the poor'.[48] On this head he thought it evident that 'a benevolent Physician will not restrict his attendance on the poor to those whom the bounty of the public brings before him',[49] but rather would make regular provision for such folk, by 'setting apart an appointed time in every week for giving gratuitous advice to the indigent'.[50]

Discussion of the poor naturally led to the new and vexacious question of the ethics governing hospital practice. In this regard, Gisborne – here, unlike Percival – issued a strongly-worded 'caution against making unnecessary or rash experiments in the treatment of the patients'. Doubtless, experimentation was not to be altogether excluded, for[51]

> The science of medicine undoubtedly derives continual accession of improvement from the inventive genius of its followers. New substances are introduced into the materia medica; new modes are discovered of preparing and of combining drugs already in use; and new applications of antient remedies to the cure of diseases, in which recourse was never had to them before.

Nor, of course, was it the high-minded Gisborne's intention to wag the finger of blame, explaining that it was 'not meant by these remarks to censure experiments designed to lessen the danger, or the sufferings, of the individual, when founded on rational analogies; commenced after mature deliberation; conducted by upright and skilful men; watched during the whole progress with circumspect attention; and abandoned in time when unfavourable appearances take place'.[52] Nevertheless, he certainly did not mince his words:[53]

> it is meant strongly to reprobate every experiment rashly or hastily adopted; or carried on by the selfish, the ignorant, the careless, or the obstinate. Proceedings of this nature are highly criminal, partly because they involve the health and life of the sufferers in great and needless hazards; and partly because they tend to confirm an opinion already too prevalent in some places in the minds of the poor, that such is the general conduct of Hospital Physicians.

Here as elsewhere, this highlighting of ethical dilemmas was symptomatic of Gisborne's anxiety that scientific medicine was posing genuine threats to the humane and pious practice of healing:[54]

> Experiments are not unfrequently made upon living animals by Physicians, in the course of their private researches, for the purpose of ascertaining the properties of drugs, or other facts of importance in medical and anatomical science. Neither the right nor the propriety of making these experiments on reasonable occasions can be disputed: but every degree of needless and inconsiderate cruelty in prosecuting them will be avoided with scrupulous care by men of feeling and reflection.

Alongside the common people, and experimental animals, Gisborne felt the physician needed advice in regard to one final sort of 'Other': 'the inferior members of the medical profession', to say nothing of his own 'competitors'.[55] What were the protocols here? With regard to all such fellow labourers, the physician 'will conduct himself ... under all circumstances on Christian principles; with Christian temper; and with a scrupulous regard to the attentions which they may reasonably expect, and the privileges which they may justly claim, in consequence of their respective situations'.[56]

Above all, respecting fellow physicians:[57]

> He will study to preserve that amicable intercourse between his medical brethren and himself, which may lead to an habitual, free, and mutually beneficial communication of interesting facts, which may occur to them in the circle of their practice. He will refrain from every approach towards obtrusive interference with respect to a case already under the management of another.

If fraternal accord should properly govern dealings with fellow physicians, defining relations with inferior practitioners obviously posed slightly more ticklish problems. On the one hand, there must be no hint of snobbish disdain:[58]

> Nor will he scornfully exclude from all the privileges of fellowship intelligent medical practitioners, who have not been fortunate enough to receive a degree from any university; when they give proofs of actually possessing those attainments, of which an academical education is considered as the basis, and a degree regarded as presumptive evidence.

At the same time, the physician must keep a certain distance from lesser practitioners, whose sights and scruples were likely to be lower, and who might drag him down to their level. Gisborne was rather scandalized by the prospects looming here for collusion and corruption – for (added the upright provincial), 'it is said to have happened more than once in London, that an old and established Apothecary has received half of a Physician's fees in return for his indiscriminate recommendation'.[59]

One key duty of the physician was to advance the public stake in health care:[60]

> By taking an active part in promoting and superintending useful medical institutions, a Physician may render essential services to the community. To his zeal and industry may be owing the erection or the good management of hospitals, of dispensaries, of asylums for lunatics, and the establishment of societies for the relief of decayed members of the medical profession, their widows, and their orphans.

Not least, medical knowledge itself had to be promoted. To that end, 'the Medical Journals of eminence published in foreign countries, as well as those established in his own, will properly engage his attention. From the one and the other he will probably derive very important assistance in the discharge of his duty as a Physician'.[61] Nevertheless, Gisborne warned against infatuation with novelties and book learning. 'Particular caution however may be requisite in the practical application of the intelligence which he gains from the former source; as remedies and modes of treatment which are crowned with success in one country, may prove by no means suited to patients who live in another climate, and in very different habits of life.'[62] And once again, here as elsewhere, the thirst for personal glory must be tempered:[63]

> He will not subject himself, by committing his thoughts to the press without sufficient previous enquiry, to the charge of purloining the discoveries of others; nor of being vain of communicating what is either unworthy of notice, or as yet but feebly and imperfectly developed, or hastily inferred from few and inadequate trials.

Indeed, when considering such innovations, Gisborne fretted over the danger of rampant disputatiousness, recommending, 'if in consequence of any thing which he has done, or of any thing which he has published, he should find himself driven into a controversy; let him conduct the literary warfare with becoming temper'.[64]

As will be evident, Gisborne saw medical ethics as a code governing the duties of doctors, and these duties were derived from an anterior body of moral laws guaranteed by Christian philosophy. As viewed by Gisborne, medical ethics ought not to be route-maps to professional advancement, still less handbooks of excuses and special pleading. Here, as throughout his *oeuvre*, he deplored the Paleyan calculus of expediency, while, even more fiercely, denouncing the excesses of the old, secular, aristocratic code of honour.

In the event, the medical profession got off rather lightly in Gisborne's dressing-down of professional values. Accustomed to Percival's somewhat anodyne view of medical practice, what strikes us about Gisborne is his scrupulous concern about the pomp and mercenariness of doctors. But these failings were mere peccadilloes compared to the shortcomings Gisborne lashed in other professions. Barristers readily slipped into the unforgivable and conscience-destroying habit of telling bare-faced lies in court, preferred interest or vengeance to justice, and displaying an '*esprit de corps* which so often leads professional men into unjustifiable and disgraceful practices'.[65] Military officers too often succumbed to unchristian bloodthirstiness and blasphemy, and gloried in that pagan abomination, duelling.[66] The established nature of the Church of England tempted the Anglican clergy into idleness, especially those numerous Oxbridge dons whose lifestyles were all too liable to convince the public that *all* ministers were as 'irreligious and time-serving' as themselves.[67] And, finally, merchants and bankers frequently fell short of the 'strict rules of integrity' required of them.[68] To return to an earlier observation of Gisborne's, it may in the end be no coincidence that the profession which 'does not possess so many splendid prizes as the Church and the Bar; and on that account perhaps is rarely if ever pursued by young men of noble families'[69] was viewed, for that very reason, as offering mercifully few opportunities for gross abuse.

Conclusion

It is unlikely that Gisborne's text was fundamentally important in shaping the future development of medical ethics.[70] Nevertheless, through its platitudes, it does offer an interesting commentary on contemporary affairs and provoke some intriguing questions. For one thing, behind the veneer and the pieties, it is clear that Gisborne believed much was worryingly wrong – much was *unethical* – about contemporary medical practice. He lambasted ambition, vanity, and greed. More significantly, perhaps, he was troubled lest certain recent developments – the hospital, experimentation, science, opportunities for swelling profits and social advancement – should jeopardize properly humane outlooks. It may not be surprising to find such high-minded admonitions in a book penned by an evangelical minister; but, *mutatis mutandis* – change the idiom, the prejudices, the standpoint, and the solutions somewhat – and one can discern in the *Enquiry* a critique of the 'sick trade' not altogether different from Thomas Beddoes' almost contemporary (radical) anatomy of abuses. Though Gisborne acknowledged Percival's help and friendship, his work was differently slanted from Percival's arguably rather complacent account of the workings of the profession. Whereas, for instance, Percival was adamant against waiving fees, even to the poor, on the grounds that the profession of physic could not be supported except 'as a lucrative one', Gisborne commended charity.[71]

Gisborne was, of course, writing from a different angle – that of a parson not a physician. Even so, it is worth noting that the outcome is a corpus of medical ethics (or, better, perhaps, a bundle of advice) with a different emphasis. For Percival, the crucial task was to establish and uphold a professional *esprit de corps,* to provide doctors with a practical, shop-floor handbook. Gisborne was no casuist. He aimed to fire young practitioners with idealistic zeal: his message was that medical practice must never deviate from the straight-and-narrow of the Christian gentleman.

In so far as late Georgian medicine followed any 'ethics' at all, one may surmise that it was more in the Percivalian than the Gisbornian mould.[72] But dogmatism would be premature. Pre-Victorian earnestness galvanized at least large sections of the professional classes. Some read Gisborne, most did not. Many young doctors were, however, probably imbued, by their family and their schooling, with broadly Gisbornian precepts. The religious imputs into medical practice need much further study.[73] Historians have been so concerned with questions such as the secularization of the medical world-view that they have neglected to study the continuing religious motivations for medical practice. Works such as Gisborne's may have had a profound influence not upon 'medical ethics' narrowly conceived, but upon the ethics behind medicine.

Notes

1. On the sociology of the professions see E. Freidson, *Profession of Medicine: A Study of the Sociology of Applied Knowledge* (New York: Dodd, Mead, 1970); T. J. Johnson, *Professions and Power* (London: Macmillan, 1972); R. Dingwall and P. Lewis (eds), *The Sociology of the Professions* (London: Macmillan, 1983); I. Waddington, 'The Development of Medical Ethics – A Sociological Analysis', *Medical History*, 19 (1975), 36–51. On social differentiation, see Pierre Bourdieu, *Distinction: A Social Critique of the Judgement of Taste*, trans. by Richard Nice (Cambridge, Mass.: Harvard University Press, 1984). For important historical views of the status of doctors in early modern England, see M. Pelling, 'Medical Practice in Early Modern England: Trade or Profession?', in W. Prest (ed.), *The Professions in Early Modern England* (London: Croom Helm, 1987), 90–128; G. Holmes, *Augustan England: Professions, State and Society, 1680–1730* (London: George Allen & Unwin, 1982); I. S. L. Loudon, *Medical Care and the General Practitioner 1750–1850* (Oxford: Clarendon Press, 1986).
2. John Gregory, *Observations on the Duties of a Physician* (London: Strahan & Cadell, 1770); Thomas Percival, *Medical Ethics; or, A Code of Institutes and Precepts Adapted to the Professional Conduct of Physicians and Surgeons* (Manchester: J. Johnson & R. Bickerstaff, 1803); on Gregory see L. McCullough, 'John Gregory's Medical Ethics and Humean Sympathy: A Closer Look', in Robert Baker, Dorothy Porter and Roy Porter (eds), *The Codification of Medical Morality in the Eighteenth and Nineteenth Centuries*, vol i (Dordrecht: Kluwer, 1993), 145–60. On Percival, see Robert Baker, 'Deciphering Percival's Code', in *ibid.*, 179–212; J. V. Pickstone, 'Thomas Percival and the Production of Medical Ethics', in *ibid.*, 161–78.
3. This kind of context is surveyed in Roy Porter, 'Plutus or Hygeia? Thomas Beddoes and Medical Ethics', in Robert Baker, Dorothy

Porter and Roy Porter (eds), *The Codification of Medical Morality in the Eighteenth and Nineteenth Centuries,* vol i (Dordrecht: Kluwer, 1993), 73–92.

4. Mary Fissell, 'Innocent and Honourable Bribes: Medical Manners in Eighteenth Century Britain', in Robert Baker, Dorothy Porter and Roy Porter (eds), *The Codification of Medical Morality in the Eighteenth and Nineteenth Centuries,* vol. i (Dordrecht: Kluwer, 1993), 19–46; see also Bonamy Dobrée (ed.), *The Letters of Philip Dormer Stanhope, Fourth Earl of Chesterfield,* 6 vols (London: Eyre and Spottiswoode, 1932); and Fenella Childs, 'Prescriptions for Manners in Eighteenth Century Courtesy Literature' (D. Phil. thesis, Oxford University, 1984). For the standing of medical ethics in England in the previous era, see the essay by Andrew Wear in this volume. For discussions of earlier medical ethics, see D. W. Amundsen, 'Medical Deontology and Pestilential Disease in the Late Middle Ages', *Journal of the History of Medicine,* xxxii (1977), 403–21; *idem,* 'Casuistry and Professional Obligations; The Regulation of Physicians by the Court of Conscience in the Late Middle Ages', *Transactions and Studies, College of Physicians of Philadelphia,* s. 5, iii (1981), 22–39; H. J. Cook, 'The Rose Case Reconsidered: Physicians, Apothecaries and the Law in Augustan England', *Journal of the History of Medicine,* vl (1990), 527–55; *idem,* 'Intellectual Property and Propriety: Professional "Monopolies" and the Physicians of Early Modern England' (paper presented to Clark Library Seminar, 1990).
5. Chauncey Leake (ed.), *Percival's Medical Ethics* (Baltimore: Williams and Wilkins, 1927); Jeffrey Berlant, *Profession and Monopoly. A Study of Medicine in the United States and Great Britain* (Berkeley: University of California Press, 1975); I. Waddington, 'The Development of Medical Ethics – A Sociological Analysis', *Medical History,* 19 (1975), 36–51.
6. Robert Baker, 'Deciphering Percival's Code', in Robert Baker, Dorothy Porter and Roy Porter (eds), *The Codification of Medical Morality in the Eighteenth and Nineteenth Centuries,* vol i 179–211 (Dordrecht: Kluwer, 1993); J. V. Pickstone, 'Thomas Percival and the Production of Medical Ethics', in *ibid.*
7. H. Perkin, *The Origins of Modern English Society 1780–1880* (London: Routledge and Kegan Paul, 1969).
8. Catherine Crawford, 'Malpractice and Bad Manners: Disputes over Professional Conduct in 18th Century England' (unpublished paper delivered to the Symposium on the History of Medical Ethics, Wellcome Institute, London, 1989); David Harley, 'Ethics and Dispute Behaviour in the Career of Henry Bracken of Lancaster, Surgeon, Physician and Manmidwife', in Robert Baker, Dorothy Porter and Roy Porter (eds), *The Codification of Medical Morality in the Eighteenth and Nineteenth Centuries,* vol i (Dordrecht: Kluwer, 1993), 47–72.

9. Thomas Gisborne, *An Enquiry into the Duties of Men in the Higher and Middle Classes of Society in Great Britain, Resulting from their Respective Stations, Professions and Employments*, 2 vols (London: B. and J. White, 1794). Subsequent editions were published in 1795 (2 editions), 1797, 1800, and 1811. Quotations below will be from the 1797 edition published by White. Note that Gisborne wrote a companion volume for women: *Inquiry into the Duties of the Female Sex* (London: T. Cadell, Jr, and W. Davies, 1797). This went through nine editions.
10. For the life of Gisborne, see *The Gentleman's Magazine*, xxv (n.s.), (1846), 643–5; J. C. Colquhoun, *William Wilberforce: His Friends and His Times*, 2nd ed (London: Longman 1867); on his connexion with Percival, see Gisborne, *An Enquiry into the Duties of Men*, vol ii, 132. This fact explains the close congruence between Percival's and Gisborne's accounts on many points, thereby making the divergences the more significant.
11. Gisborne, *An Enquiry into the Duties of Men*, vol ii, 132. Gisborne was very much the kind of conservative prominenced in J. C. D. Clark, *English Society, 1688–1832: Ideology, Social Structure and Political Practice During the Ancien Régime* (Cambridge: Cambridge University Press, 1985); and *idem*, *Revolution and Rebellion: State and Society in England in the Seventeenth and Eighteenth Centuries* (Cambridge: Cambridge University Press, 1986). For his Evangelicalism, see F. K. Brown, *Fathers of the Victorians: The Age of Wilberforce* (Cambridge: Cambridge University Press, 1961).
12. Roy Porter, 'Plutus or Hygeia? Thomas Beddoes and Medical Ethics', in Robert Baker, Dorothy Porter and Roy Porter (eds), *The Codification of Medical Morality in the Eighteenth and Nineteenth Centuries*, vol i (Dordrecht: Kluwer, 1993), 73–92, attempts to show how one contemporary of Gisborne's offered a far more pessimistic reading of contemporary medical failings.
13. Gisborne, *An Enquiry into the Duties of Men*, vol ii, 135.
14. Gisborne, *An Enquiry into the Duties of Men*, vol ii, 137.
15. Gisborne, *An Enquiry into the Duties of Men*, vol ii, 139.
16. Gisborne, *An Enquiry into the Duties of Men*, vol ii, 139.
17. Gisborne, *An Enquiry into the Duties of Men*, vol ii, 142; see T. R. Forbes, *Surgeons at the Bailey: English Forensic Medicine to 1878* (New Haven, Conn.: Yale University Press, 1986).
18. Gisborne, *An Enquiry into the Duties of Men*, vol ii, 140.
19. Gisborne, *An Enquiry into the Duties of Men*, vol ii, 140. For the survival of Latin as a scholarly lingua franca see Peter Burke, 'Eheu, Domine, Adsunt Turcae', in Peter Burke and Roy Porter (eds), *Language, Self and Society* (Cambridge: Polity, 1991), 23–50.
20. Gisborne, *An Enquiry into the Duties of Men*, vol ii, 141.
21. Gisborne, *An Enquiry into the Duties of Men*, vol ii, 143.
22. Gisborne, *An Enquiry into the Duties of Men*, vol ii, 145–6.

23. Gisborne, *An Enquiry into the Duties of Men,* vol ii, 146.
24. Gisborne, *An Enquiry into the Duties of Men,* vol ii, 147.
25. Gisborne, *An Enquiry into the Duties of Men,* vol ii, 148.
26. Gisborne, *An Enquiry into the Duties of Men,* vol ii, 148. One is reminded here of the fact that Gisborne's contemporary, Jane Austen, made 'ordination' the subject of *Mansfield Park.* Austen, herself of some Evangelical leanings, was fascinated by the tests of fitness to be undergone by the young clergyman, rather as Gisborne sees the junior physician being tested and exposed to moral danger.
27. Gisborne, *An Enquiry into the Duties of Men,* vol ii, 148–9. Some account of the medical market-place is offered in Dorothy Porter and Roy Porter, *Patient's Progress: Doctors and doctoring in eighteenth-century England* (Cambridge: Polity Press, 1989), chs 1 and 2. For medical ambitiousness, see ch. 7.
28. Gisborne, *An Enquiry into the Duties of Men,* vol ii, 150.
29. Gisborne, *An Enquiry into the Duties of Men,* vol ii, 151.
30. Gisborne, *An Enquiry into the Duties of Men,* vol ii, 150. For the operation of an aristocratic patronage system in medicine see N. Jewson, 'Medical Knowledge and the Patronage System in Eighteenth Century England', *Sociology,* viii (1974), 369–85; for Thomas Beddoes' critiques of its evils, not least the other Gisborne's sycophancy, see Roy Porter, 'Plutus or Hygeia? Thomas Beddoes and Medical Ethics', in Robert Baker, Dorothy Porter and Roy Porter (eds), *The Codification of Medical Morality in the Eighteenth and Nineteenth Centuries,* vol i (Dordrecht: Kluwer, 1993), 73–92; and Roy Porter, 'Reforming the Patient. Thomas Beddoes and Medical Practice', in Roger French and Andrew Wear (eds), *Medicine in the Age of Reform* (London: Routledge, 1991), 9–44. For Warren's rapacity see Dorothy Porter and Roy Porter, *Patient's Progress: Doctors and Doctoring in Eighteenth-century England* (Cambridge: Polity Press, 1989), 130.
31. Gisborne, *An Enquiry into the Duties of Men,* vol ii, 151. For Evangelical values see E. J. Bristow, *Vice and Vigilance: Purity Movements in Britain Since 1700* (Dublin: Gill and Macmillan, 1977); F. K. Brown, *Fathers of the Victorians: The Age of Wilberforce* (Cambridge: Cambridge University Press, 1961); M. Jaeger, *Before Victoria: Changing Standards and Behaviour, 1787–1837* (London: Chatto & Windus, 1956).
32. Gisborne, *An Enquiry into the Duties of Men,* vol ii, 154. For background see Andreas-Holger Maehle and Ulrich Troehler, 'Animal Experiments from Antiquity to the End of the Eighteenth Century: Attitudes and Arguments', in N. A. Rupke, *Vivisection in Historical Perspective* (London: Croom Helm, 1987), 14–47.
33. Gisborne, *An Enquiry into the Duties of Men,* vol ii, 155–6.
34. Gisborne, *An Enquiry into the Duties of Men,* vol ii, 151. On the mercenariness of contemporary medicos, see C. H. Brock, 'The

Happiness of Riches', in W. F. Bynum and R. Porter (eds), *William Hunter and the Eighteenth Century Medical World* (Cambridge: Cambridge University Press, 1985), 35–56; Roy Porter, 'William Hunter: A Surgeon and a Gentleman', in W.F. Bynum & Roy Porter (eds), *William Hunter and the Eighteenth Century Medical World* (Cambridge University Press, 1985), 7–34.

35. Gisborne, *An Enquiry into the Duties of Men,* vol ii, 157.
36. Gisborne, *An Enquiry into the Duties of Men,* vol ii, 157.
37. Gisborne, *An Enquiry into the Duties of Men,* vol ii, 157.
38. Gisborne, *An Enquiry into the Duties of Men,* vol ii, 158.
39. Gisborne, *An Enquiry into the Duties of Men,* vol ii, 158. Supporting evidence is provided in J. S. Lewis, *In the Family Way: Childbearing in the British Aristocracy 1760–1860* (New Brunswick, N.J.: Rutgers University Press, 1986).
40. Gisborne, *An Enquiry into the Duties of Men,* vol ii, 159. For contemporary allegations that regulars indulged in quackish theatrical display see Roy Porter, *Health for Sale: Quackery in England 1650–1850* (Manchester: Manchester University Press, 1989).
41. Gisborne, *An Enquiry into the Duties of Men,* vol ii, 159.
42. Gisborne, *An Enquiry into the Duties of Men,* vol ii, 160–1. See Dorothy Porter and Roy Porter, *Patient's Progress: Doctors and Doctoring in Eighteenth-century England* (Cambridge: Polity Press, 1989), ch. 8 for analysis of such 'authority'.
43. Gisborne, *An Enquiry into the Duties of Men,* vol ii, 162. On the etiquette regarding informing the patient of terminal conditions, see the discussion in Dorothy Porter and Roy Porter, *Patient's Progress: Doctors and Doctoring in Eighteenth-century England* (Cambridge: Polity Press, 1989), 144f.
44. Gisborne, *An Enquiry into the Duties of Men,* vol ii, 167. For Percival's view, see Thomas Percival, *Medical Ethics; or, A Code of Institutes and Precepts Adapted to the Professional Conduct of Physicians and Surgeons* (Manchester: J. Johnson & R. Bickerstaff, 1803), 172. See Roy Porter, 'Death and the Doctors in Georgian England', in R. Houlbrooke (ed.), *Death, Ritual and Bereavement* (London: Routledge, 1989), 77–94.
45. Gisborne, *An Enquiry into the Duties of Men,* vol ii, 164–5.
46. Gisborne, *An Enquiry into the Duties of Men,* vol ii, 166. On the abuse of watering places, see Roy Porter, *Doctor of Society: Thomas Beddoes and the Sick Trade in Late Enlightenment England* (London: Routledge, 1991), 123f.
47. Gisborne, *An Enquiry into the Duties of Men,* vol ii, 168.
48. Gisborne, *An Enquiry into the Duties of Men,* vol ii, 169.
49. Gisborne, *An Enquiry into the Duties of Men,* vol ii, 172.
50. Gisborne, *An Enquiry into the Duties of Men,* vol ii, 187.
51. Gisborne, *An Enquiry into the Duties of Men,* vol ii, 168–9. Some of the special issues raised by the hospital for medical ethics are covered

in I. Waddington, 'The Development of Medical Ethics – A Sociological Analysis', *Medical History,* 19 (1975), 36–51. The question of the hospital as a site of experimentation is briefly discussed in Roy Porter, 'The Gift Relation: Philanthropy and Provincial Hospitals in Eighteenth Century England', in Lindsay Granshaw and Roy Porter (eds), *The Hospital in History* (London, Routledge, 1989), 149–78. For Thomas Beddoes's sturdy defence of medical experimentation, see Roy Porter, *Doctor of Society: Thomas Beddoes and the Sick Trade in Late Enlightenment England* (London: Routledge, 1991), 37.

52. Gisborne, *An Enquiry into the Duties of Men,* vol ii, 170.
53. Gisborne, *An Enquiry into the Duties of Men,* vol ii, 171.
54. Gisborne, *An Enquiry into the Duties of Men,* vol ii, 170–1.
55. Gisborne, *An Enquiry into the Duties of Men,* vol ii, 174.
56. Gisborne, *An Enquiry into the Duties of Men,* vol ii, 174.
57. Gisborne, *An Enquiry into the Duties of Men,* vol ii, 176–7.
58. Gisborne, *An Enquiry into the Duties of Men,* vol ii, 178.
59. Gisborne, *An Enquiry into the Duties of Men,* vol ii, 179. For suchlike allegations, see Dorothy Porter and Roy Porter, *Patient's Progress: Doctors and Doctoring in Eighteenth-century England* (Cambridge: Polity Press, 1989), ch. 7.
60. Gisborne, *An Enquiry into the Duties of Men,* vol ii, 185.
61. Gisborne, *An Enquiry into the Duties of Men,* vol ii, 185. For Thomas Beddoes' parallel thoughts, see Roy Porter, 'Doctor of Society', ch. 4.
62. Gisborne, *An Enquiry into the Duties of Men,* vol ii, 187.
63. Gisborne, *An Enquiry into the Duties of Men,* vol ii, 184. Contemporary priority disputes are discussed in Roy Porter, 'William Hunter: A Surgeon and a Gentleman', in W. F. Bynum & Roy Porter (eds), *William Hunter and the Eighteenth Century Medical World* (Cambridge University Press, 1985), 7–34.
64. Gisborne, *An Enquiry into the Duties of Men,* vol ii, 184–5.
65. For lawyers, see especially Gisborne, *An Enquiry into the Duties of Men,* vol i, 339ff. and 354. For the wider questions of professional vocations, see W. Prest (ed.), *The Professions in Early Modern England* (London: Croom Helm, 1987).
66. For military and naval officers, see especially Gisborne, *An Enquiry into the Duties of Men,* vol i, 297ff. For Evangelical loathing of the duel, see V. Kiernan, *The Duel in European History* (Oxford: Oxford University Press, 1988), 182, 212, 221.
67. Gisborne, *An Enquiry into the Duties of Men,* vol ii, 89.
68. Gisborne, *An Enquiry into the Duties of Men,* vol ii, 207.
69. Gisborne, *An Enquiry into the Duties of Men,* vol ii, 135.
70. Though it is interesting that his recommendations for doctors were separately reprinted as *On the Duties of Physicians Resulting from their Profession,* edited by W. A. Greenhill (Oxford: Parker, 1847).
71. Thomas Percival, *Medical Ethics; or, A Code of Institutes and Precepts*

Adapted to the Professional Conduct of Physicians and Surgeons (Manchester: J. Johnson & R. Bickerstaff, 1803),

72. But see, for a somewhat different reading of early nineteenth century developments, Robert Baker, 'Deciphering Percival's Code', in Robert Baker, Dorothy Porter and Roy Porter (eds), *The Codification of Medical Morality in the Eighteenth and Nineteenth Centuries*, vol i (Dordrecht: Kluwer, 1993), 179–212.
73. For a good, though slightly later, example – the case of a Quaker – see A. M. Kass and E. H. Kass, *Perfecting the World: The Life and Times of Dr Thomas Hodgkin 1798–1866* (Boston: Harcourt, Brace, Jovanovich, 1988).

10

Does a Certificate of Lunacy Affect a Patient's Ethical Status?

Psychiatric Paternalism and its Critics in Victorian England

Michael J. Clark

Throughout the modern period many of the classical problems of medical ethics, such as truth-telling and informed consent to treatment – to say nothing of the injunction to do the sick no harm – have been posed in especially acute and intractable forms in the context of psychiatric practice. Indeed, given the ubiquity of ethical problems in psychiatric practice, it is perhaps surprising that psychiatrists have not made a greater contribution to the literature of general medical ethics than in fact they have.[1] In this chapter, however, I do not intend to discuss any particular ethical problem or problems of psychiatric practice so much as the altogether more general, and more elusive, notion of the *ethical status* ascribed to the mental patient – that is, the idea of the patient's moral status implicit or, very occasionally, explicit in psychiatric discourse and practice[2] – in relation to one of the most important and ubiquitous features of Victorian psychiatric practice, namely, the certification of insanity. Most discussions of ethical problems in psychiatry (and in psychoanalysis too, for that matter) have tended to concentrate on what one might term 'downstream' aspects of psychiatric practice – that is to say, problems which normally arise *after* a person has entered upon the status of patient and a doctor–patient relationship has, at least in principle, already been formed.[3] However, I would wish to argue that the ethical status ascribed to the mental patient logically precedes, and in practice powerfully conditions, any particular ethical prescription regarding his or her care and treatment; and that, at least in the practice of what Thomas Szasz would call 'institutional' or non-contractual psychiatry,[4] much of what happens 'downstream' cannot fully be understood without some prior appreciation of the important modifications which the patient's legal and, by implication, ethical status has already undergone 'upstream' at the stage of diagnosis and referral – or, in the Victorian context, of certification. Certification subjected the Victorian mental patient to an elaborate system of medical, legal and administrative restraint, which effectively reduced his or her status from that of responsible adult to dependent minor. Viewed in this light, certification assumes great importance not just for the fate of the individual patient, but for the legal rights and ethical status of Victorian mental patients in general. In this chapter, I shall be concentrating mainly on the ethical implications of certification and on the closely-related question of patients' legal rights. However, Victorian psychiatry and lunacy administration generally afford numerous opportunities for historical studies of the ethical implications of psychiatric theory and practice, and this chapter offers no more than a brief glimpse of a very large field of historical inquiry, of which the greater part as yet remains unexplored.

The implications of the practice of certification need to be examined, however, in the broader context of the treatment of ethical questions in nineteenth-century English psychiatry generally. Whereas in the earlier part of the century, English psychiatry had seen a number of lively debates of a primarily theoretical character,[5] after about 1840 general ethical and moral issues began to play an increasingly important part in professional debates, even those ostensibly concerned with detailed technical or practical questions. Indeed, as Roger Smith has recently pointed out, what chiefly characterized Victorian psychiatry as a specialty was not so much any special body of knowledge or technique related to particular bodily organs or functions, but rather its distinctive medico–legal, social-administrative and institutional – to which one might add, ethical – frameworks and contexts of practice.[6] In the context of Victorian psychiatry, only the most relative and contingent distinctions can be drawn between 'technical' problems of the specialty and general political, socio-economic, religious and philosophical issues of the day, many of which found their way into 'core debates' on apparently special aspects of psychiatric theory and practice, such as the causes and classification of mental disorders, the organization of psychiatric care for the insane poor, and the ideal composition of asylum dietaries. Moreover, some of the most keenly-debated technical questions, such as the controversies over the use of 'mechanical' and 'chemical' restraint in asylums, largely turned upon what were in fact professional or general-ethical questions, while in practice many of the controversies which most seriously called psychiatry's professional credibility and standing into question, such as the 'wrongful confinement' controversies or the debate over the merits of general hospital treatment for acute cases of insanity, had, or were alleged to have had, important ethical dimensions.[7] Finally, the persistence of a substantial 'trade in lunacy' – that is, of a considerable number of private asylums for fee-paying patients run essentially as commercial enterprises rather than as charities or public utilities – meant that the conflicting ideals and ethical values of medicine as a trade, and medicine as a vocation, co-existed uneasily in the same specialty throughout the Victorian period.[8]

Yet, despite the apparent ubiquity of ethical questions in Victorian psychiatry, in the course of their ordinary professional activities psychiatrists seldom addressed themselves directly to the ethical implications of their practice, much less to questions concerning the ethical status of their patients. This was an issue far more often raised by ex-patients such as Thomas Mulock, J. T. Perceval and Richard Paternoster in relation to their own former treatment than by asylum doctors themselves.[9] Nineteenth-century psychiatric literature contains many unflattering allusions to the forms of thought, feeling and conduct to be met with in the insane but little explicit discussion of their moral or ethical status, and much of what psychiatrists (and, for that matter, the general public) thought about such questions has to be inferred from other kinds of evidence, such as the use and abuse of certification.

But the failure to formulate any consistent view of the patient's ethical status was only one aspect of a more general omission. One of the most striking features of nineteenth-century English psychiatric practice was the absence of anything resembling a systematic professional deontology or code of practice. Nineteenth-century psychiatric texts contain many idealized descriptions of the mental and moral qualities required of the good 'psychological physician',[10] as well as a good deal of practical advice as to how physicians should behave in certain delicate situations, such as the treatment of female hysterics, or when testifying to the sanity or insanity of an accused person. But, except obliquely in connection with certain practical questions, notably the 'restraint' of patients in asylums, there are no attempts to form any broad, general overview of ethical questions in psychiatric practice, much less any authoritative guidelines or recommended solutions to everyday problems of practice. Rather, psychiatrists saw 'ethical' problems as essentially the result either of individual character defects on the part of asylum doctors, superintendents or attendants, or of dysfunction of the asylum system, to be resolved by legislative, institutional and practical reforms rather than by concerted professional stocktaking or public debate.

In his wide-ranging study of the development of English lunacy law and practice during the past 100 years, Clive Unsworth has remarked that:

> The history of legal provision for the mentally disordered [in England and Wales] since the early nineteenth century has consisted of the construction within the context of a legal order based upon ... formal freedom and equality of a limited status [for the mental patient] composed of ... '*something more subtle than rights*'.[11]

But however much this may coincide with the characteristic English preference for unwritten constitutions and ambiguous precedents, the historian may well wonder whether this arrangement really served the best interests of either the sane or the insane public, or whether, in the absence of any agreed code of practice or professional deontology, both mental patients and asylum doctors did not sometimes find this 'limited status' altogether too subtle for their own good. A closer examination of certification, the principal medico-legal instrument whereby this status was conferred, may, however, help to clarify its implications for the patient's ethical status and shed light upon some of the functions which involuntary psychiatric commitment performed in nineteenth-century society. Similarly, a brief survey of some of the major criticisms made of institutional psychiatric practice by Victorian patients' rights organizations, and of the reasons for their comparative lack of success, may help us better to understand some of the wider socio-cultural and social-administrative constraints affecting Victorian psychiatric practice and the lives of Victorian mental patients.

Although there were, no doubt, in practice many partial exceptions to this rule, following the passage of the Madhouse Act of 1828 (9 Geo.IV, c.41) and the Lunatics Act of 1845 (8 and 9 Vict., c.100) Victorian psychiatric care and treatment was very largely based upon the principle and practice of involuntary commitment to asylums by medical certificate.[12] In 1853, provision was made for the informal readmission, without certification, of some former patients to private licensed houses as voluntary boarders, while throughout the Victorian period there was an unknown number of 'Chancery patients' found 'lunatic by inquisition' living in single private lodgings, for the most part without certificates.[13] But for the great majority of Victorian mental patients, both private and pauper, psychiatric care and treatment meant involuntary confinement under certificates in some public asylum, private licensed house or registered hospital for the insane. The insane, it was widely accepted, were best treated away from their homes and families, in special institutions or 'receptacles'; and the need for early treatment while there was still a chance of cure, together with the burden which the insane placed upon their families and the potential nuisance or danger which they represented both to themselves and to others, was generally held to justify their certification and commitment to an asylum at the earliest possible moment.[14]

The original purpose of the lunacy certificate had been to serve as a legal safeguard against improper detention.[15] By the Victorian period, its medical-diagnostic content was becoming increasingly important, but it remained primarily a legal and administrative document, and insofar as it authorized drastic restrictions on patients' freedom of movement, access to due process of law and freedom to dispose of their own property and persons, it clearly signalled a fundamental change in their *legal* status. Certification effectively reduced the patient's status to that of a minor, and placed him or her under a complex medico-legal and administrative tutelage or 'guardianship' for which asylum doctors and superintendents, visiting magistrates, the Commissioners in Lunacy, the patient's family or friends, Poor Law overseers and Guardians and, in the case of Chancery patients, Committees of the Body and Estate, the Lord Chancellor's Visitors in Lunacy and the Lord Chancellor himself all shared some responsibility. While 'under certificates', mental patients in asylums or private lodgings could not marry, vote, enter into contracts, or be held liable for contractual obligations entered upon before their certification, nor could they embark upon any legal action on their own behalf, though they could make wills and could testify in legal actions brought by the Lunacy Commissioners on behalf of other patients. The ethical implications of this regime were somewhat less clear-cut, but in a society whose conception of individual rights was highly legalistic, and whose whole concept of citizenship was based on the notion of individual responsibility, it was hard to avoid the conclusion that certification seriously detracted from the patient's *moral* status as well.

Certification also entailed a whole series of practical consequences which further emphasized the patient's loss of status. As J. T. Perceval and other ex-patients forcefully complained, not only did certification legitimate involuntary confinement in an asylum, but the mere fact of thus being 'under restraint' was further held to justify many practices which would otherwise have been regarded as unacceptable behaviour towards mature adults. These included being held, for the most part, under lock and key; being liable to both compulsory 'treatment' and physical coercion by asylum attendants; surveillance and denial of privacy; censorship of correspondence; denial of free access to one's family and friends, and (for the most part) segregation from persons of the opposite sex; subjection to prescribed dietaries and fixed diurnal routines, and often neither having access to full information nor being told the whole truth about one's medical condition and remaining legal rights.[16] Admittedly, certification also entitled patients to regular, if perfunctory, medical attention, and to the protection of various legal persons and statutory bodies against physical neglect, abuse or exploitation. But, despite these provisions, there could be little doubt that certification entailed a *de facto* loss or downgrading of the patient's legal and ethical status. Just as the mere fact of being 'under restraint' was held to justify the many exceptional features of asylum life,[17] so the mere fact of being certifiably insane was generally held to justify, or at least to render unproblematic, a drastic reduction in the patient's moral or ethical status and a corresponding curtailment of his or her legal rights. Such was the stigma frequently attached to an episode of mental disorder that even recovery and discharge often failed to make good this loss of credibility and status, as many ex-patients found to their dismay and indignation.

Even when regarded from a highly paternalistic standpoint, this state of affairs might have been expected to give rise to some unease among practitioners. But instead of critically appraising the implications of certification and commitment for the ethics of their own practice, Victorian psychiatrists largely ignored these more problematic aspects of the asylum doctor–patient relationship, preferring to stress the special mental and moral qualities required in an asylum doctor, and the quasi-religious character of what Forbes Winslow called 'The Vocation of the Psychological Physician'.[18] Within what one might call the English lunacy establishment, proposals for reform of the asylum system focused largely on detailed aspects of the internal regime of asylums, such as the use and abuse of mechanical restraint and seclusion, or the pros and cons of redistributing 'chronic' and 'harmless' patients from the county asylums to Poor Law infirmaries or other, less costly, 'receptacles'.[19] Almost no one, certainly not the Commissioners in

Lunacy, seriously doubted that, whatever its precise institutional make-up, the system as a whole would, for the most part, continue to be based on the practice of involuntary confinement. For more radical civil-libertarian perspectives on certification and psychiatric practice, it is necessary to look beyond the ranks of asylum doctors and lunacy administrators at some of the rather more original ideas and colourful personalities to be found in lay patients' rights organizations, such as the Alleged Lunatics' Friend Society.[20]

In October 1838, Richard Paternoster, a former East India Company clerk in the Madras Civil Service, was released from a private asylum in Kensington on the orders of the Metropolitan Lunacy Commissioners. On securing his release, Paternoster brought a legal action against his father (at whose instance he had been confined) for false imprisonment, and placed an advertisement in *The Times* inviting other former mental patients and members of the public concerned with the defects of English lunacy administration to join him in a campaign to reform what, in a book published in 1841, he was to call *The Madhouse System*.[21] Paternoster received half-a-dozen serious replies, and he and this small group of fellow-sufferers and sympathizers, among whom were John Thomas Perceval (1803–76), fifth son of the assassinated Prime Minister Spencer Perceval and soon to become well known as the author of *A Narrative of the Treatment Experienced by a Gentleman During a State of Mental Derangement* (1838–40) and Admiral Richard Saumarez (1791–1866), a distinguished ex-naval officer, magistrate and sometime Mayor of Bath, were to form the core of what, in 1845, eventually became known as the Alleged Lunatics' Friend Society (hereafter the A.L.F.S.).[22]

The A.L.F.S. was an unlikely but surprisingly effective mixture of apparently contradictory elements. It probably never had more than 50–60 members, of whom the vast majority seem to have belonged to the wealthy middle and upper classes, but it had no less than 17 directors, 18 vice-presidents, and, for much of the 1840s and 1850s, boasted a dozen or so MPs among its members, as well as a number of sympathizers in the House of Lords.[23] The Society was supposed to be non-sectarian and apolitical in character, and in fact its Parliamentary representation was about evenly divided between Whigs, Liberals and Radicals, on the one hand, and Conservatives and Peelites, on the other. However, Perceval's evangelical fervour made a deep impression on the Society, while the intense activism of its politically most radical supporters, notably the Radical MPs Thomas Wakley, Thomas Duncombe and

William Sharman Crawford, gave the Society as a whole an unmistakably radical-libertarian character.[24]

During its effective life, spanning roughly the years 1841 to 1865, the Society was active both as a pressure-group and as a support organization in individual cases in many different ways, and at several quite distinct levels of the English governmental, judicial and political systems. At a local, as well as national level, it took up specific cases of ill-treatment or violation of patients' legal rights and malpractice or maladministration by local asylum superintendents, visiting magistrates and madhouse proprietors. Between 1845 and 1863 the Society took up more than 70 individual cases in this way, many of them pauper lunatics.[25] In Parliament and in the courts, it took advantage of the quite disproportionate numbers of MPs, solicitors and barristers among its members to agitate for lunacy law reform, contest court cases on behalf of patients and press for the simplification of civil legal procedures in lunacy,[26] while at the level of national government it used its upper-class members' extensive social connections and political influence to lobby successive Liberal and Conservative Home Secretaries and Lord Chancellors and to counteract the rigid, bureaucratic-centralist mentality of the Lunacy Commissioners. In 1847, 1848, 1851 and 1853 the Society presented a series of draft Bills to the Home Office, intended to improve various aspects of patient care and patients' legal rights in both public and private asylums.[27] In 1845 its then principal Parliamentary spokesman, the Radical Thomas Duncombe, secured important concessions by way of enhanced legal protection of patients' rights during the passage of the Care and Treatment of Lunatics Act through Parliament, despite fierce opposition from Lord Shaftesbury, the Chairman of the Metropolitan Lunacy Commissioners.[28] In 1859–60 Perceval, Saumarez and Gilbert Bolden, the Society's organizing Secretary, gave extensive evidence on the Society's behalf to the House of Commons Select Committee on the operation of the Lunacy Laws, whose appointment was itself in part the result of the Society's persistent lobbying of the Home Office and pressure in Parliament over nearly two decades.[29] In addition, the Society made effective use of its good offices with the Law Amendment Society and its leading spokesmen, the former Whig and Conservative Lord Chancellors Lord Brougham and Lord Lyndhurst, indirectly to secure a number of substantive and procedural reforms to the lunacy laws and the separate issue of civil lunacy inquisitions in Chancery between 1848 and 1862.[30] Among the Society's specific proposals were the following: that a magistrate should examine either the certificates or the patient in question in every proposed committal proceedings, and that no patient, whether private or pauper, should be admitted to an asylum unless the magistrate had satisfied himself of the legality and necessity of the proceedings; that patients and their friends and relations should not be denied access to the courts, and that the Commissioners in Lunacy should lose their statutory monopoly on legal actions brought under the lunacy laws; that it should be possible for persons to become voluntary patients, or boarders, without having to be certified and subject to legal restraint; that men and women should be allowed greater freedom of association in asylums, and individual patients be given more opportunities for contact with sane visitors; that patients' personal property should be placed under seal for the duration of their confinement; that every asylum should have a sealed postbox to ensure the privacy of patients' correspondence; and finally, that copies of the clauses of the Lunacy Acts relating to patients' legal rights should be displayed prominently in every asylum ward.[31] Though very few of these suggestions found favour in official circles at the time, quite a number, such as the proposals for judicial authorization of all commitments and the safeguarding of patients' personal belongings, were subsequently taken up by the Home Office and even by the Lunacy Commissioners and incorporated into later-nineteenth-century lunacy legislation.[32]

In addition, the Society's increasingly wide-ranging concern with patients' rights and the quality of patient care led it to criticize many aspects of contemporary psychiatric theory and practice, and to advocate radical reforms to the institutional structure of psychiatric care and treatment. Thus in defiance of the prevailing psychiatric orthodoxy, Perceval attacked the ideology of moral treatment as a monstrous imposition of society's values on the individual, and denounced the implication in moral treatment's emphasis on the sentimental re-education of the insane that mental patients should be treated as children of a larger growth, rather than as responsible adults.[33] The Society also attacked the growth of large, impersonal asylums or 'warehouses for the insane', especially in the public sector, and in contrast to the Lunacy Commissioners' obsession with the need for strict certification and control of admissions to and discharges from asylums, urged that provision be made for the informal admission of middle- and upper-class patients to private asylums and single lodgings as voluntary boarders, and similarly for the boarding out of chronic pauper patients in ordinary private homes.[34] But in thus attempting to ensure treatment regimes better adapted to the needs of individual patients, the A.L.F.S. found itself advocating the transfer of patients from an institutional sector with at least some built-in safeguards against physical abuse and violation of rights to non-institutional settings with few, if any, such safeguards,[35] and they were to be no more successful in resolving this dilemma than modern-day advocates of 'decarceration' and the 'community care' of mental patients have been.

After the Society's failure to secure anything very tangible from the 1859 Select Committee by way of enhanced statutory protection for patients' rights, it slowly began to decline.[36] It was not very long, however, before a new lunacy law reform organization was to appear in somewhat similar circumstances to those which attended the A.L.F.S's birth. In 1871 Mrs Louisa Lowe, an Anglican clergyman's wife, was admitted to a private asylum at the urgent insistence of her husband, apparently for no better reason than that she had embraced a radically anti-Christian form of spiritualism.[37] On her release later the same year, she began legal proceedings against her husband and his doctors for false imprisonment, began to compose an elaborate denunciation of the private asylum system, eventually published in 1883 as *The Bastilles of England*,[38] and founded the Lunacy Law Reform Association, whose permanent Secretary she became. Unfortunately, not much is known about this organization. The militant and uncompromising tone of its publicity seems closely to have reflected its founder's personality, experiences and prejudices, and the Association seems to have been mostly preoccupied with the question of enhanced legal safeguards against wrongful confinement, rather than with the much wider range of patients' rights issues taken up by the A.L.F.S.[39]

In 1876, a number of the Association's members broke away to form a separate Lunacy Law Amendment Society, not, it seems, out of any real disagreement with the Association's aims and methods so much as from fear that Lowe's fervent identification with spiritualism might discredit the cause of lunacy law reform.[40] Both the Association and the Society probably had many more members on paper than the A.L.F.S., but seem altogether to have lacked its formidable Parliamentary representation and numerous channels of influence, and no connection has yet been shown between them and the efforts of successive Liberal and Unionist Lord Chancellors to revise the lunacy laws during the 1880s, culminating in the Lunacy Act of 1890.[41] Both James Billington, secretary of the Lunacy Law Amendment Association, and Louisa Lowe gave evidence to the

1879 Select Committee on the Lunacy Laws, and both presented the Committee with a formidable set of proposals for reform. Some of these, including the opening of private asylums to inspection by patients' friends, the removal of the Lunacy Commissioners' veto over private prosecutions under the lunacy laws, and the prominent display of notices advertising patients' legal rights in asylum wards, harked back to the earlier demands of the A.L.F.S. However, neither Billington nor Lowe obtained any more satisfaction from the Committee than the A.L.F.S. had done from its predecessor of 1859, while Billington failed to substantiate certain allegations he had made about the extent and frequency of wrongful confinement.[42] In 1884, Louisa Lowe and her Association strongly supported Lowe's fellow-spiritualist Mrs Georgina Weldon in the series of actions which she brought first against her husband and his doctors, and then against a number of other parties, including the management of the Covent Garden Opera House and the French composer Gounod, in connection with an unsuccessful attempt to commit her to a private asylum.[43] But after this, little more is known about either the Association or the Lunacy Law Amendment Society, and both organizations seem to have ceased to function before the end of the decade.

Why was the cause of patients' rights not more effectively represented in Victorian England? Certainly, both the A.L.F.S. and its successor organizations suffered from persistent stigmatization and trivialization of their aims simply because they had been founded by ex-patients and numbered many former patients among their principal spokespersons,[44] and neither the A.L.F.S., the Lunacy Law Reform Association nor the Lunacy Law Amendment Society were at all well organized for sustained political agitation and campaigning, as opposed to Parliamentary or Whitehall lobbying. There was, however, a more fundamental reason for their lack of success. In discussing the A.L.F.S.'s work on behalf of pauper patients, Nicholas Hervey remarks that:

> The Society spent a lot of time representing pauper [lunatics'] interests ... most often through the global rights [which] it advocated. *The difficulty [was] that these rights were located at the interface of medical professionalism, government growth and individual freedoms.*[45]

Hervey goes on to say of the Lunacy Commissioners that:

> The Commission, although ceding a large measure of control to the [county asylum] superintendents, was anxious to retain an ultimate

> veto on medical activities. This should have given it some sympathy with the [Alleged Lunatics' Friend Society's] views. *But whilst ... individual Commissioners supported aspects of the Society's programme, the Lunacy Board was wary of alienating the medical profession by curbing its powers in favour of patients' rights.*[46]

This, I believe, gets close to the heart of the matter. Patients' rights, and the ethical conceptions which sustained them, were victims of the in-fighting among the various professional and social-administrative interest groups which made up the Victorian lunacy establishment. Though otherwise deeply divided among themselves, asylum doctors were almost unanimous in opposing any break-up of the public asylum system and in resisting the kind of lay (and, for that matter, ecclesiastical) interference in the management of asylums advocated by some lunacy reformers, while for the Lunacy Commissioners, patients' rights organizations were at best irrelevant distractions and at worst bands of dangerous cranks intent on destroying the delicate balance of English lunacy administration. But it was government growth, in the shape of the Lunacy Commission, rather than medical professionalism or psychiatric imperialism, which constituted the chief obstacle to the more effective advocacy of patients' rights.[47] Jealous of its powers, mistrustful of would-be critics, and committed to one, effectively timeless blueprint for English lunacy administration, the Commissioners under Shaftesbury followed a policy of divide and rule and were in large measure able to impose their own narrow vision on the English asylum system at the expense of both patients' rights and the progress of psychological medicine.[48] Hence paradoxically, one of the conditions which had to be fulfilled before the cause of patients' rights could more effectively be advocated was to be the decline and eventual demise of the very statutory body which was supposed to constitute their principal safeguard – namely, the Lunacy Commission.

But why should patients' rights and liberties have posed such intractable problems for Victorian psychiatry in the first place? Part of the answer surely lies in the complex and often contradictory attitudes towards merely eccentric or mildly deviant behaviour of any kind revealed time and again by the various 'Wrongful Confinement' controversies which punctuated the whole period down to 1890 and beyond.[49] As contemporary critics such as John Stuart Mill were well aware, Victorian England was a society which exalted individual liberty in the abstract, and was horrified at the thought of sane persons being wrongfully confined in asylums, yet which also suffered from a pervasive, indeed oppressive, conformism of dress, manners, social behaviour, expectations and values, and where the vigorous defence of *individual property rights* co-existed with a usually tacit belief that the *'interests' of property,* especially dynastic wealth, might be held to justify the most drastic and far-reaching restrictions of personal freedom.[50] Against this background, it was hardly surprising if, from time to time, some well-to-do persons who indulged overmuch in independent thought and conduct, or in immoral and profligate behaviour, should have found themselves, as Mill put it, '... in peril of a commission de lunatico, and of having their property taken from them and given to their relations';[51] or, less spectacularly but just as effectively, of being certified and confined in an asylum or hospital for the insane.

Many Victorian clinical-psychiatric texts devoted a great deal of space to the problem of merely 'eccentric' or 'immoral' behaviour not amounting to insanity, and stressed the practical difficulty of distinguishing such conduct from insanity proper.[52] Yet, as Peter McCandless has observed, the whole system of Victorian institutional psychiatric care and treatment was based on the assumption of an abrupt discontinuity between sanity and insanity, the everyday world and that of the asylum,[53] and the practice of certification, which marked the divide between them, itself seemed to confirm and sanction this discontinuity. One response might have been for psychiatrists to adopt a more cautious and pragmatic approach to the practical problems posed by mental disorder. Yet, far from acknowledging the need for a more flexible approach, some eminent Victorian psychiatrists actually favoured the progressive extension of the boundaries of certifiable insanity to include much of what had hitherto been regarded merely as the 'borderlands' of insanity. This paradox was perfectly exemplified as early as 1830 by John Conolly in his *Indications of Insanity.* After discussing some of the many slight or temporary exaggerations of normal feelings, disturbances of the intellect and aberrations of conduct to be met with along the transition from sanity to insanity, and warning of the danger of over-reacting to trifling or fleeting deviations from the norm by certifying the patient, Conolly nevertheless goes on to advocate the creation of a sliding scale of legal 'restraint' corresponding to the various degrees of mental disorder from mere eccentricity to raving lunacy.[54] Given the existence of such tendencies among even the more enlightened members of the profession, it is hardly surprising that the certification of 'borderline' cases should frequently have been contested, and that the public should have come to regard the certificate-happy psychiatrist as a threat to civil liberties. But the system of involuntary psychiatric hospitalization itself, and the lunacy certificate which served to police its boundaries, remained indispensable, since they served to maintain the all-important normative and cultural distinctions between sanity and insanity, order and disorder, moral responsibility and moral anarchy. In this charged situation, psychiatrists were tacitly required to be both the mediators and the scapegoats for the contradictions involved in these ideologies, and patients' rights were an almost inevitable casualty of this non-rational way of dealing with conflicting social and moral values.

Yet if, on the one hand, patients' rights were in part sacrificed to overriding social pressures, on the other they may equally have been a victim of the growth of nineteenth-century scientific rationalism. Though usually associated with 'progress' and the rise of enlightened, humane treatment programmes, the rise of 'scientific naturalism' in nineteenth-century psychiatry may actually have been partly at the expense of respect for both the ethical status and the civil rights and liberties of mental patients. Though without many of the legal safeguards and organizational resources at least potentially available to the modern mental patient, in some ways early nineteenth-century mental patients were perhaps in a better position to affirm their human dignity and demand, if not exercise, their 'rights' *vis-à-vis* their medical masters than were many of their successors. Not only were early nineteenth-century 'mad-doctors' among the most reviled members of a profession still widely regarded as little or no better than tradesmen or quacks, but as yet the scientific naturalism with which psychiatry was increasingly associated from the 1850s onwards exercised none of the ideological hegemony it was to enjoy during the late nineteenth and much of the twentieth centuries.[55] Patients, especially wealthy, well-educated private patients, were not, therefore, at any great intellectual or social disadvantage *vis-à-vis* their doctors and 'keepers' and could dispute the ethical, philosophical and medical bases of their treatment with relative ease and impunity. To the newly-fashionable clichés of such exponents of 'moral management' as Dr Fox of Brislington, wealthy and determined private patients like Perceval were able to oppose a potent but historically very contingent mixture of Evangelical Christianity and upper-class self-esteem.[56] From an Evangelical perspective, both mad-doctors and their patients were sinners in need of grace and equals in the sight of God, to whom alone knowledge, wisdom and authority could properly be ascribed, while to minds formed in the belief that class distinctions were divinely ordained and immutable it was intolerable that mere mad-doctors and lower-class 'keepers' should presume to exercise arbitrary power over persons of gentle birth and refined natures. However, for many patients less fortunate than Perceval both in respect of their social rank and the strength of their religious convictions, the task of maintaining their self-esteem and demanding that their rights be respected must have been far more difficult; and as time passed, public opinion became increasingly inured to both madhouses and mad-doctors, and scientific naturalism and psychological medicine commanded more and more intellectual assent, the struggle was to become too much for even the most articulate and socially privileged patients – as the case of Virginia Woolf demonstrates.[57] It was not so very difficult to sustain a dissident voice against the new-fangled quackery of upstart mad-doctors and the ignorant brutality of unenlightened keepers, but it was to prove well-nigh impossible in the face of the esoteric science and professional humanitarianism of consultant psychiatrists and trained mental nurses, backed up by the full authority of modern medical science.

In the late twentieth century, religious belief is no longer generally considered to provide a viable justification for individual self-esteem, while class membership and privilege are no longer seen as acceptable bases for demanding rights. But during the past twenty years or so, organizations like MIND have succeeded in mounting highly-effective critiques of modern mental health legislation and practice from purely secular and egalitarian standpoints. Modern scientific humanism and pseudo-egalitarianism may largely have undermined traditional religious belief and class consciousness, but a combination of secular human rights ideology and neo-liberal legal activism – themselves, ironically, part of the same complex and often contradictory intellectual heritage of the Enlightenment as psychiatric paternalism – has proved as effective a vehicle for affirming and enhancing patients' legal rights as was the Evangelical and Quaker philanthropy which inspired 'moral management' and 'non-restraint'. Johanna Geyer-Kordesch has recently argued that 'The development of natural law theory and the involvement of positive law and medicine with its agenda created modern professional ethics.'[58] But where, as in the case of psychiatry, the ethical implications of scientific naturalism have failed to measure up to expectations based on ideas of 'natural rights', natural law philosophy, far from providing a harmonious context for the development of professional ethics, has tended rather to heighten the tensions and multiply the points of conflict between legal and medical, lay and professional perspectives on ethical problems of medical practice.

Notes

1. For a typically controversial exception, see, however, Thomas S. Szasz, *The Theology of Medicine: The Political-Philosophical Foundations of Medical Ethics* (Baton Rouge:Louisiana University Press, 1977). A recent example in a quite different vein is K. W. M. Fulford, *Moral Theory and Medical Practice* (Cambridge: Cambridge University Press, 1989). During the past two decades, psychiatrists have, in fact, engaged in extensive ethical reflection upon their practice, which has increasingly impacted on general medical-ethical debate. See especially American Psychiatric Association Ethics Committee, *Principles of Medical Ethics with Annotations Applicable to Psychiatry* (Washington, D.C.: American Psychiatric Press, 1986) [first issued in 1973], and Allen Dyer, *Ethics and Psychiatry: Towards Professional Definition* (Washington, D.C.: American Psychiatric Press, 1988).
2. The implicit attribution to mental patients of a certain definite moral or 'ethical' status in Victorian psychiatric discourse and practice may perhaps best be understood by analogy with the more explicit attribution – or denial – of distinct moral statuses to human beings and animals in contemporary ethical and philosophical debate. See, for example, S. R. L. Clark, *The Moral Status of Animals* (Oxford: Clarendon Press, 1977).
3. This is clearly the case, for example, with regard to truth-telling, the avoidance of interventions and procedures likely to harm the patient, and informed consent to treatment.
4. For Szasz' distinction between 'contractual', or voluntary, and 'institutional' or involuntary psychiatry, see especially his *The Manufacture of Madness: A Comparative Study of the Inquisition and the Mental Health Movement* (New York and London: Harper and Row, 1970), xvii, xxii–iii, 101.
5. See W. F. Bynum, 'Rationales for Therapy in British Psychiatry, 1780–1835', *Medical History*, xviii (1974), 317–34, and Roger Cooter, 'Phrenology and British Alienists, c.1825–1845', *Medical History*, xx (1976), 1–21, 135–51.
6. Roger Smith, 'The Law and Insanity in Great Britain, with Comments on Continental Europe', in F. Koenraadt, (ed.), *Ziek of schuldig? Twee eeuwen forenssische psychiatrie en psychologie* (Utrecht: Willem Pompe Instituut, 1991), 247–81.
7. On the controversies surrounding 'mechanical' and 'chemical' restraint, see especially Nancy Tomes, 'The Great Restraint

Controversy: A Comparative Perspective on Anglo-American Psychiatry in the Nineteenth Century', in W. F. Bynum, Roy Porter and Michael Shepherd, (eds), *The Anatomy of Madness: Essays in the History of Psychiatry* (3 Vols) (London and New York: Tavistock Publications/Routledge, 1985–88), Vol III (1988), 190–225. On the 'wrongful confinement' controversies, see especially Peter McCandless, 'Liberty and Lunacy: The Victorians and Wrongful Confinement', *Journal of Social History*, xii, No. 3 (Spring 1978), 366–85, reprinted in Andrew T. Scull, (ed.), *Madhouses, Mad-Doctors and Madmen: The Social History of Psychiatry in the Victorian Era* (Philadelphia and London: University of Pennsylvania Press/Athlone Press, 1981), 338–62. For the debate over the merits of general hospital treatment for acute cases of insanity, see David Yellowlees, 'Presidential Address delivered at the Annual Meeting of the Medico-Psychological Association, ... July 24th., 1890', *Journal of Mental Science*, xxxvi (1890), 473–89.

8. William Ll. Parry-Jones, *The Trade in Lunacy: A Study of Private Madhouses in England in the Eighteenth and Nineteenth Centuries* (London: Routledge and Kegan Paul, 1972); Charlotte MacKenzie, *Psychiatry for the Rich: A History of Ticehurst Private Asylum* (London and New York: Routledge, 1992).
9. For Mulock's case, see especially his *British Lunatic Asylums* (Stafford, 1858); see also McCandless, 'Liberty and Lunacy', in Scull, (ed.), *Madhouses, Mad-Doctors and Madmen*, 340–41. For Perceval and Paternoster, see below, in this chapter, 280–1
10. See, for example, John Conolly, *On the Construction and Government of Lunatic Asylums and Hospitals for the Insane* (London: John Churchill, 1847); W. A. F. Browne, *What Asylums Were, Are, and Ought to Be: Five Lectures Delivered Before the Managers of the Royal Montrose Lunatic Asylum* (Edinburgh: Adam and Charles Black, 1837); *idem, Religio Psycho-Medici* (London: Baillière, Tindall and Cox, 1877). For Conolly, see especially Andrew T. Scull, 'A Victorian Alienist: John Conolly, FRCP, DCL (1794–1866)', in Bynum, Porter and Shepherd, (eds), *The Anatomy of Madness*, Vol I, 103–50. For Browne, see Scull, 'Introduction', in Andrew Scull, ed. and introd., *The Asylum as Utopia: W.A.F. Browne and the Mid-Nineteenth Century Consolidation of Psychiatry* (London and New York: Tavistock/Routledge, 1991), vii–lxxvii.
11. Clive Unsworth, *The Politics of Mental Health Legislation* (Oxford: Clarendon Press, 1985), 44 [Emphasis added]. The phrase 'something more subtle than rights' is attributed to H. P. Macmillan, Chairman of the Royal Commission on Lunacy and Mental Disorder (1924–6), in *Royal Commission on Lunacy and Mental Disorder: Minutes of Evidence* (1926), Vol I, Para. 900.
12. The clearest account of the development of the legal framework of nineteenth-century psychiatric practice is still that given in Kathleen

Jones, *Lunacy, Law and Conscience 1744–1845* (London: Routledge and Kegan Paul, 1955). See also McCandless, 'Liberty and Lunacy', and for the later nineteenth century, Unsworth, *Politics of Mental Health Legislation*, chs 1, 2.

13. For the readmission of former private patients to 'half- way' houses as voluntary boarders, see 16 and 17 Vict., c.96, Section 6. For Chancery patients, see Kathleen Jones, *Mental Health and Social Policy, 1845–1959* (London: Routledge and Kegan Paul, 1960), 13, 35–6, and note 35, below.
14. The initial elaboration and growing influence of what was to become the standard nineteenth-century rationale for the asylum treatment of insanity is described in Andrew T. Scull, *Museums of Madness: The Social Organization of Insanity in Nineteenth-Century England* (London: Allen Lane, 1979), chs 3, 4.
15. See especially Jones, *Mental Health and Social Policy*, ch. 1, 'Public Opinion and the Liberty of the Subject'; McCandless, 'Liberty and Lunacy' and Unsworth, *Politics of Mental Health Legislation*, 66–7, 87–95.
16. For all these aspects of institutional psychiatric practice in the Victorian era, as seen from the patient's standpoint, see John Thomas Perceval, *A Narrative of the Treatment Experienced by a Gentleman ...* [see Note 22, below, for full reference].
17. See John Conolly, *An Inquiry Into the Indications of Insanity, with Suggestions for the Better Protection and Care of the Insane* (London: John Taylor, 1830), 4–6.
18. Conolly, *On the Construction and Government of Lunatic Asylums*; Browne, *What Asylums Were, Are, and Ought to Be*; Forbes Benignus Winslow, 'The Mission of the Psychologist', *Journal of Psychological Medicine*, x (1857), 611–22.
19. See, for example, William Ll. Parry-Jones, 'The Model of the Geel Lunatic Colony and its Influence on the Nineteenth-Century Asylum System in Britain', in Scull, (ed.), *Madhouses, Mad-Doctors and Madmen*, 202–17, especially 207–12; Peter McCandless, '"Build! Build!" The Controversy Over the Care of the Chronically Insane in England, 1855–1870', *Bulletin of the History of Medicine*, liii (1979), 553–74; and Tomes, 'The Great Restraint Controversy'.
20. Until recently, apart from a few dismissive asides, the Alleged Lunatics' Friend Society had attracted very little attention from historians of psychiatry. Thanks, however, to Nicholas Hervey, historians now have a wealth of materials to draw upon in presenting the complex and often fierce debates surrounding law, liberty and psychiatry in early- and mid-Victorian England. See Nicholas Hervey, 'Advocacy or Folly: The Alleged Lunatics' Friend Society, 1845–63', *Medical History*, xxx (1986), 245–75. The following brief account of the Society and its work is very largely based on Hervey's work.

21. Richard Paternoster, *The Madhouse System* (London: for the author, 1841).
22. John Thomas Perceval, *A Narrative of the Treatment Experienced by a Gentleman, During a State of Mental Derangement; Designed to Explain the Causes and the Nature of Insanity, and to Expose the Injudicious Conduct Pursued towards Many Unfortunate Sufferers under that Calamity* (2 Vols) (London: Effingham Wilson, 1838–40). For Perceval himself, see Richard Hunter and Ida Macalpine, 'John Thomas Perceval (1803–1876), Patient and Reformer', *Medical History*, vi (1962), 391–5; Hervey, 'Advocacy or Folly', and Roy Porter, *A Social History of Madness: Stories of the Insane* (London: Weidenfeld and Nicolson, 1987), ch. 9. For Saumarez, see Hervey, *art. cit.*, 252, 265–6, 269, 272.
23. Hervey, 'Advocacy or Folly', pp. 254–5.
24. *Ibid.*, 254–5.
25. *Ibid.*, 256, 262.
26. *Ibid.*, 262, 264–6.
27. *Ibid.*, 257, 258–9, 264–5, 275.
28. *Ibid.*, 257–8.
29. *Ibid.*, 259, 274, note 170.
30. *Ibid.*, 265–6.
31. *Ibid.*, 258–9, 273.
32. *Ibid.*, 256, 257, 258, 260.
33. *Ibid.*, 253–4.
34. *Ibid.*, 256, 259, 268, 275.
35. On the position of single patients in private lodgings at this time, see Jones, *Mental Health and Social Policy*, 7, 16, and Hervey, 'A Slavish Bowing Down: The Lunacy Commission and the Psychiatric Profession 1845–60', in Bynum, Porter and Shepherd, (eds), *The Anatomy of Madness*, Vol II, 98–131, especially 105, 115–18.
36. Hervey, 'Advocacy or Folly', 259, 271–2.
37. Jones, *Mental Health and Social Policy*, 32; Unsworth, *Politics of Mental Health Legislation*, 67, 93; Hervey, 'Advocacy or Folly', 245, note 2.
38. Louisa Lowe, *The Bastilles of England; or, The Lunacy Laws at Work*, (London: Crookenden, 1883).
39. See Unsworth, *Politics of Mental Health Legislation*, 80, 94–6.
40. *Ibid.*, 95.
41. On these attempts to revise the lunacy laws and on the Act of 1890, see Jones, *Mental Health and Social Policy*, 26–37, and Unsworth, *Politics of Mental Health Legislation*, 87–93 and ch. 4.
42. Unsworth, *Politics of Mental Health Legislation*, 93–4.
43. Jones, *Mental Health and Social Policy*, 168; Unsworth, *Politics of Mental Health Legislation*, 95–6.
44. See, for example, Hervey, 'Advocacy or Folly', 245, 270, note 151.
45. Hervey, *art. cit.*, 256. [Emphasis added.]

46. *Ibid.*, 256. [Emphasis added.]
47. The Lunacy Commission has largely been ignored in the many studies of nineteenth-century government growth which have appeared in the last 30 years. See, however, D. J. Mellett, 'Bureaucracy and Mental Illness: The Commissioners in Lunacy 1845–90', *Medical History*, xxv (1981), 221–50; Hervey, 'A Slavish Bowing Down', 98, 103–4, 108, 113–14, 119, and Notes 141 and 142; *idem*, 'Advocacy or Folly', 249–50, 253.
48. This interpretation is all but explicit in Hervey, 'A Slavish Bowing Down', 112, 118–19.
49. On the 'Wrongful Confinement' controversies of the period, see especially McCandless, 'Liberty and Lunacy'.
50. John Stuart Mill, *On Liberty* (Everyman edn), 126. See also McCandless, 'Liberty and Lunacy', 350–7.
51. Mill, *On Liberty*, 126.
52. See, for example, Conolly, *Indications of Insanity*, especially 172–3; Charles Mercier, *A Text-Book of Insanity* (London: Swan Sonnenschein, 1902), ch.1, 96–7; *idem*, 'Vice, Crime and Insanity', in Thomas Clifford Allbutt and Humphry Davy Rolleston, (eds), *A System of Medicine ...* (2nd revd edn), Vol 8, 842–74.
53. McCandless, 'Liberty and Lunacy', 340–1.
54. Conolly, *Indications of Insanity*, especially 172–4, 176, 431–3.
55. On 'scientific naturalism' and its contributions to the authority of mid- and late-Victorian psychiatry, see especially L. Stephen Jacyna, 'The Physiology of Mind, the Unity of Nature and the Moral Order in Victorian Thought', *British Journal of the History of Science*, xiv (1981), 109–32; *idem*, 'Somatic Theories of Mind and the Interests of Medicine in Britain, 1850–1879', *Medical History*, xxvi (1982), 233–58; Michael J. Clark, 'The Data of Alienism; Evolutionary Neurology, Physiological Psychology and the Reconstruction of British Psychiatric Theory, *c.*1850–*c.*1900' (Unpubld. D.Phil. Thesis, Oxford, 1983).
56. On this point, see especially Porter's account of Perceval's confinement, in Porter, *Social History of Madness*, ch.9.
57. See Stephen Trombley, *'All That Summer She Was Mad'; Virginia Woolf and her Doctors* (London: Junction Books, 1981), especially Pt. II.
58. Johanna Geyer-Kordesch, 'Infanticide and Medico-legal Ethics in Eighteenth Century Prussia', in this vol, 181–202, especially 181–2.

Index

H

K

L

M

Printed in the United Kingdom
by Lightning Source UK Ltd.
106167UKS00001B/225

9 789051 835533